STUDY GUIDE FOR

KOZIER & ERB'S FUNDAMENTALS OF NURSING

Concepts, Process, and Practice

8TH EDITION

BERMAN ■ SNYDER ■ KOZIER ■ ERB

STUDY GUIDE FOR

KOZIER & ERB'S FUNDAMENTALS OF NURSING

Concepts, Process, and Practice

8TH EDITION

MICHELLE BUCHMAN, RN, BSN, BC
Manager, Educational Support Services
Springfield, Missouri

DEBORAH RUSHING, RN, MSN
Assistant Professor
Troy University School of Nursing
Troy, Alabama

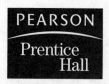

PEARSON

Prentice
Hall

Upper Saddle River, New Jersey

Pearson Education Ltd.
Pearson Education Australia Pty, Limited
Pearson Education Singapore, Pte. Ltd.
Pearson Education North Asia Ltd.
Pearson Education Canada, Ltd.

Pearson Educación de Mexico, S.A. de C.V.
Pearson Education—Japan
Pearson Education Malaysia, Pte. Ltd
Pearson Education, Upper Saddle River, NJ

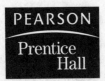

10 9 8 7 6 5 4 3
ISBN 0-13-188938-9
ISBN 978-0-13-188938-5

CONTENTS

PREFACE

Students entering the field of nursing have a tremendous amount to learn in a very short time. This concise study guide has been developed to help you learn and apply key concepts and procedures, and master critical-thinking skills based on *Kozier & Erb's Fundamentals of Nursing, eighth edition.*

At the beginning of each chapter in this study guide, you will find a MediaLink box. Just as in the main textbook, this box identifies the specific media resources and activities available for that chapter on the *Prentice Hall Nursing MediaLink DVD-ROM* that accompanies the main textbook and the Companion Website at www.prenhall.com/berman. You will find references to animations and videos clips on the *Prentice Hall Nursing MediaLink DVD-ROM* that will help you visualize and comprehend difficult concepts. On the Companion Website you will find a variety of activities such as Case Studies and Application Activities that help you apply concepts to clinical scenarios. Chapter by chapter, this MediaLink box guides you to hone your critical-thinking skills and apply concepts.

In addition, each chapter of this study guide includes a variety of questions and activities to help you comprehend difficult concepts and reinforce basic knowledge gained from textbook reading assignments. Following is a list of features included in this edition that will enhance your learning experience:

- **Learning Outcomes** summarize the objectives of each chapter.
- **Chapter Outlines** help you follow lectures and organize your notes.
- **Key Topic Review** exercises contain matching, fill-in-the-blank, and true/false questions on key terms and key topics from each chapter.
- **Focused Study Tips** help you recall the important nursing concepts from each chapter.
- **Case Studies** provide clinical settings for critical thinking and the opportunity to apply learned processes and procedures.
- **Review** questions are NCLEX®-style questions to help you prepare for the NCLEX®.
- **Answers** with complete rationales are included in the Appendix to provide immediate reinforcement and to permit you to check the accuracy of your work.

It is our hope that this study guide will serve as a valuable learning tool and will contribute to your success in the nursing profession.

CHAPTER 1

HISTORICAL AND CONTEMPORARY NURSING PRACTICE

CHAPTER OUTLINE

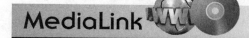

MediaLink

www.prenhall.com/berman

DVD-ROM
- Audio Glossary
- NCLEX® Review
- Video: History of Nursing

Companion Website
- Additional NCLEX® Review
- Case Study: Evolution of Nursing
- MediaLink Activities:
  - Florence Nightingale
  - American Association of Colleges of Nursing
  - Sigma Theta Tau
- Links to Resources

C. Teacher
D. Client Advocate
E. Counselor
F. Change Agent
G. Leader
H. Manager
I. Case Manager
J. Research Consumer
K. Expanded Career Roles

IV. Criteria of a Profession
A. Specialized Education
B. Body of Knowledge
C. Service Orientation
D. Ongoing Research
E. Code of Ethics
F. Autonomy
G. Professional Organization

V. Socialization to Nursing
A. Critical Values of Nursing

VI. Factors Influencing Contemporary Nursing Practice
A. Economics
B. Consumer Demands
C. Family Structure
D. Science and Technology
E. Information and Telecommunications
F. Legislation
G. Demography
H. The Current Nursing Shortage
I. Collective Bargaining
J. Nursing Associations

VII. Nursing Organizations
A. American Nurses Association
B. Canadian Nurses Association
C. National League for Nursing
D. International Council of Nurses
E. National Student Nurses' Association
F. International Honor Society: Sigma Theta Tau

KEY TOPIC REVIEW

1. The four functions identified within the scope of nursing practice are:
   a.
   b.
   c.
   d.

2. The role of religious orders on the development of nursing include:
   a. instilling the values of hard work.
   b. influencing the image of nursing.
   c. identifying an increased need for nurses.
   d. imprinting the profession as involving hard work.
   e. improving the status of nursing.

3. The contemporary nursing leader who defined nursing is:
   a. Clara Barton.
   b. Florence Nightingale.
   c. Linda Richards.
   d. Virginia Henderson.

4. A nurse registered to practice in one state is relocating to another neighboring state. What should this nurse do to ensure the ability to work as a nurse in the new state?
   a. Nothing. The nurse is registered as a nurse.
   b. Contact the state's department of nursing.
   c. Enroll in a school of nursing in the new state.
   d. File the paperwork to take the new state's nursing licensing examination.

5. From the following list, select the definition that best defines the following:
   a. Caregiver   _____ Helps the client modify behaviors.
   b. Communicator   _____ This can be provided by the nurse or delegated to someone else.
   c. Teacher   _____ Supervises and evaluates performance.
   d. Client advocate   _____ Sensitive to protecting the rights of human subjects.
   e. Counselor   _____ Acts to protect the client.
   f. Change agent   _____ Influences others to work together to reach a common goal.
   g. Leader   _____ Done verbally or written.
   h. Manager   _____ Care is oriented to the client and controls costs.
   i. Case manager   _____ Helps promote personal growth.
   j. Research consumer   _____ Assess readiness to learn.

6. The terms used to identify the recipients of nursing are:
   a.
   b.
   c.
7. Of the following nursing roles, select the ones that provide more autonomy within the practice of nursing.
   a. Nurse anesthetist
   b. Staff nurse on an orthopedic unit
   c. Operating room nurse
   d. Clinical nurse specialist
   e. Nurse in a physician's office
8. The process a nurse undergoes in effort to be viewed as an integral member of the discipline of nursing is termed _____.
9. A nurse is interested in participating with the American Nurses Association. Participating with this organization is an example of:
   a. autonomy.
   b. governance.
   c. extended education.
   d. service.
10. The purpose of nursing students working together on projects is to:
    a. begin the process of socialization into the profession.
    b. get more work done faster.
    c. help each other through difficult courses.
    d. make new friends.
11. The payments for hospital services implemented by Medicare are termed _____ (DRGs).
12. A nurse who provides care to a patient over the telephone will need to:
    a. obtain licensure in the patient's state of residence.
    b. take a course in telenursing.
    c. find out if the patient's state is one of mutual recognition for licensure.
    d. do nothing.
13. The Patient Self-Determination Act requires that every patient be provided with _____ and _____.

FOCUSED STUDY TIPS

1. Why is it important to review the history of nursing as one of the first steps in the education of a new nurse? What value does understanding the history of nursing provide to the contemporary nursing student?

2. What are the characteristics of a profession? How does nursing address each of these characteristics?

3. What are Benner's five stages of nursing practice? In which stage is a nurse considered proficient? Why?

4. How have economics, consumer demands, and the family structure impacted the profession of nursing?

5. A nurse who has been in the profession for over 25 years does not know how to operate a computer. What suggestions do you have to help this nurse? Why should this nurse be concerned with the inability to utilize current technology?

6. Identify the reasons for the current nursing shortage. How will this affect the future education of new nurses entering the profession?

7. The nurses in a hospital are contacting a labor union. Why do you think the nurses are contacting this union? What benefits will be gained by working with a union? What disadvantages are associated with nurses working with a union?

8. Go to the Companion Website (www.prenhall.com/berman) and click on the Sigma Theta Tau and the American Association of Colleges of Nursing (AACN) weblinks. What do these two organizations represent in nursing? What are the differences between the two sites and what are the similarities? Is there information that you could refer to if you wanted to continue your education in nursing? Which site offers continuing education units (CEUs) for nurses? Explore other nursing sites such as American Nursing Association (ANA) and American Academy of Colleges in Nursing (AACN).

CASE STUDY

A client with adult-onset asthma is attempting to quit his two-pack-per-day tobacco habit. The nurse, who has been practicing for 4 years, is assisting the client with supportive measures to improve his health status. The nurse is discussing the plan of care with the physician.

1. *What role is the nurse acting in by representing the client's needs and wishes and assisting the client in behavior modification plans?*
2. *The nurse is in the process of assisting the client to recognize and cope with both the asthma condition and the tobacco cessation program. The nurse is acting as a change agent, and what other role is the nurse representing?*
3. *According to Benner's stages of nursing expertise, in what stage is the nurse functioning?*

REVIEW QUESTIONS

1. A female is considering a career as a nurse because of the aspects of caring and nurturing. This individual is using which factor of nursing to base her decision?
   1. Women's roles
   2. Religion
   3. War
   4. Economics

2. A registered nurse is considering additional education so that she can provide non-emergent acute care in an ambulatory clinic. This nurse is considering which expanded career role?
   1. Nurse anesthetist
   2. Clinical nurse specialist
   3. Nurse practitioner
   4. Nurse administrator

3. A nurse is able to provide care to several complex clients and focuses on those items that are the most important. Within which stage of Benner's stages of nursing expertise is this nurse functioning?
   1. Stage II
   2. Stage III
   3. Stage IV
   4. Stage V

4. The health care organization is having difficulty recruiting and retaining nurses. Which of the following nursing shortage factors is this organization experiencing?
   1. Aging workforce
   2. Aging population
   3. Increased demand for nurses
   4. Workplace issues

5. Which of the following can be viewed as an effort by an organization to improve the image of nursing?
   1. Offering scholarships to high school students to attend nursing school
   2. Television commercials showing nurses and doctors providing care together
   3. A print advertisement with the statement "Nursing—The hardest job you'll ever love"
   4. An ANA-sponsored radio commercial explaining the role of nurses in society today

6. A nurse providing care in a well-baby clinic is practicing within which area of nursing practice?
   1. Promoting health and wellness
   2. Preventing illness
   3. Restoring health
   4. Providing care to the dying

7. While attending a continuing education seminar, several nurses from different states are discussing their individual state requirements for nursing licensure. Which of the following is the one common thread between all of the states' departments of nursing?
   1. Protect the public.
   2. Further nursing education.
   3. Obtain continuing education contact hours.
   4. Gain specialization.

8. A new nursing student is disappointed because classes so far are focused on topics such as communication and planning, and she wanted to be a nurse to "provide care." This nursing student is describing which role of the nurse?
   1. Teacher
   2. Client advocate
   3. Caregiver
   4. Counselor

9. A graduate nurse is learning different aspects of the nursing profession while maintaining a sense of responsibility and accountability. The process this nurse is learning is:
   1. case manager.
   2. professionalization.
   3. socialization.
   4. governance.

10. An article appears in a nursing journal identifying one area of the United States with unusually high numbers of individuals with type 2 diabetes. This information would be considered:
    1. news.
    2. health statistics.
    3. a targeted area of study.
    4. demography.

CHAPTER 2

NURSING EDUCATION, RESEARCH, AND EVIDENCE-BASED PRACTICE

CHAPTER OUTLINE

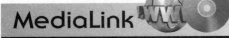

MediaLink

www.prenhall.com/berman

DVD-ROM
- Audio Glossary
- NCLEX® Review
- Video: LPN/LVN
- Video: Nursing Assistants
- Video: The Health Care Team

Companion Website
- Additional NCLEX® Review
- Case Study: Nursing Profession
- Application Activity: Entry into Practice
- Links to Resources

KEY TOPIC REVIEW

1. _____ are responsible for supervising the work of the licensed practical nurse/licensed vocational nurse.
2. The four rights of human subjects that nurses must safeguard are:
    a.
    b.
    c.
    d.
3. The term _____ means that any information a client relates will not be made public or available to others without the patient's consent.
4. What is the definition of research?

5. According to the "Standards of Clinical Nursing" published by the ANA (1998), _____ is included as one of the standards of professional performance.
6. Select and mark either (1) for quantitative research or (2) for qualitative research from the following items in regards to research:
    a. _____ associated with naturalistic inquiry that explores subjective and complex experiences of human beings
    b. _____ data collection and analysis occur concurrently
    c. _____ a systematic, logical sequence based on a specific plan designed to collect information in controlled conditions; analyzed using statistical procedures
    d. _____ theory or framework is developed after the data is analyzed to identify patterns and/or themes
    e. _____ viewed as "hard science"
7. CEUs meet the following needs of the nurse: (Select all that apply.)
    a. assists nurses in enriching their professional careers through networking.
    b. assists nurses in attaining expertise in a specific area of nursing (i.e., wound care).
    c. provides nurses with information essential to nursing practice.
    d. provides nurses with opportunities to travel to different areas of the world.
    e. keeps nurses up to date on new techiques and/or knowledge.
8. Correctly identify the order of the steps in conducting quantitative research:
    a. Review the related literature.
    b. Communicate conclusions and implications.
    c. Define the study's purpose or rationale.
    d. Conduct a pilot study.
    e. Analyze the data.
    f. Formulate hypotheses and define variables.
    g. Collect the data.
    h. Select the population, sample, and setting.
    i. State a research question or problem.
    j. Select a research design to test the hypothesis.
9. From the following list, select the definition that best defines the elements to consider in conducting a research critique.
    a. Substantive and theoretical dimensions
    b. Methodologic dimensions
    c. Ethical dimensions
    d. Interpretive dimensions
    e. Presentation and stylistic dimensions

    _____ The nurse must determine whether the rights of human subjects were protected during the course of the study and whether any ethical problems compromised the scientific merit of the study or the well-being of the subjects.

    _____ For these dimensions, the nurse needs to ascertain the accurancy of the discussion, conclusions, and implications of the study results. The findings must be related to the original hypotheses and the conceptual framework of the study. The implications and limitations of the study should be reviewed, together with the potential for replication or generalizability of the findings to similar populations.

_____ The nurse needs to evaluate the significance of the research problem, the appropriateness of the conceptualizations and the theoretical framework of the study, and the congruence between the research question and the method used to address it.

_____ The dimensions pertain to the appropriateness of the research design, the size and representativeness of the study sample as well as the sampling design, validity and reliability of the instruments, adequacy of the research procedures, and the appropriateness of data analysis techniques used in the study.

_____ The manner in which the research plan and results are communicated refers to the presentation and stylistic dimensions. The research report must be detailed, logically organized, concise, and well written.

10. Measures of central tendency describe the center of a distribution of data, denoting where most of the subjects lie, and variability, which indicates the degree of dispersion or spread of the data. Define the following terms that describe these measures.
    a. mean
    b. median
    c. mode
    d. range
    e. variance
    f. standard deviation

11. The Bachelor of Science in nursing (BSN) is the usual degree awarded to participants that have taken courses and:
    a. successfully completed a basic 2-year degree in a community college as an associate science of nursing.
    b. successfully completed a 4- to 5-year program that offered courses in liberal arts, sciences, humanities, and nursing.
    c. successfully completed 3 years in a hospital-based educational program.
    d. successfully completed a 9- to 12-month program and can work under the supervision of registered nurses.

12. According to the "Standards of Clinical Nursing" published by the ANA (1998), research is included as one of the standards of professional performance.
    a. True
    b. False

13. It is the responsibility of the employer to provide all CEUs for the nursing personnel.
    a. True
    b. False

14. _____ pertains to the availability of time as well as the material and human resources needed to investigate a research problem or question.

15. A _____ _____ is conducted prior to the actual study to assess the adequacy of the data collection plan and to identify any potential flaws in the study.

FOCUSED STUDY TIPS

1. What is the NCLEX®? How is it administered? Who takes the NCLEX®?

2. Describe three educational routes to be eligible for the RN licensure review (NCLEX®). List the major emphasis of each of the programs.

3. List three examples of documented nursing research in nursing magazines or refer to the weblinks for this chapter on the Companion Website.

4. Which level of nursing do you think should be the entry level into professional practice? Discuss the debate over entry and defend your choice for the entry level for professional practice. Cite two resources in your response using APA style. Refer to the Application Activity: Entry into Practice on the Companion Website.

5. List four ways for a nurse to provide for patient confidentiality.

CASE STUDY

Go to the Companion Website at www.prenhall.com/berman and locate and read the student research provided. Then answer the following critical thinking questions.

1. *Which theorist and theory is used as a framework to explore the concept of spirituality? Why do you think that the author used that theorist?*
2. *What was the purpose of this pilot study? Why did the authors use a pilot study instead of doing a more in-depth research study?*
3. *What were the indications for further study?*
4. *What tools were used in this pilot study? What was the reliability of this study?*

REVIEW QUESTIONS

1. A licensed practical nurse can perform which of the following functions?
   1. Assess the client's condition.
   2. Develop a care plan or concept map for the client.
   3. Provide basic care to the client.
   4. Evaluate the outcomes of the nursing plan and revise the care accordingly.

2. Upon successful completion of the NCLEX-RN®, the registered nurse is asked to participate in a research study on the coping and adjustment skills of a newly graduated registered nurse. The plan is to use an oral, recorded interview with a grounded theory. What type of research study is being conducted?
   1. Pilot study
   2. Quantitative study
   3. Qualitative study
   4. Ethnographic study

3. Which of the following activities are examples of how a professional nurse may participate in research? (Select all that apply.)
   1. Critiquing research for application to practice
   2. Identifying clinical problems suitable for nursing research
   3. Encouraging patient participation in a study without informed consent
   4. Using research findings in the development of policies, procedures, and practice guidelines for patient care

4. A nursing student documents the client's full name and date of birth on the required paperwork for the clinical course and turns it in to the instructor. Which of the following client rights is being violated?
   1. Right not to be harmed
   2. Right to full disclosure
   3. Right of self-determination
   4. Right of privacy and confidentiality

5. Which of the following topics would be considered an in-service educational opportunity?
    1. PowerPoint—Tips for Successful Presentations
    2. How to Knit a Sweater in 3 Hours
    3. Fire Safety
    4. New Techniques to Promote Continence in Older Adults

6. An RN manager is making assignments for an RN and LPN on the unit. Which of the following clients would the manager assign to the RN? (Select all that apply.)
    1. A newly diagnosed diabetic patient who needs education on foot care, diabetic injections, and a 1,800-calorie ADA diet
    2. A patient who is 2 days postop and needs assistance with ambulation in the hallway and to the restroom
    3. A patient receiving total parental nutrition (TPN)
    4. A patient who is undergoing a 24-hour urine collection

7. What are the reasons for continually revising nursing education curricula? (Select all that apply.)
    1. New scientific knowledge acquired with new discoveries regarding health
    2. Cultural changes that are continuously changing as time progresses
    3. New nursing instructors began their career in nursing and continuously change the curriculum
    4. Socioeconomic changes that occur in society

8. Continuing education is the responsibility of the nurse to keep abreast of _____ and _____ changes and also changes within the nursing profession.
    1. Scientific and technological
    2. Medical and technological
    3. Scientific and human responses
    4. Cardiac and neurological

9. As a nurse researcher, what is involved in the research project? (Select all that apply.)
    1. Identifying a research question or problem
    2. Writing a thesis paper
    3. Collecting data using various means such as computer searches and/or questionnaires
    4. Analyzing the data and writing up the results
    5. Publishing or presenting the research findings to expand the body of nursing knowledge

10. One of the major nursing responsibilities of nursing research that the nurse has is:
    1. encouraging participation of the clients in nursing research.
    2. being aware of and advocating on behalf of the client's rights.
    3. exposing the client to the possibility of injury from the research.
    4. pressuring the client into participating in the study.

CHAPTER 3

NURSING THEORIES AND CONCEPTUAL FRAMEWORKS

CHAPTER OUTLINE

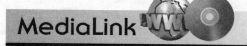

MediaLink

www.prenhall.com/berman

DVD-ROM
- Audio Glossary
- NCLEX® Review

Companion Website
- Additional NCLEX® Review
- Case Study: Theories
- Application Activities:
  - The Growth of Nursing Theory
  - Shaping Watson's Theory
- Links to Resources

KEY TOPIC REVIEW

1. Define theory. List two characteristics of a theory.

2. What is the main function of theory (and research) in a practice discipline?

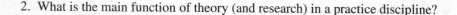

3. During the latter half of the 14th century, disciplines seeking to establish themselves in universities had to demonstrate something that Nightingale had not envisioned for nursing—a unique body of theoretical knowledge.
   a. True   b. False

4. Disciplines without a strong theory and research base were referred to as "_____," a negative comparison with the "_____" natural sciences.

5. What is the term encompassing the "building blocks" of theories? _____

6. A _____ _____ is a group of related ideas, statements, or concepts. It may also be called _____ theories or _____ _____.

7. _____ refers to a pattern of shared understandings and assumptions about reality and the world. It includes a person's notions of reality that are largely unconscious or taken for granted.

8. What four major concepts are related to the metaparadigm for nursing?

9. According to Figure 3-1 in your textbook, what are some foundational theories prevalent in nursing?

10. Match each theorist with the appropriate term: philosophies, conceptual models, or midlevel theories.
   a. Philosophies   _____ Orem
   b. Conceptual Models   _____ Nightingale
   c. Midlevel Theories   _____ Peplau
                                _____ Parse
                                _____ Henderson
                                _____ Roy
                                _____ Neuman
                                _____ Rogers
                                _____ Leininger
                                _____ Watson
                                _____ King

11. Who is considered to be the first nurse theorist?

12. An early effort to define nursing phenomena, _____ serves as the basis for later theoretical formulations.

13. Debates about the role of theory in nursing practice provide evidence that nursing is maturing as both an academic discipline and a clinical profession.
   a. True   b. False

14. Define the following terms:
   a. Client (person)
   b. Environment
   c. Health
   d. Nursing

15. Why is nursing considered to be a practice discipline?

FOCUSED STUDY TIPS

1. Describe the two paradigms of nursing theories.

2. List the major points of the following nursing theories:
   a. Nightingale's Environmental Theory

   b. Peplau's Interpersonal Relations Model

   c. Henderson's Definition of Nursing

    d. Roger's Science of Unitary Human Beings

    e. Orem's General Theory of Nursing

    f. King's Goal Attainment Theory

    g. Neuman's Systems Model

    h. Roy's Adaptation Model

    i. Leininger's Cultural Care Diversity and Universality Theory

    j. Watson's Human Caring Theory

    k. Parse's Human Becoming Theory

3. Read the "Research Note" on "*How can the use of a nursing model affect patient's condition?*" that is in this chapter in the textbook. Identify the implications for nursing practice.

CASE STUDY

The chief executive officer (CEO) has requested that the director of nursing (DON) revise the current philosophy of nursing that is being used for both a long-term care facility and an assisted living facility. The DON wants to develop the philosophy based on a nursing theory that adequately reflects both the healthy and ill clients housed in the facilities. The facilities' mission statements embrace the ideal of clients improving and sustaining independent functions, and encourage individualized goals for all clients to meet their individual needs. The DON wants to emphasize the nurses' responsibilities during the process of nurse-client interactions as well as the outcomes of nursing care.

1. *Choose the best nursing theory on which to base the revised philosophy of nursing for this particular facility.*
2. *Explain your rationale for using the theory that you have choosen.*

REVIEW QUESTIONS

1. A supposition or system of ideas that is proposed to explain a given phenomenon or something significant is called a:
   1. concept.
   2. theory.
   3. paradigm.
   4. conceptual model.

2. Some examples of concepts, which are defined as labels given to ideas, objects, or events, are:
   1. intelligence, motivation, and obesity.
   2. comfort, fatigue, pain, depression, and/or environment.
   3. self-care, adaptation, caring, behavioral system, and/or nurse-client transactions.
   4. humanistic endeavors, unitary man, and/or learned helplessness.

3. Which theorist addresses hospice nursing issues during end-of-life care?
   1. Imogene King
   2. Callista Roy
   3. Dorothea Orem
   4. Jean Watson

4. An example of a middle-range nursing theory is:
   1. Peplau's psychodynamic nursing model.
   2. Jean Watson's model of human caring.
   3. Roy's adaptation model.
   4. Imogene King's theory of goal attainment.

5. This theorist based her theory of nursing on the principle that nursing assists clients with 14 essential functions that move them toward independence.
   1. Myra Estrin Levine
   2. Dorethea Orem
   3. Madeline Leininger
   4. Virginia Henderson

6. One of the goals of Betty Neuman's health care systems model is:
   1. maintenance of system equilibrium.
   2. assisting the client to achieve the highest level of self-care.
   3. promoting internal and external stimuli that influence the client's well being.
   4. to heal the client and make the bed available for sicker clients.

7. Nightingale, Henderson, and Watson developed philosophies of nursing. Why are their works considered philosophies when discussed in nursing?
   1. Because they were the first three nursing theorists.
   2. Because it was an early effort to define nursing phenomena that serves as the basis for later theoretical formulations.
   3. Because they had grand theories of nursing and not middle-level theories.
   4. Because it was a late effort to define nursing.

8. Disciplines without a strong theory and research base were historically referred to as:
   1. hard.
   2. concrete.
   3. soft.
   4. medium.

9. A conceptual framework is considered to be:
   1. a group of related ideas, statements, or concepts.
   2. a pattern of shared understandings and assumptions about reality and the world.
   3. the way to elucidate how social structures affect a wide variety of human experiences, from art to social practices.
   4. a belief system, often an early effort to define nursing phenomena that serves as the basis for later theoretical formulations.

10. In the late 20th century, much of the theoretical work in nursing focused on articulating relationships among four major concepts. (Select the major concepts.):
    1. person.
    2. environment.
    3. nursing.
    4. professionalism.
    5. health.

CHAPTER 4

LEGAL ASPECTS OF NURSING

CHAPTER OUTLINE

I. General Legal Concepts
- A. Functions of the Law in Nursing
- B. Sources of Law
  - 1. Constitutional Law
  - 2. Legislation (Statutory Law)
  - 3. Administrative Law
  - 4. Common Law
- C. Types of Laws
- D. Kinds of Legal Actions
- E. The Civil Judicial Process
- F. Nurses as Witnesses

II. Regulation of Nursing Practice
- A. Nurse Practice Acts
- B. Credentialing
  - 1. Licensure
  - 2. Mutual Recognition Model
  - 3. Certification
  - 4. Accreditation/Approval of Basic Nursing Education Programs
- C. Standards of Care

III. Contractual Arrangements in Nursing
- A. Legal Roles of Nurses
  - 1. Provider of Service
  - 2. Employee or Contractor for Service
  - 3. Citizen
- B. Collective Bargaining

IV. Selected Legal Aspects of Nursing Practice
- A. Informed Consent
  - 1. Exceptions
  - 2. Nurse's Role
- B. Delegation
- C. Violence, Abuse, and Neglect
- D. The Americans with Disabilities Act
- E. Controlled Substances
- F. The Impaired Nurse

MediaLink

www.prenhall.com/berman

DVD-ROM
- Audio Glossary
- NCLEX® Review
- Video:
  - Collective Bargaining
  - Understanding Legal and Ethical Issues

Companion Website
- Additional NCLEX® Review
- Case Study: Legal Aspects of Obstetrics
- Application Activities:
  - Nurse Practice Act
  - Collective Bargaining
  - Good Samaritan Act
- Links to Resources

G. Sexual Harassment
H. Abortions
  I. Death and Related Issues
    1. Advance Health Care Directives
    2. Autopsy
    3. Certification of Death
    4. Do-Not-Resuscitate Orders
    5. Euthanasia
    6. Inquest
    7. Organ Donation
  V. Areas of Potential Liability in Nursing
    A. Crimes and Torts
      1. Unintentional Torts
      2. Intentional Torts

B. Privacy of Clients' Health Information
C. Loss of Client Property
D. Unprofessional Conduct
VI. Legal Protections in Nursing Practice
  A. Good Samaritan Acts
  B. Professional Liability Insurance
  C. Carrying Out a Physician's Orders
  D. Providing Competent Nursing Care
  E. Documentation
  F. The Incident Report
VII. Reporting Crimes, Torts, and Unsafe Practices
VIII. Legal Responsibilities of Students

KEY TOPIC REVIEW

1. Why is it important for nurses to know the basics of legal concepts?
2. What is accountability, and what are two reasons it is needed in nursing?
  a.
  b.
3. Name two functions of laws in nursing.
  a.
  b.
4. The Constitution of the United States is the supreme law of the state.
  a. True   b. False
5. Regulation of nursing is a function of state law.
  a. True   b. False
6. List two types of laws and give the definition of each type.
  a.
  b.
7. There are two types of legal actions: civil action and criminal action. Choose the correct definition of criminal action, the correct example of criminal action, and the potential results if a person is found guilty in a criminal trial.
  a. Deals with the relationships among individuals in society.
  b. Deals with disputes between an individual and the society as a whole.
  c. If found guilty, the defendant may have to pay a sum of money.
  d. If found guilty, the defendant may lose money, be jailed, be executed, and/or lose any professional licenses.
  e. One example of this type of legal infraction is a nurse who deliberately delivers a lethal dose of medication to a client.
  f. One example of this type of legal action is a malpractice suit.
8. The action of a lawsuit is called _____.
9. Organize the following five steps in the civil judicial process according to the procedural rules.
  a. A document, called a complaint, is filed by a person referred to as the plaintiff, who claims that his or her legal rights have been infringed on by one or more other persons or entities, referred to as defendants.
  b. In the trial of the case, all the relevant facts are presented to a jury or only to a judge.
  c. The judge renders a decision, or the jury renders a verdict. If the outcome is not acceptable to one of the parties, an appeal can be made for another trial.
  d. Both parties engage in pretrial activities, referred to as discovery, in an effort to obtain all the facts of the situation.
  e. A written response, called an answer, is made by the defendants.

10. What is the legal purpose for defining the scope of nursing, licensing requirements, and standards of care? (Select all that apply.)
    a. For the protection of the nurse
    b. For the protection of the client
    c. For the protection of the public
    d. Maintain client confidentiality
    e. For the protection of the physician

11. Each state has an obligation to define its scope of nursing practice and licensing requirements in accordance with the neighboring states.
    a. True   b. False

12. The name of the newly developed regulatory model is the _____ _____ model. It allows for multistate licensure for nurses. Nurses can practice in states bordering their own state if both states have an _____ compact.

13. _____ is the voluntary practice of validating that an individual nurse has met minimum standards of nursing competence in specialty areas such as maternal-child health, pediatrics, metal health, gerontology, and school nursing.

14. Define standards of care and list the two classifications.
    a.
    b.

15. List four examples of external standards of care:
    a.
    b.
    c.
    d.

16. A written contract cannot be changed legally by an oral agreement.
    a. True   b. False

17. Describe the difference between an expressed contract and an implied contract. Give an example of each type.

18. Explain the difference between a right and a responsibility and give an example of each.

19. A _____ is an organized work stoppage by a group of employees to express a grievance, enforce a demand for changes in conditions of employment, or solve a dispute with management. Usually, it is a result of failed collective bargaining between the parties.

20. What are the two types of informed consent?
    a.
    b.

21. It is the nurse's responsibility to have the informed consent form signed prior to an invasive procedure.
    a. True   b. False

22. What three things does the nurse's signature confirm with the signed consent form?
    a.
    b.
    c.

23. If a client refuses to sign the consent form, what actions does the nurse need to take?

24. What are two reasons for nurses to be knowledgeable regarding the Nurse Practice Act in their state of practice?

25. Nurses may be included as mandated reporters of violence, abuse, and/or neglect.
    a. True   b. False

26. How is the nurse involved in the Americans with Disabilities Act? Explain your answer.

27. State laws regulate the distribution and use of controlled substances such as narcotics, depressants, stimulants, and hallucinogens.
    a. True   b. False

28. _____ is cited as one of the main reasons for chemical dependence in health care workers.

29. Define the terms and list any nursing responsibilities about the following legal issues surrounding death:
    a. Advance directives:
    b. Autopsies:
    c. Certification of death:
    d. Do-Not-Resuscitate orders (DNRs):
    e. Euthanasia:
    f. Inquests:
    g. Organ donation:
30. _____ law is usually involved with nursing liability.
31. Choose the types of invasion that the client must be protected from:
    a. Reporting the number of births that occurred in the hospital for statistical analysis.
    b. Reporting of infections and communicable diseases.
    c. Taking photographs or having nursing students observe the client's care without the client's consent.
    d. Revealing the name of a client who was treated for domestic violence.
    e. Reporting violent incidents to the local authorities.
32. What is the Health Insurance Portability and Accountability Act of 1996 (HIPAA), and why is it important? What are the four specific areas of HIPAA? Refer to the HIPAA website found on the Companion Website.
33. What are four categories that nurses must question to protect themselves legally when carrying out physician's orders?

FOCUSED STUDY TIPS

1. Define and give an example of the following laws. Which is the highest level of law? Refer to the Prentice Hall Nursing MediaLink DVD-ROM that accompanies the textbook or the Companion Website for definitions:
    a. Civil law:

    b. Common law:

    c. Contract law:

    d. Law:

    e. Private law:

    f. Public law:

    g. Statutory law:

    h. Tort law:

2. Refer to Figure 4-1 in the textbook. Describe how laws are created from constitutions, statutes, administrative agencies, and decisions of courts.

3. Why is it important to know the state legislators that represent your state? Name the state legislators for your state. How do you contact your legislators, and why is it necessary to contact the legislators regarding nursing issues?

4. State your position on having malpractice insurance as a registered nurse. Is it your responsibility or the responsibility of your employer? Under what circumstances could you use the malpractice insurance? Refer to the Application Activity: Nurse Practice Act on the Companion Website.

5. What are the procedures that occur when a nursing license is revoked in the state that you will practice?

6. Go to the NCSBN website and list the states that have passed the NLC legislation. Refer to Box 4–1 in the textbook for additional information.

7. What are the statutes in your state for "consent"? What is considered the legal age of consent?

8. Discuss the areas of potential liablity in nursing and define the following terms: malpractice, intentional torts, crime, felony, manslaughter, misdemeanors, duty, and torts. Refer to the Application Activity: Liability on the Companion Website.

9. Determine the difference between defamation and slander. Give an example of each that might occur in the health care setting. Who could bring a defamation/slander lawsuit?

10. What are some legal protections in nursing practice to protect the nurse from litigation? Is the Good Samaritan Act designed for nurses? What are the responsibilites of nurses who choose to render emergency care? Is it required in your state for nurses to assist in emergencies?

11. Discuss and defend your position on professional liablity insurance. Is it a requirement for all nurses? List the advantages of maintaining professional liablity insurance.

12. Why is nurse documentation so important? What is the purpose of nurse documentation? How can it be used in a court of law? Does the nurse need to document if an incident report is filled out in the client's chart? Refer to the textbook, Chapter 4, Figure 4-5 for additonal information.

13. What are measures that nursing students may implement in order to fulfill responsibilites to clients and to minimize the chances for liability? Refer to Boxes 4–4 and 4–5 in Chapter 4 of the textbook.

CASE STUDY

A client was scheduled for the surgical removal of the left ovary. During the surgery, the surgeon noticed that the appendix of the client was inflamed. He decides to remove it to prevent further problems. The client's consent for surgery only listed removal of the left ovary.

1. *Did the surgeon adhere to the signed consent form that the client signed before the surgery?*
2. *Under the circumstances, what type of tort is the surgeon liable for?*
3. *What was the operating nurse's role in this incident?*

REVIEW QUESTIONS

1. Which nurse would be considered to be the "best expert witness" for the defense in a case regarding an obsterical patient who died after delivery complications?
   1. A nurse who holds a bachelor's degree in nursing and has been practicing for 2 years
   2. A nurse who holds a master's degree in nursing and has a certification in emergency nursing
   3. A nurse who holds a doctorate of nursing science in pediatric care
   4. A nurse who holds a master's degree in nursing and a state certification in maternal infant nursing

2. Which of the following clients could make decisions regarding health care? (Select all that apply.)
   1. A woman who arrives in the emergency department with an altered mental state and the aroma of ethyl alcohol
   2. The parents of a 14-year old girl involved in a car collision
   3. A middle-aged man who has the mental capacity of an 8-year old
   4. A 10-year old boy who has arrived with friends and has a shallow laceration needing three sutures
   5. A compentent older adult that requries surgery on a prolapsed bladder

3. A client was discharged after having a 1-day surgery on her gallbladder. The nurse discharging the client failed to give her oral or written discharge instructions. This failure to carry out the provision of discharge instructions could result in charges of:
   1. malpractice.
   2. negligence.
   3. assault.
   4. battery.

4. For the nurse, which of the following statements indicates that the client understands informed consent of a surgical procedure?
   1. The nurse discovers the signed informed consent form on the bedside table before the surgeon discusses the procedure with the client.
   2. The client's oldest son stated that he explained the procedure to the client and the client told him that he wanted the surgery.
   3. The client states that the surgeon explained the procedure to him, allowed him to ask questions, and explained the risks of not permitting the surgery.
   4. The client is obviously operating at a 10-year-old mental capability but has never been declared legally incompetent.

5. A nurse is caring for an 89-year old client who has severe chronic obstructive pulmonary disease and was transferred from a long-term care facility. While reviewing the transfer papers, she notes that the client has both a living will and a durable power of attorney. A living will differs from a durable power of attorney in that a living will:
   1. describes how the client wants his wishes carried out in the event of a terminal illness.
   2. is an example of an advanced medical directive.
   3. determines which relative gets the house.
   4. allows a designated person to make decisions if the client is unable to make decisions.

6. A nurse threatens to give a loud, disruptive client an injection that will "knock him or her out." The nurse follows through on the threat and gives the injection without the client's consent. In which of the following orders did the nurse have liablity?
   1. Battery, assault
   2. Battery, invasion of privacy
   3. Assault, invasion of privacy
   4. Assault, battery

7. A nurse documents in the client's chart that the physician is incompetent because he did not respond promptly to the nurse's call regarding the client. This is an example of _____ and _____ .
   1. defamation
   2. slander
   3. libel
   4. battery
   5. unprofessional conduct

8. Conviction for practicing nursing without a license, incompetence or gross negligence, falsification of client records, and illegally obtaining, using, or possessing controlled substances is called:
   1. libel.
   2. slander.
   3. unprofessional conduct.
   4. assault.

9. Most statutes include conscience clauses that are designed to protect hospitals and nurses in matters dealing with abortion services. These clauses allow the nurse to be protected from:
   1. prejudicial statements.
   2. discrimination or retaliation.
   3. defamation or unjust prejudice.
   4. legal liability.

10. Identify the element that is *not* one of the functions of the law in the nursing environment.
    1. Accountability helps to maintain a minimum standard of nursing practice.
    2. Law differentiates nurses' responsibilities from those of other health care professionals.
    3. Law specifies which nursing actions are legal in caring for clients.
    4. Law specifies which nursing actions and hospital policies are legal in caring for clients.

CHAPTER 5

VALUES, ETHICS, AND ADVOCACY

CHAPTER OUTLINE

MediaLink

www.prenhall.com/berman

DVD-ROM
- Audio Glossary
- NCLEX® Review
- End-of-Unit Concept Map Activity

Companion Website
- Additional NCLEX® Review
- Case Study: Ethics Committee
- Application Activities:
  - AIDS Resources
  - Privacy
- Links to Resources

V. Advocacy
   A. The Advocate's Role
      1. Advocacy in Home Care
      2. Professional and Public Advocacy

KEY TOPIC REVIEW

1. Define values and describe why they are important in nursing.
2. Describe the difference between values and beliefs.
3. _____ are mental positions or feelings toward a person, object, or idea.
4. List five values identified by the American Association of Colleges of Nursing (AACN, 1998). Refer to Table 5–1 in the textbook.
   a.
   b.
   c.
   d.
   e.
5. When should the nurse use values clarification as a nursing intervention?
6. When nurses make decisions regarding their participation in the acts of abortion or euthanasia, they are using which type of ethics?
7. What is the term that is similar to *ethics* and often used interchangeably?
8. Moral development is the process of learning to tell the difference between right and wrong. It begins in young adulthood and continues through life.
   a. True   b. False
9. Match the following three moral framework theories with the correct descriptive terms.
   A. Consequence-based (teleological) theories   a. _____ involve logical and formal processes.
   B. Principles-based (deontological) theories   b. _____ look to outcomes or consequences of an action.
   C. Relations-based (caring) theories   c. _____ promote the common good or the welfare of the group.
                                                   d. _____ stress individual rights.
                                                   e. _____ one form of this theory is called utilitarianism.
                                                   f. _____ these theories focus on issues of fairness.
                                                   g. _____ stress courage, generosity, commitment, and the need to nurture and maintain relationships.
                                                   h. _____ involve logical, formal processes and emphasize individual rights, duties, and obligations.
10. Within recent years, what statements regarding ethics have been made broader in scope or added to the "Code of Nurses"? Refer to Box 5–4 and Box 5–5 in the textbook.
11. What is the goal of ethical reasoning within the context of nursing?
12. As a nurse, what are three functions of the advocacy role?
13. _____ means "doing good."
14. _____ is often referred to as fairness.
15. _____ refers to telling the truth.
16. _____ means "answerable to oneself and others for one's own actions," while _____ refers to "the specific accountability or liability associated with the performance of duties of a particular role."

FOCUSED STUDY TIPS

1. What are your values regarding life, death, health, and illness?

2. Practice assisting someone (a friend, parent, significant other, etc.) in clarifying their values and identifying behaviors that may need further clarification by using the seven steps listed in Table 5–3 of the textbook.

3. What are some factors that have led to increased ethical concerns? Why do ethical concerns even exist?

4. List 6 of the 12 rights of the *Bill of Rights* for clients receiving health care. As a nurse, what are your responsibilities in promoting the *Bill of Rights*?

5. What common ethical issues currently face health care professionals? How do some hospitals resolve ethical issues?

6. Define harm. What is nonmaleficence? Give one example of unintentional harm and one example of intentional harm.

7. When caring for a client with acquired immune deficiency syndrome (AIDS), what is the moral obligation of the nurse according to the ANA position statement?

8. Explore your values on assisted abortion. What is your perception of the "morning after" pill? How do you plan on handling these issues in the workplace? What are your options if you choose not to participate in such actions?

CASE STUDIES

1. *You are the nurse caring for a 45-year-old client who is in the end stages of acquired immune deficiency syndrome (AIDS). She is married and has two children, ages 14 and 17. The client is unable to perform the care needed by her children and spouse and she had to take a leave of absence from employment 8 months ago due to her advanced AIDS. Her family is experiencing emotional turmoil and financial stress due to her prognosis and inability to fully function in her roles as a contributor to income, a mother, and a wife. The client requests your assistance in deciding what actions should be taken to prolong her life. Her family and friends want her to do everything in her power to survive; however, she tells you that she is "so tired."*
   a. *What considerations should you take into account in assisting the client to make those decisions?*
   b. *In what way could you assist the client in reaching decisions about further health care?*
   c. *Would an ethics committee be involved in this matter?*
   d. *What principles of autonomy are applied to this situation?*

2. A well-known government official is in the hospital for cosmetic surgery. A story and photograph of the client and his medical information appears in the local paper. The client feels that his privacy has been invaded.
   a. *What are his rights as a client?*
   b. *Could he take legal actions?*

REVIEW QUESTIONS

1. When distinguishing between morality and law, the nurse should identify which indicators may reflect morality: (Select all that apply.)
   1. an awareness of feelings such as guilt, shame, or hope.
   2. that certain laws reflect the moral values of an individual, and actions can be illegal but remain moral but usually just concern trivial matters.
   3. the tendency to respond to the situations with words such as ought, should, right, wrong, good, and bad.

2. What is the "best" example of altruism exhibited by a nurse?
   1. Turning the bed-bound client every 4 hours
   2. Withholding scheduled pain medication to a client that has a level 6 pain scale rating
   3. Insisting that a client use the bedpan instead of assisting the client to the restroom because it is easier for the nurse
   4. Allowing a Catholic client to keep his rosary beads within reach as a comfort measure

3. What behavior exhibited by the client might indicate unclear self-values?
   1. A client with coronary heart disease who follows the recommended diet plan to reduce cholesterol and fat
   2. A mother with a child diagnosed with asthma stops smoking tobacco
   3. A client who has multiple admissions to the chemical dependency program
   4. A diabetic client who monitors finger-stick blood sugars and other health concerns relating to the diabetic condition

4. Choose the correct statement regarding ethical committees and the role they play in dealing with health care conflicts regarding treatments.
   1. The ethical committees have no legal authority.
   2. The ethical committees are necessary to take an activist role for health care providers.
   3. The ethical committees decide when laws or regulations are being violated.
   4. Nurses usually do not serve as team members on ethical committees.

5. What moral framework is the nurse operating under if she refuses to participate in a surgery for a 93-year-old client who has stated on numerous occasions that he does not want further surgery? His family and surgeon are insisting on the client having the surgery. The nurse's rationale is that the nurse-client relationship commits her to protecting him and meeting his needs.
   1. Relationships-based theory
   2. Consequences-based theory
   3. Deontological-based theory
   4. Principles-based theory

6. Which of the following is an example of nonmaleficence and unintentional harm?
   1. Not locking a wheelchair and transferring a client into the wheelchair
   2. Catching a client who is falling and bruising the client's arm
   3. A client's allergic reaction to a prescribed medication
   4. Administering oxygen at 6 L/min to a client when the order is for 2 L/min

7. Identify behaviors that would be classified as an invasion of privacy for a client. (Select all that apply.)
   1. A nurse that removes articles from a bedside table in order to "clear out some of that junk."
   2. A middle-aged, mentally alert client that requests a nursing assistant to "get rid of a bedpan, used ketchup container, and other unused items."
   3. A nursing student that documents the client's name and address on paperwork to hand into the clinical faculty member.
   4. A cousin that wants to review the chart for lab results and the physicians' orders.

8. What is the correct response (actions) by the nurse if a physician asks a nurse to perform a task and the nurse has a lack of education or experience in performing that task?
   1. Inform the physician about the lack of education and experience, and then perform the task.
   2. Do not inform the physician and carry out the task.
   3. Inform the physician regarding the lack of education and/or experience necessary to safely perform the task. Refuse to do the task.
   4. Inform the physician, and then both parties can attempt to figure it out.

9. What is the best example of documentation by the nurse in the client's record?
   1. All facts and information regarding a person's condition, treatment, care, progress, any refusal or consent of treatment, and response to illness and treatment are noted.
   2. All facts and information regarding a person's condition, treatment, care, progress, and response to illness and treatment are noted.
   3. All facts and information regarding a person's condition, treatment, care, progress, any refusal or consent of treatment, physician's competence, and response to illness and treatment are noted.
   4. Chart as little as possible and the nurse will have no reason to fear lawsuits.

10. Organ donation prohibits the (select all that apply):
    1. donation of clients with brain death.
    2. sale of body organs.
    3. marketing of body organs.
    4. donation of cartilage and bones.

CHAPTER 6

HEALTH CARE DELIVERY SYSTEMS

CHAPTER OUTLINE

I. Types of Health Care Services
  A. Primary Prevention: Health Promotion and Illness Prevention
  B. Secondary Prevention: Diagnosis and Treatment
  C. Tertiary Prevention: Rehabilitation, Health Restoration, and Palliative Care

II. Types of Health Care Agencies and Services
  A. Public Health
  B. Physicians' Offices
  C. Ambulatory Care Centers
  D. Occupational Health Clinics
  E. Hospitals
  F. Subacute Care Facilities
  G. Extended Care (Long-Term Care) Facilities
  H. Retirement and Assisted Living Centers
  I. Rehabilitation Centers
  J. Home Health Care Agencies
  K. Day-Care Centers
  L. Rural Care
  M. Hospice Services
  N. Crisis Centers
  O. Mutual Support and Self-Help Groups

III. Providers of Health Care
  A. Nurse
  B. Alternative (Complementary) Care Provider
  C. Case Manager
  D. Dentist
  E. Dietitian or Nutritionist
  F. Occupational Therapist
  G. Paramedical Technologist
  H. Pharmacist
  I. Physical Therapist
  J. Physician
  K. Physician Assistant
  L. Podiatrist
  M. Respiratory Therapist
  N. Social Worker
  O. Spiritual Support Personnel
  P. Unlicensed Assistive Personnel

IV. Factors Affecting Health Care Delivery
  A. Increasing Number of Elderly
  B. Advances in Technology

MediaLink

www.prenhall.com/berman

DVD-ROM
- Audio Glossary
- NCLEX® Review
- Videos:
  - Long-Term Care Facilities
  - Using Health Care Technology Systems

Companion Website
- Additional NCLEX® Review
- Case Study: Delivery Systems
- Application Activities:
  - Where Do Elders Live?
  - Issues Plaguing Women and Children
  - Health Care and Indigents
  - The Competent Case Manager
- Links to Resources

C. Economics
D. Women's Health
E. Uneven Distribution of Services
F. Access to Health Insurance
G. The Homeless and the Poor
H. Health Insurance Portability and Accountability Act (HIPAA)
I. Demographic Changes
V. Frameworks for Care
A. Managed Care
B. Case Management
C. Patient-Focused Care
D. Differentiated Practice
E. Shared Governance

F. Case Method
G. Functional Method
H. Team Nursing
I. Primary Nursing
VI. Financing Health Care
A. Payment Sources in the United States
1. Medicare and Medicaid
2. Supplemental Security Income
3. State Children's Health Insurance Program (SCHIP)
4. Prospective Payment System
B. Insurance Plans
1. Private Insurance
2. Group Plans

KEY TOPIC REVIEW

1. What are the three types of health care services?
   a.
   b.
   c.
2. What is the purpose of primary prevention health care systems?
   a. Health promotion and illness prevention
   b. Rehabilitation, health restoration, and palliative care
   c. Diagnosis and treatment
   d. To promote the World Health Organization
3. What is the purpose of secondary prevention?
   a. Health promotion and illness prevention
   b. Rehabilitation, health restoration, and palliative care
   c. Diagnosis and treatment
   d. To promote the World Health Organization
4. What is the purpose of tertiary prevention?
   a. Health promotion and illness prevention
   b. Rehabilitation, health restoration, and palliative care
   c. Diagnosis and treatment
   d. To promote the World Health Organization
5. What are the primary goals of *Healthy People 2010*?
   a.
   b.
6. What is an example of a secondary prevention?
   a. Physicians' offices
   b. Weight control programs
   c. Blood pressure clinics
   d. Rehabilitation hospitals
7. _____ is the official agency at the federal level for public health.
8. What is the function of occupational health clinics? Give some examples of the types of roles that a nurse might perform in that environment.
9. Name four factors affecting health care delivery in today's health care environment.
   a.
   b.
   c.
   d.
10. According to the U.S. Census, the expected number of frail elderly (people over age 85) will be the _____ growing population segment in the United States and will number over _____ million by 2020 and _____ million by 2030.

11. What impact does the Health Insurance Portability and Accountability Act of 1996 (HIPAA) have on the health care system?
12. What is the definition of critical pathways, and how are critical pathways used in case management and managed care?

FOCUSED STUDY TIPS

1. Discuss the World Health Organization (WHO) project and *Healthy People 2010*.

2. Differentiate between the hospital classification systems. What role does the federal government have in providing care to veterans and merchant mariners?

3. Define the roles of the following providers of health care.
   a. Registered nurse

   b. Licensed vocational nurse or licensed practical nurse

   c. Advanced practice nurse

   d. Complementary care provider

   e. Case manager

   f. Dentist

   g. Dietitian

   h. Occupational therapist

   i. Paramedical technologist

   j. Pharmacist

   k. Physical therapist

   l. Physician

   m. Physician assistant

     n. Podiatrist

     o. Respiratory therapist

     p. Social worker

     q. Spiritual support personnel

     r. Unlicensed assistive personnel

4. Discuss in depth the uneven distribution of health services in the United States. What are the two facets of this problem?

CASE STUDIES

1. *You are taking the health and physical assessment for an 80-year-old blind client who has just been admitted to the unit.*
   a. *What type of health care coverage could she have at this point?*
   b. *If the client's income is below the poverty level, what type of coverage could also be included in the health care coverage plan?*

2. *After caring for the client for 3 days, she is getting ready for discharge. The physician has written an order for physical therapy after discharge. In addition, he requests that a dietitian follow up with additional education regarding the client's newly diagnosed type II diabetes.*
   a. *What roles do the two providers fulfill?*
   b. *Where could the client receive the services, and what type of coverage could possibly pay for these services?*

3. *Refer to the "Research Note" in the textbook to answer the following questions regarding the types of nurses and delivery models in hospitals and how those factors influence patient outcomes.*
   a. *How was the quality of care measured?*
   b. *What types of models were used? Define each of those models.*
   c. *How was quality, coordination, and communication in the units affected?*
   d. *Why is this research important in today's health care delivery systems?*

REVIEW QUESTIONS

1. Choose two frameworks for care that are used for the delivery of nursing care that supports continuity of care and cost-effectiveness:
   1. managed care.
   2. nonfunctional method.
   3. secondary nursing.
   4. team nursing.

2. Medicare is divided into two divisions, Part A and Part B. Another plan was added in January 2006. Part A is the:
   1. voluntary prescription drug plan that began in January 2006.
   2. voluntary plan that provides partial coverage of outpatient and physician services to those who are eligible.
   3. plan section providing insurance toward hospitalization, home care, and hospice care.
   4. plan section providing very limited financial coverage to low-income persons.

3. Medicare is divided into two divisions, Part A and Part B. Another plan was added in January 2006. Part B is the:
    1. voluntary prescription drug plan that began in January 2006.
    2. voluntary plan that provides partial coverage of outpatient and physician services to those who are eligible.
    3. plan section providing insurance toward hospitalization, home care, and hospice care.
    4. plan section providing very limited financial coverage to low-income persons.

4. Medicare is divided into two divisions, Part A and Part B. Another plan was added in January 2006. Part D is the:
    1. voluntary prescription drug plan that began in January 2006.
    2. voluntary plan that provides partial coverage of outpatient and physician services to people eligible.
    3. plan section providing insurance toward hospitalization, home care, and hospice care.
    4. plan section providing very limited financial coverage to low-income persons.

5. Medicaid is described as:
    1. a voluntary prescription drug plan that began in January 2006.
    2. a voluntary plan that provides partial coverage of outpatient and physician services to those who are eligible.
    3. a plan providing insurance toward hospitalization, home care, and hospice care.
    4. a plan providing very limited financial coverage to low-income persons.

6. Choose the person(s) eligible for Supplemental Security Income.
    1. Blind
    2. Persons not eligible for Social Security
    3. Children from low-income families that are covered under Medicaid
    4. Anyone over age 65
    5. Has recognized disablities

7. What is the name of the classification system that prospective payment systems utilize?
    1. Medicare
    2. Medicaid
    3. State Children's Health Insurance Program (SCHIP)
    4. Diagnosis-related groups (DRGs)

8. Third-party reimbursement refers to the insurance company that pays the client's (first party) bill to the provider (second party). This component is part of the:
    1. private health insurance plan.
    2. diagnosis-related group (DRG).
    3. group health insurance plan.
    4. preferred provider organization.

9. Prepaid group plans for insurance include:
    1. Medicare and Medicaid
    2. Blue Cross and Blue Shield
    3. HMOs, PPOs, PPAs, IPAs, and PHOs
    4. Social Security and Supplemental Security Income

10. What is an example of health promotion?
    1. Immunizing children against chickenpox
    2. Caring for a dying client
    3. Assisting a stroke victim to highest rehabilitation possible
    4. Secondary prevention

CHAPTER 7

COMMUNITY NURSING AND CARE CONTINUITY

CHAPTER OUTLINE

I. The Movement of Health Care to the Community
   A. Primary Health Care and Primary Care
II. Community-Based Health Care
III. Community Health
   A. Community-Based Frameworks
   B. Community-Based Settings
      1. Community Nursing Centers
      2. Parish Nursing
      3. Telehealth
IV. Community-Based Nursing
   A. Competencies Required for Community-Based Care
   B. Collaborative Health Care
      1. The Nurse as a Collaborator
      2. Competencies Basic to Collaboration
V. Continuity of Care
   A. Care Across the Life Span
   B. Discharge Planning
   C. Preparing Clients to Go Home
   D. Home Health Care Teaching
   E. Referrals

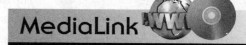

MediaLink

www.prenhall.com/berman

DVD-ROM
• Audio Glossary
• NCLEX® Review

Companion Website
• Additional NCLEX® Review
• Case Studies:
   • The Amish
   • Community Health Nursing
• Application Activities:
   • Community Nursing Standards
   • Government Services
• Link to Resources

KEY TOPIC REVIEW

1. What are three of the factors motivating change in the health care system?
   a. Escalating health care costs
   b. Decreasing technology
   c. Definite patterns of demographics
   d. Shorter hospital stays
   e. Decreased patient acuity
   f. Limited access to health care

2. List four characteristics of primary care.
   a.
   b.
   c.
   d.
3. List four characteristics of primary health care.
   a.
   b.
   c.
   d.
4. Define community-based health care (CBHC). Where is the care directed, and what is involved in CBHC?
5. A _____ is a collection of people who share some attribute of their lives and interact with each other in some way. It is also defined as a social system in which the members interact formally or informally and form networks that operate for the benefit of all people in the community.
6. A _____ is composed of people who share some common characteristic but who do not necessarily interact with each other.
7. List six types of community-based frameworks and give the definition of each.
   a. Type:
      Definition:
   b. Type:
      Definition:
   c. Type:
      Definition:
   d. Type:
      Definition:
   e. Type:
      Definition:
   f. Type:
      Definition:
8. Easy access is needed for an effective community-based health care system.
   a. True   b. False
9. Choose the community-based settings for nursing practice.
   a. Community nursing centers
   b. Long-term care facilities
   c. Parish nursing
   d. Telehealth
   e. Hospitals
10. Community-based nursing focuses on care of individuals in geographically local settings, whereas community health nursing emphasizes the promotion and preservation of the health of groups.
    a. True   b. False

FOCUSED STUDY TIPS

1. What does the Pew Commission competencies for future practitioners include? What are the competencies (listed in the textbook) that the health care practitioner would require?

2. How does the future practitioner obtain these competencies?

3. Primary health care involves five principles. List and explain the five principles in detail.

4. Identify the essential aspects of home health nursing. What makes this community-based role especially challenging?

5. How does the community health care setting differ from traditional settings?

CASE STUDY

A nurse has been working as the case manager in a pediatric unit and decides that she wants to be involved in community nursing.

1. *What are some types of community nursing that could be considered?*
2. *What skills would be needed for the community nursing that might not be used in the pediatric ward?*

REVIEW QUESTIONS

1. The competencies necessary for collaboration between health care providers include:
   1. mutual respect, trust, and negotiation.
   2. communication skills, trust, and decision making.
   3. negotiation, conflict management, and mutual respect.
   4. conflict management, trust, and decision making.

2. As a nurse collaborator, the nurse will perform these actions:
   1. share personal expertise with other nurses and elicit the expertise of others to ensure quality client care.
   2. seek opportunities to collaborate with and within professional organizations.
   3. offer expert opinions on legislative initiatives related to health care.
   4. collaborate with other health care providers and consumers on health care legislation to best serve the needs of the public.

3. Which roles, besides educator, does the nurse need to have in community-based nursing in order to meet the challenges?
   1. Manager, collaborator, advocate, and clinician
   2. Advocate, clinician, decision maker, and empowerment
   3. Advocate to heighten degree of awareness of being a rural nurse, advocate, and enforcer
   4. Enforcer of health policies, clinician, and team nurse

4. When does discharge planning begin for a client?
   1. Prior to discharge
   2. At admission
   3. Two days after admission
   4. Two hours before discharge

5. While doing a home health appraisal, the home health nurse notes the following conditions. Which are potential hazards? (Select all that apply.)
   1. Adequate lighting in the rooms, hallways, stairways, and night lights in the hallways
   2. Stairs without handrails
   3. Grab bars near toilet and tub
   4. Unsecured throw rugs
   5. No fire alarm or extinguisher
   6. Running water and electricity

6. Which of the following populations would possibly be identified before discharge as needing a referral to a long-term nursing facility?
   1. An elderly client who has no caregivers to provide the necessary oversight of care
   2. A child who has had an uncomplicated removal of the tonsils
   3. A mother who delivered a 7-pound baby vaginally the previous day
   4. A client who has a well-healed surgical wound to the abdomen

7. What is the major responsibility of community nursing?
   1. Primary health care in the event of an emergency
   2. Health promotion and disease prevention
   3. Being dependent in their practice
   4. Practices in an institutional setting

8. Choose the correct responses that identify a healthy community.
   1. The members are aware that they belong to and participate in a community.
   2. There are closed channels of communication that do not allow information to flow among the citizens.
   3. Legitimate and effective ways to settle disputes that arise within the community exist.
   4. A decreased level of wellness is promoted among some of its members.

9. One community-based program is parish nursing; identify one of the following roles that the parish nurse may perform.
   1. Establish an abuse program.
   2. Serve as an outreach coordinator.
   3. Serve as faith healer.
   4. Serve as a personal health counselor.

10. One group that benefits from having advanced practice nurses within the community is:
    1. institutionalized persons.
    2. school-age children.
    3. homeless persons.
    4. socially adept individuals.

CHAPTER 8

HOME CARE

CHAPTER OUTLINE

I. Home Health Nursing
  A. Unique Aspects of Home Health Nursing
  B. Practice of Home Health Nursing
II. The Home Health Care System
  A. Referral Process
  B. Home Health Agencies
  C. Private Duty Agencies
  D. Durable Medical Equipment Companies
  E. Reimbursement
III. Roles of the Home Health Nurse
  A. Advocate
  B. Caregiver
  C. Educator
  D. Case Manager or Coordinator
IV. Perspectives of Home Care Clients
V. Selected Dimensions of Home Health Nursing
  A. Client Safety
  B. Nurse Safety
  C. Infection Control
  D. Caregiver Support
VI. The Practice of Nursing in the Home
  A. Establishing Health Issues
  B. Planning and Delivering Care
VII. The Future of Home Health Care

KEY TOPIC REVIEW

1. Identify factors that have contributed to the increase and growth in home health care.
2. What does home care involve in today's health care system?
3. _____ nursing is support and care of the dying person and his or her family and is considered a subspecialty of home health nursing.
4. What are the advantages of home health nursing?
5. What are the disadvantages of home health nursing?

6. List four of the duties that a home health nurse might perform in the home setting.
   a.
   b.
   c.
   d.
7. Any person involved with the client may identify the need for home health.
   a. True   b. False
8. How is home health reimbursed?
9. Match the following types of home health agencies with their descriptions.
   a. Official or public agencies
   b. Voluntary or private not-for-profit agencies
   c. Private, proprietary agencies
   d. Institution-based agencies

   _____ These institutions rely on private pay sources or "third-party" reimbursement
   _____ United Way
   _____ Hospital home health agencies
   _____ State health department

FOCUSED STUDY TIPS

1. Refer to the Visiting Nurses Associations of America website (go to the Companion Website). What is this agency's definition of a home health nurse?

2. Describe the unique aspects of home health nursing. What is involved in the practice of home health nursing? List additional providers in home health and describe their duties or roles.

3. What does the referral process entail? What is necessary from the physician in order to begin home health care? What are the nurse's responsibilities?

4. How is home health reimbursed? What criteria or guidelines for reimbursement are followed by Medicare or Medicaid?

5. Why is documentation especially critical in home health?

6. Explain the concept of infection control in the home setting. What is the nurse's major role? How can the nurse minimize risk of infection?

CASE STUDY

Refer to the Research Note in Chapter 8 of the textbook regarding the nurse's safety during home health visits.

1. *What were the community concerns with the nurse's safety?*
2. *What are some additional measures that could be carried out in order to promote the safety of the home health personnel?*

REVIEW QUESTIONS

1. What type of company provides health care equipment for home health clients?
   1. Hospice
   2. Private home health agency
   3. Durable medical equipment (DME)
   4. Durable equipment

2. The home health nurse is functioning as an educator during a home health visit. Which of the following is the best example of that role?
   1. Changing an indwelling Foley catheter
   2. Discussing living wills and durable power of attorney and obtaining a social work consult
   3. Instructing a client on a diabetic diet
   4. Documentation of care provided by the agency

3. The home health nurse is functioning as an advocate during an initial assessment. Which of the following is the best example of that role?
   1. Changing an indwelling Foley catheter
   2. Discussing living wills and durable power of attorney
   3. Instructing a client on a diabetic diet
   4. Documentation of care provided by the agency

4. The home health nurse is functioning as a caregiver (provider of direct care) during a home health visit. Which of the following is the best example of that role?
   1. Changing an indwelling Foley catheter
   2. Discussing living wills and durable power of attorney
   3. Instructing a client on a diabetic diet
   4. Documentation of care provided by the agency

5. What is considered to be the crux of home health care?
   1. Being an advocate
   2. Being a caregiver
   3. Being a case manager
   4. Being an educator

6. In home health nursing, family members are considered as _____ clients because they are associated with caregiving and have a major impact on the client's wellness status.
   1. primary
   2. secondary
   3. tertiary
   4. isolated

7. Identify the signs of caregiver role strain. (Select all that apply.)
   1. Complains of decreasing energy and not enough time to perform tasks
   2. Has anxiety about ability to meet future needs
   3. Has feelings of joy and happiness
   4. Has difficulty performing routine tasks for the client

8. An example of a home health service provided by nurses is:
   1. housekeeping duties for the client.
   2. providing a hospital bed for the client.
   3. daily wound care for the client.
   4. writing the living will for the client.

9. Hospice nursing provides:
   1. intravenous therapy for nutrition such as total parental nutrition (TPN).
   2. tracheotomy care for a chronic COPD client.
   3. care to the terminally ill client.
   4. education about acute conditions such as diabetes.

10. When is the most appropriate time for the client and family members to be involved in obtaining home health services?
    1. During the initial home health assessment visit by the registered nurse
    2. On admission to the hospital
    3. Prior to discharge from the hospital
    4. While the client is terminally ill

CHAPTER 9

NURSING INFORMATICS

CHAPTER OUTLINE

I. General Concepts
  A. Computer Hardware
    1. Central Processing Unit
    2. Computer Memory and Storage
    3. Input Devices
    4. Output Devices
    5. Communications Devices
  B. Computer Software
    1. Word Processing
    2. Databases
    3. Spreadsheets
    4. Communications
    5. Presentation Graphics Programs
  C. Computer Systems
    1. Management Information Systems
    2. Hospital Information Systems
    3. World Wide Web and the Internet
II. Computers in Nursing Education
  A. Teaching and Learning
    1. Literature Access and Retrieval
    2. Computer-Assisted Instruction
    3. Classroom Technology
    4. Distance Learning
  B. Testing
  C. Student and Course Record Management
III. Computers in Nursing Practice
  A. Documentation of Client Status and Medical Record Keeping
    1. Bedside Data Entry

2. Computer-Based Client Records
    3. Data Standardization and Classifications
    4. Tracking Client Status
  B. Electronic Access to Client Data
    1. Client Monitoring and Computerized Diagnostics
    2. Telemedicine/Telehealth
  C. Practice Management
  D. Specific Applications of Computers in Nursing Practice
    1. Community and Home Health
    2. Case Management

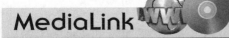

MediaLink

www.prenhall.com/berman

DVD-ROM
• Audio Glossary
• NCLEX® Review
• End of Unit Concept Map Activity

Companion Website
• Additional NCLEX® Review
• Case Study: Computerizing Clinical Documentation
• Application Activities:
  • Confidentiality Laws
  • Working on the Hospital Informatics Committee
  • Informatics Certification Exam
• Links to Resources

IV. Computers in Nursing Administration
   A. Human Resources
   B. Medical Records Management
   C. Facilities Management
   D. Budget and Finance
   E. Quality Assurance and Utilization Reviews
   F. Accreditation

V. Computers in Nursing Research
   A. Problem Identification
   B. Literature Review
   C. Research Design
   D. Data Collection and Analysis
   E. Research Dissemination
   F. Research Grants

KEY TOPIC REVIEW

1. List the parts of computer hardware.
   a.
   b.
   c.
   d.
   e.
2. Client concerns regarding _____ and _____ of health records have arisen as electronic databases and communications have proliferated.
3. What are the most common computer software programs used in nursing?
4. Define the following terms associated with computer hardware:
   a. Hardware
   b. Central processing unit (CPU)
   c. Peripherals
   d. Random-access memory (RAM)
5. Give two examples of a personal computer.
6. The term _____ refers to a computer being connected to other computers in a _____.
7. Indicate one type of computer software used in nursing and list one application used with that software.
8. A hospital information system (HIS) organizes data from various areas in the hospital. Give four examples of where this information may be gathered.
   a.
   b.
   c.
   d.
9. _____ established legal requirements for the protection, security, and appropriate sharing of patient personal health information (referred to as Protected Health Information or PHI).
10. What are the four ways that computers have enhanced nursing education?
    a.
    b.
    c.
    d.

FOCUSED STUDY TIPS

1. Discuss the criteria for evaluating Internet health information. How has the widespread availability of information impacted health care today?

2. What is the difference between distance education courses and Web-enhanced or hybrid courses?

3. What are the advantages of taking the National Council Licensure Examination (NCLEX®) on a computer? When did the test change from pen-and-paper administration to computer administration?

4. Telemedicine (or telehealth) uses technology to transmit electronic data about clients to persons at distant locations. What are some of the advantages of telemedicine? What are the disadvantages?

5. One of the main concerns with health care and information technology is privacy issues. Refer to the Companion Website for links to confidentiality laws. As a nurse, how can you impact changes on the state and federal level regarding privacy? Refer to the ANA position statement on privacy. What is the nurse's role in the privacy issue?

CASE STUDY

A 45-year-old client is scheduled to have a hysterectomy later this week. She is at the hospital to get her preoperative nursing assessment, several laboratory exams, and chest x-ray. The nurse and laboratory technologist are using a computerized data entry system that is managed on a handheld device.

1. *If the client's results are entered into computer-based patient records (CPRs), who would be able to legally access her medical information?*
2. *The chest x-ray is abnormal and the primary care provider wishes to consult a respiratory specialist. If he sends the x-ray film electronically to the consulting primary care provider that is an example of what type of medicine?*
3. *What are the advantages of this type of consultation?*
4. *Does the client have to sign any consent forms in regard to her electronic medical records?*

REVIEW QUESTIONS

1. What is an advantage of having "paper" medical records for clients?
   1. There are legal standards that have been tested for the paper medical record and there are years of cost analysis for the financial aspects of having paper medical records.
   2. The paper medical records are often illegible and incomplete.
   3. Paper medical records take up a lot of storage space due to the required time to keep the records on file.
   4. Records are shared only through hard copy and thus are difficult to locate and provide copies to the various agencies requiring records for review.

2. The World Wide Web (WWW) refers to:
   1. wrestling team.
   2. complex links among Web pages or websites.
   3. universal resource locators.
   4. a network designed to facilitate the organization and application of data.

3. Universal resource locators (URLs) are also called:
   1. television stations.
   2. addresses.
   3. links among Web pages or websites.
   4. rural addresses.

4. Which of the following computerized systems would assist a physician in Russia to consult with a physician in the United States?
   1. Distance learning
   2. Computer-based client records
   3. Telemedicine
   4. Local area network

5. What does the designation of ".org" denote?
   1. Commercial sites
   2. Organizations
   3. Educational institutions
   4. Government sites

6. A group of nursing students located in different sites for a nursing class are participating in classes through two-way audio and video transmissions. In addition, they use chat and instant messaging. This is an example of which type of distance learning model?
   1. Asynchronous distance learning
   2. Synchronous distance learning
   3. Computer-assisted instruction in distance learning
   4. Self-study distance learning

7. What is one way that a nurse administrator might use a computer?
   1. To follow client's health status during the hospital stay
   2. To manage a budget
   3. To obtain the latest information on cardiac diseases
   4. To participate in a research study

8. How is computer-based instruction (CAI) used by nurses to further their education?
   1. It allows nurses to further their education and also demonstrate continuing education units required for license renewal.
   2. It allows the nurses to share health care information with clients.
   3. It is used to test nursing students for the NCLEX.
   4. It is used as a bookkeeping system.

9. Nurses play a critical role in preserving client privacy and confidentiality. What role does the Health Insurance Portability and Accountability Act (HIPAA) play in client confidentiality?
   1. It provides a database for insurance agencies to utilize.
   2. It provides for data standardization.
   3. It provides for data classifications.
   4. It provides for privacy and confidentiality for clients in health care.

10. Electronic medical records (EMRs) or computer-based records (CPRs) permit electronic client data retrieval by caregivers, administrators, creditors, and other persons who require the data. Who sets the national standards to protect the identity of the clients?
    1. The federal government sets the standards.
    2. There are no national standards.
    3. The different states set the standards.
    4. HIPAA sets the standards.

CHAPTER 10

CRITICAL THINKING AND THE NURSING PROCESS

CHAPTER OUTLINE

I. Critical Thinking
II. Skills in Critical Thinking
III. Attitudes that Foster Critical Thinking
    A. Independence
    B. Fair-Mindedness
    C. Insight into Egocentricity
    D. Intellectual Humility
    E. Intellectual Courage to Challenge the Status Quo and Rituals
    F. Integrity
    G. Perseverance
    H. Confidence
    I. Curiosity
IV. Standards of Critical Thinking
V. Applying Critical Thinking to Nursing Practice
    A. Problem Solving
        1. Trial and Error
        2. Intuition
        3. Research Process and Scientific/Modified Scientific Method
    B. Decision Making
VI. Developing Critical-Thinking Attitudes and Skills
    A. Self-Assessment
    B. Tolerating Dissonance and Ambiguity
    C. Seeking Situations Where Good Thinking Is Practiced
    D. Creating Environments that Support Critical Thinking

MediaLink

www.prenhall.com/berman

DVD-ROM
- Audio Glossary
- NCLEX® Review
- Video: Thinking Critically

Companion Website
- Additional NCLEX® Review
- Case Study: Examining an Increase in Pressure Ulcers
- Application Activity: Practicing Critical Thinking
- Links to Resources

KEY TOPIC REVIEW

1. Critical thinking consists of high-level cognitive processes that include _____ _____ and _____ _____ .

2. Define the following problem-solving methods:
    a. Trial and error
    b. Intuition
    c. Nursing process
    d. Scientific method
    e. Modified scientific method
3. _____ _____ is a purposeful mental activity that guides beliefs and actions.
4. What is meant by inductive and deductive reasoning in critical thinking?
5. _____ _____ is a technique one can use to look beneath the surface, recognize and examine assumptions, search for inconsistencies, examine multiple points of view, and differentiate what one knows from what one merely believes.
6. List five or more characteristics that most critical thinkers have.
7. _____, at every step of critical thinking and nursing care, helps examine the ways in which the nurse gathers and analyzes data, makes decisions, and determines the effectiveness of interventions.
8. Identify the sequential steps to the decision-making process.
    a.
    b.
    c.
    d.
    e.
    f.
    g.
    h.
9. What is the definition of decision making? Give one example of the decision-making process as a critical-thinking process for choosing the best actions to meet a desired goal.
10. Critical thinkers are unwilling to admit what they do not know; they are willing to seek new information and to rethink their conclusions in light of new knowledge.
    a. True   b. False

FOCUSED STUDY TIPS

1. What are the four stages of critical thinking?

2. Describe Maslow's hierarchy of basic human needs. Why is this concept important to nursing?

3. List the characteristics of critical thinking. What are the skills needed by one who uses critical thinking?

4. List and describe the three methods used with critical thinking that is used to problem-solve during the nursing process.

5. Why must the nursing process occur in chronological order of assessment, analyzing, planning, implementing, and evaluating?

CASE STUDY

The student nurse should begin using critical thinking in daily life. By doing this, the student nurse will practice using critical thinking in the clinical environment and in everyday situations. In order to clarify the critical-thinking process for a beginning nursing student, a non-nursing case study will be used for this case study.

A close friend states that she is habitually overdrawing her bank checking account. She has asked you for advice with this problem. Using the Socratic questions listed in Box 10–2 of the textbook, analyze this problem.

    a. *Questions about the question or problem:*

    b. *Questions about assumptions:*

    c. *Questions about point of view:*

    d. *Questions about evidence and reasons:*

    e. *Questions about implications and consequences:*

REVIEW QUESTIONS

1. In critical thinking, the least effective decision-making process is:
   1. analyzing the data.
   2. formulating conclusions.
   3. establishing assumptions.
   4. synthesizing information.

2. When discussing the trial-and-error method of problem solving, it is understood that this method lacks:
   1. emphasis.
   2. order.
   3. efficiency of time.
   4. precision.

3. The scientific method of problem solving is:
   1. most effective in controlled situations.
   2. least effective in controlled situations.
   3. illogical.
   4. lacking in precision.

4. The modified scientific method is used in nursing because it (select all that apply):
   1. does not involve the interaction between the client and nurse as they work together.
   2. does involve the interaction between the client and nurse as they work together.
   3. is used to identify potential or actual health care needs, set goals, devise a plan to meet the client's needs, and evaluate the plan's effectiveness.
   4. deals with stressful environments.

5. During emergency situations, critical thinking enables nurses to:
   1. delay response.
   2. underreact to the problem.
   3. meet the physician's needs.
   4. recognize important cues.

6. In the pediatric unit, a nurse tries to have a young child use the incentive spirometer. The child is refusing to use the equipment and the nurse encourages the child to inhale slowly and steadily to maintain constant flow through the unit, then hold her breath for 2–3 seconds, and then exhale slowly. If the child cannot grasp the mechanics behind using the incentive spirometer, the nurse could give the client balloons and/or a jar of bubbles to blow. This is an example of:
   1. modified scientific method.
   2. scientific method.
   3. creativity.
   4. critical thinking.

7. While working in the critical care unit, a nurse is caring for a client after cardiac bypass. The nurse gets a gut feeling "that something is wrong" even though the client has no outward signs or symptoms. This is an example of:
   1. intuition.
   2. trial and error.
   3. research process.
   4. scientific method.

8. In the emergency department, the nurse observes that a client is actively bleeding from an abdominal gunshot wound. The nurse assumes that the client is at an increased risk for hypovolemic shock. The nurse bases her viewpoint after viewing the outpouring of frank, red bleeding and reasoning that shock may occur if fluids or blood is not replaced. This is an example of:
   1. creativity.
   2. deductive reasoning.
   3. inductive reasoning.
   4. critical analysis.

9. While attending a nursing educator's conference, a nursing instructor obtains information about the use of concept maps and clinical pathways. The nursing instructor returns to work at the university and discusses the new techniques with the other instructors. This is an example of:
   1. creating an environment to support critical thinking.
   2. seeking information regarding new educational promotions.
   3. intellectual humility.
   4. judgment.

10. The definition of the nursing process is:
    1. essential to safe, competent, skillful nursing practice.
    2. thinking that results in the development of new ideas and products.
    3. a critical-thinking process for choosing the best actions to meet a desired goal.
    4. a systematic, rational method of planning and providing individualized nursing care.

CHAPTER 11

ASSESSING

CHAPTER OUTLINE

MediaLink

www.prenhall.com/berman

DVD-ROM
- Audio Glossary
- NCLEX® Review

Companion Website
- Additional NCLEX® Review
- Case Study: Down Syndrome Client
- Application Activity: Care of a Disorganized Elderly Client
- Links to Resources

KEY TOPIC REVIEW

1. What is the purpose of the nursing process?
2. The nursing process is both interpersonal and collaborative between the nurse and the client.
   a. True   b. False

3. Assessing is a continuous process carried out though all the phases of nursing.
    a. True   b. False
4. What are the four different types of assessment?
    a.
    b.
    c.
    d.
5. According to the Joint Commission on Accreditation of Healthcare Organizations (JACHO), each client must have an initial assessment within _____ hours of admission.
6. What are the four activities involved in the nursing process?
    a.
    b.
    c.
    d.
7. Determine if the following information is subjective or objective assessment data.
    (S) Subjective   (O) Objective
    a. _____   "I feel tired all the time."
    b. _____   Skin warm and dry to touch
    c. _____   "I am itching all over."
    d. _____   Smell of ammonia in urine
    e. _____   Purplish discoloration on left forearm
    f. _____   Temperature of 102 degrees orally
8. Distinguish between the primary and secondary (indirect) sources of data in the assessment process.
    (P) Primary   (S) Secondary
    a. _____   "My son has vomited for 3 days."
    b. _____   "I have been coughing for 2 weeks."
    c. _____   45-year-old female
    d. _____   "I have a rash."

9. When does the observation portion of data collection occur?
    a. On the initial assessment
    b. Immediately
    c. It is an ongoing process.
    d. Observation is not part of data collection.
10. _____ is planned communication or conversation with a purpose.

FOCUSED STUDY TIPS

1. Explain the difference between the medical model of problem solving and the nursing process. What are the parallels between the two models?

2. Why would it be important to review data from client records such as occupation, religion, marital status, and so on before beginning the nurse health history?

3. Why is sharing of information important in health care? What is pertinent information that needs to be relayed between nursing shifts?

CASE STUDY

A client is being transferred to the unit from the recovery room after having an abdominal tumor removed. The recovery room nurse gives an oral report on the client's condition stating that the dressing is dry and intact, vital signs stable, IV of RL infusing at 100 mL per hour in the left forearm, intact and patent, medications given, and that the client has no complaints of pain. During the initial assessment, the medical surgical nurse notes that the abdominal dressing has bright red drainage. The client stated, "I am really hurting bad!" The vital signs are 140/86, RR 24, T 98.2 orally, and pulse of 90 beats per minute.

1. *What is the objective data?*
2. *What is the subjective data?*
3. *Who is considered the primary source?*
4. *Who is considered the secondary source?*

REVIEW QUESTIONS

1. The nurse is assessing the sputum characteristics of a client with pneumonia. What are the senses that the nurse may use in the assessment of the sputum? (Select all that apply.)
   1. Vision
   2. Smell
   3. Hearing
   4. Touch

2. What are two coping mechanisms that clients may exhibit during hospitalization?
   1. Micromanaging and/or anger
   2. Macromanaging and/or anger
   3. Misery and/or aggression
   4. Anger and/or mismanagement

3. During the process of data collection, the nurse must be cognizant of the different cultural aspects in health care. In the interview phase, what should the nurse consider that might have a cultural aspect?
   1. Time of the interview
   2. Setting of the interview
   3. Distance between nurse and client
   4. Seating arrangement

4. What is an example of an open-ended question that the nurse may use in the interview process?
   1. "What medication did you take today?"
   2. "What surgeries have you had in the past?"
   3. "Are you a student at the local college?"
   4. "How have you been feeling lately?"

5. What is the name of the head-to-toe approach that usually begins the nurse physical examination?
   1. Review of systems
   2. Screening examination
   3. Cephalocaudal
   4. Caudal approach

6. What framework is based on 11 functional health patterns and collects data about dysfunctional and functional behavior?
   1. Orem's self-care model
   2. Gordon's functional health patterns
   3. Roy's adaptation model
   4. The wellness model

7. After completing the health history and the physical assessment, the nurse identifies discrepancies in the information. What is this process called?
    1. Assessing
    2. Diagnosing
    3. Planning
    4. Evaluating

8. A client presents to the emergency department with complaints of chest pain. The nurse takes the client's vital signs. The nurse is implementing which phase of the nursing process?
    1. Assessment
    2. Diagnosis
    3. Planning
    4. Implementation

9. The nurse reassesses a client's temperature 45 minutes after administering acetaminophen. This is an example of what type of an assessment?
    1. Ongoing
    2. Intermittent
    3. Terminal
    4. Routine

10. The nurse is measuring the drainage from a Jackson Pratt drain. Which of the following should the nurse consider as objective data?
    1. The client is complaining of abdominal pain.
    2. The drainage measurement is 25 mL.
    3. The client stated, "I did not empty the drain."
    4. The client stated that he has a pain level of 5.

CHAPTER 12

DIAGNOSING

CHAPTER OUTLINE

MediaLink

www.prenhall.com/berman

DVD-ROM
- Audio Glossary
- NCLEX® Review

Companion Website
- Additional NCLEX® Review
- Case Study: Selecting Nursing Diagnoses for Client with Pneumonia
- Application Activity: Resources for a Chronically Ill Child
- Links to Resources

KEY TOPIC REVIEW

1. What is the first stage of the nursing process?
2. What is the second stage of the nursing process?
3. A _____ is a classification system or set of categories based on a single principle or set of principles.
4. What are the parts of the North American Nursing Diagnosis Association (NANDA) nursing diagnosis?
   a.   b.   c.
5. All nurses are responsible for making nursing diagnoses according to the ANA Standards of Practice.
   a. True   b. False
6. The nursing diagnosis is a judgment made only after thorough, systematic data collection.
   a. True   b. False
7. What are the five types of nursing diagnoses?
   a.
   b.
   c.
   d.
   e.
8. In order to enhance clinical usefulness, the diagnostic labels must be as _____ as possible.
9. What five words are identified as qualifiers to give additional meaning to the diagnostic statement?
   a.
   b.
   c.
   d.
   e.
10. What is the definition of etiology? What are two characteristics of etiology?
11. For risk diagnoses, there are no subjective or objective signs in the assessment phase.
    a. True   b. False

12. For actual nursing diagnoses, the defining characteristics are the client's signs and symptoms in the assessment phase of the nursing process.
    a. True   b. False

FOCUSED STUDY TIPS

1. A nursing diagnosis has three components. List the three components and give an example of each.

2. Why is it important to differentiate among the possible causes in the nursing diagnosis? (Refer to Table 12–2 in textbook.)

3. What are the differentiating factors between a nursing diagnosis and a medical diagnosis?

4. Describe characteristics of the nursing diagnosis. What is a two-part diagnostic statement? What is a three-part diagnostic statement?

5. List two examples each of a one-part, two-part, and three-part diagnostic statement. Refer to the PES diagnosis in the textbook.

CASE STUDY

A newly admitted client in the unit will be your responsibility as the registered nurse. The client is a 47-year-old male of American Indian heritage with type 2 diabetes. He stated that he hasn't been taking his medication because it does not make him feel any better; he also has difficulty remembering to take the medication. The following information pertains to this client:

- *Fingerstick blood sugar = 213 mg/dl*
- *B/P 150/90; temp 98.6 oral; respirations 24 breaths per minute; and pulse 78 beats/min.*
- *"I use the bathroom about 8 times per day."*
- *Ht 6 feet 4 inches; weight 284 pounds*

1. *What is an actual nursing diagnosis for this client?*
2. *What is a potential nursing diagnosis for this client?*
3. *Identify one subjective and one objective assessment to substantiate the nursing diagnosis.*
4. *What is the outcome goal for the patient?*

REVIEW QUESTIONS

1. The end result of data collection and analysis is:
    1. carrying out the plan of care.
    2. collecting and then analyzing the data.
    3. identifying actual or potential health concerns.
    4. identifying the client's response to care.

2. Identify the nursing diagnosis from the following medical diagnoses.
    1. Fever of unknown origin
    2. Pancreatitis
    3. Potential for sleep-pattern disturbances
    4. Congestive heart failure

3. The purpose of a nursing diagnosis is to:
    1. define taxonomy of nursing language.
    2. promote taxonomy of nursing language.
    3. identify a client's problem plus etiology.
    4. establish a set of principles.

4. Choose the appropriate activities that the nurse may perform during the diagnosing component of the nursing process. (Select all that apply.)
    1. compare data against current nursing standards.
    2. obtain a nursing health history.
    3. cluster or group the data to generate a tentative hypothesis.
    4. review the client records and nursing literature.
    5. identify gaps and inconsistencies in the data.

5. One of the nursing functions during the diagnosing phase of the nursing process is to:
    1. clarify all inconsistencies in the data before making inferences.
    2. identify Gordon's functional health patterns and compare with the client.
    3. review the literature and review professional journals and textbooks.
    4. document the health assessment in a specific form.

6. *Readiness for Enhanced Parenting* is an example of which type of diagnosis?
    1. Wellness diagnosis
    2. Health-seeking diagnosis
    3. Two-part diagnosis
    4. Three-part diagnosis

7. Which of the following nursing diagnostic statements is correct?
   1. Fluid replacement related to fever
   2. Impaired skin integrity related to immobility
   3. Impaired skin integrity related to ulceration of sacral area
   4. Pain related to severe headache

8. How does the nurse begin with a diagnostic label for a collaborative problem?
   1. Readiness for Enhanced Spiritual Well-Being
   2. Alteration of Respiratory Status
   3. Potential Complication for Pneumonia: Atelectasis
   4. Impaired Respiratory System

9. The PES format for writing a nursing diagnosis is used for which of the following?
   1. Actual nursing diagnoses
   2. Potential nursing diagnoses
   3. Risk for nursing diagnoses
   4. Wellness diagnoses

10. Choose the correct example of a qualifier.
    1. Syndrome
    2. Potential
    3. Deficient
    4. Risk for

11. Identify and select the advantages of using a taxonomy of nursing diagnoses. (Select all that apply.)
    1. A taxonomy of nursing diagnoses would promote a classification system or set of categories for a single or set of principles for professional nurses.
    2. A taxonomy of nursing diagnoses can be used by physicians to define diagnostic nursing terminology.
    3. A taxonomy of nursing diagnoses enhances the professional practice of the nurse in generating and completing a nursing care plan.
    4. A taxonomy of nursing diagnoses consists of nursing diagnoses for a single principle or set of principles that were developed by other nursing professionals.

12. Identify the components of a nursing diagnosis. (Select all that apply.)
    1. Related factors
    2. Risk factors
    3. Problem
    4. Definition
    5. Defining characteristics
    6. Medical conditions

CHAPTER 13

PLANNING

CHAPTER OUTLINE

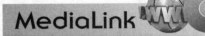

MediaLink

www.prenhall.com/berman

DVD-ROM
- Audio Glossary
- NCLEX® Review

Companion Website
- Additional NCLEX® Review
- Case Study: Client Struck by a Car
- Application Activity: Client with Peptic Ulcers
- Links to Resources

KEY TOPIC REVIEW

1. According to Dochterman and Bulechek (2004), a _____ _____ is "any treatment, based upon clinical judgment and knowledge that a nurse performs to enhance client outcomes."
2. When does planning begin?
3. Who is responsible for developing the initial comprehensive plan of care, and when is it initiated?
4. List the four purposes the nurse uses to guide daily planning by utilizing ongoing assessment data.
   a.
   b.
   c.
   d.
5. During the planning stage of the nursing process, what are four tasks that the nurse and client complete?
   a.
   b.
   c.
   d.
6. Match the four different types of nursing care plans with their correct definitions.
   a. Informal nursing care plan
   b. Standardized care plan
   c. Individualized care plan
   d. Formal nursing care plan

   _____ is tailored to meet the unique needs of a specific client—needs that are not addressed by the standardized plan.

   _____ is a strategy for action that exists in the nurse's mind.

   _____ is a written or computerized guide that organizes information about the client's care.

   _____ is a formal plan that specifies the nursing care for groups of clients with common needs.

7. Refer to Figure 13-2 in the textbook. What documents may be included in a complete plan of care?
   a.
   b.
   c.
   d.
   e.
   f.
   g.
8. Refer to the standards of care for thrombophlebits in Figure 13-3 of the textbook. How are standards of care different than individualized care plans? What are the advantages and disadvantages of standards of care?
9. Why are students asked to complete pathophysiology flow sheets or concept maps or care plans with rationales? Define concept map and rationale.
10. What do the goals or desired outcomes describe? What is the Nursing Outcomes Classification (NOC)?

FOCUSED STUDY TIPS

1. What is planning? What phase of the nursing process is planning? What is the end product of planning called? Who is involved in the planning process?

2. Discuss the three types of planning and list the significant tasks that registered nurses must do during each of the types/stages of planning.

3. Differentiate between protocols, policies, procedures, and standing orders.

4. What are the 10 guidelines for writing nursing care plans? Why is each guideline important?

5. What is meant by the activity of priority setting in the planning process? What factors need to be considered when assigning priorities?

6. What is the purpose of desired goals and/or outcomes?

CASE STUDIES

1. *A nurse is eating at a local fast food restaurant. Suddenly, another customer starts choking and clutches her throat. The nurse attempts the Heimlich maneuver and it is unsuccessful. The client becomes unresponsive and is not breathing. The customer's tray is on the table and a partially eaten hot dog is on the tray.*

   a. *What is the first action to take at this point?*
   b. *If the client does not respond, what should the next action be?*
   c. *What has the nurse done to assess the situation?*
   d. *What parts of the nursing process are being carried out?*

Outcomes should be SMART (specific, measurable, appropriate, realistic, and timely). Analyze the following nursing care plan:

2. *A client has stage 4 pressure ulcers on the coccyx, left and right mallcolus, and both heels. He is unable to turn himself in the bed. His daughter stated "This happened so suddenly; he did not have these sores until he had the stroke and quit eating." The nurse assesses the client and notes that he is an elderly, emaciated, bedfast client with the previously stated pressure ulcers.*

   a. *What is the subjective and objective data?*
   b. *What nursing diagnosis will fit this situation?*
   c. *What are the realistic short-term and long-term goals for this client?*
   d. *What are four nursing orders or interventions that can be used for this client?*

REVIEW QUESTIONS

1. "Client will walk to end of hallway without assistance by Friday" is an example of a:
   1. long-term goal.
   2. short-term goal.
   3. nursing intervention.
   4. rationale.

2. "Client will ambulate 20 yards without assistance in 8 weeks" is an example of a:
   1. long-term goal.
   2. short-term goal.
   3. nursing intervention.
   4. rationale.

3. The nurse instructs a newly diagnosed diabetes client on an 1800-calorie ADA diet. This is which type of nursing intervention?
   1. Independent intervention
   2. Dependent intervention
   3. Collaborative intervention
   4. Variable intervention

4. The nurse instructs the client on turning, coughing, and deep breathing q 2 hours. What is the relationship of nursing interventions to problem status?
   1. Health promotion interventions
   2. Treatment interventions
   3. Prevention interventions
   4. Observation interventions

5. The registered nurse needs to assign a person to insert a Foley catheter on a client. To whom can she delegate this task?
   1. Unlicensed personnel with limited training
   2. A licensed practical/vocational nurse
   3. The physician
   4. The client's daughter

6. Planning consists of which component?
   1. Reassess the client.
   2. Analyze data.
   3. Select nursing interventions.
   4. Determine the nurse's need for assistance.

7. Consider the following nursing diagnosis: "Altered nutritional status, less than body requirements related to inability to feed self." What is an example of a short-term goal for this client?
   1. The client will eat 75% of his meals by Friday (September 20) with the use of modified eating utensils to feed self with minimal assistance.
   2. The client will learn about nutritious meal planning as exhibited by choosing one correct menu.
   3. The client will acquire competence in managing cookware designed for handicapped clients.
   4. The client will learn preparation techniques that are quick and easy to manage.

8. The nurse admitted a client in active labor to the labor and delivery wing of the hospital. When does the planning for client care start?
   1. After the physician has delivered the baby
   2. After the admission process
   3. When the client is discharged to the postpartum unit
   4. During the initial meeting

9. Which of the following is part of the permanent client record?
   1. Nursing protocols
   2. Client care plan
   3. Procedures for client care
   4. The nurse's notebook of daily notes to herself

10. In caring for a client with stage 4 pressure ulcers on the coccyx, the nurse is to turn the client every 2 hours while in bed. What part of the nursing process is being carried out?
    1. Assessment
    2. Diagnosis
    3. Implementation
    4. Evaluation

11. The benefits of a nursing intervention classification system are: (select all that apply):
    1. helps demonstrate the impact that nurses have on the health care delivery system.
    2. assists educators to develop curricula that better articulates with clinical practice.
    3. standardizes and defines the knowledge base for nursing curricula and practice.
    4. facilitates the appropriate selection of a nursing intervention and communication of nursing treatments to other nurses and other providers.
    5. promotes the development of a reimbursement system for nursing services.

12. A taxonomy of nursing outcome statements were developed to describe measurable states, behaviors, or perceptions to respond to which part of the nursing process?
    1. Nursing assessments
    2. Nursing interventions
    3. Nursing goals
    4. Nursing outcomes

CHAPTER 14

IMPLEMENTING AND EVALUATING

CHAPTER OUTLINE

I. Implementing
   A. Relationship of Implementing to Other Nursing Process Phases
   B. Implementing Skills
   C. Process of Implementing
      1. Reassessing the Client
      2. Determining the Nurse's Need for Assistance
      3. Implementing the Nursing Interventions
      4. Supervising Delegated Care
      5. Documenting Nursing Activities

II. Evaluating
   A. Relationship of Evaluating to Other Nursing Process Phases
   B. Process of Evaluating Client Responses
      1. Collecting Data
      2. Comparing Data with Outcomes
      3. Relating Nursing Activities to Client Goals/Outcomes
      4. Drawing Conclusions about Problem Status
      5. Continuing, Modifying, and Terminating the Nursing Care Plan
   C. Evaluating the Quality of Nursing Care
      1. Quality Assurance
      2. Quality Improvement
      3. Nursing Audit

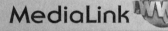

MediaLink

www.prenhall.com/berman

DVD-ROM
- Audio Glossary
- NCLEX® Review

Companion Website
- Additional NCLEX® Review
- Case Study: Treating a Client for Pain
- Application Activity:
  - Analyzing Effective Quality Insurances
- Links to Resources

KEY TOPIC REVIEW

1. The nursing process is _____ oriented, _____ _____, and _____ directed.
2. According to NIC terminology, _____ consists of doing and documenting the activities that are specific nursing actions needed to carry out the interventions.
3. _____, _____, and _____ skills are used to implement nursing strategies.
4. When does the implementing phase terminate?
5. The first three nursing phases of _____, _____, and _____ provide the basis for the nursing actions performed during the implementing step.

Match the type of skill with the following activities.

a. Cognitive skills
b. Interpersonal skills
c. Technical skills

6. _____ "May I help you to the restroom?"
7. _____ creativity
8. _____ problem solving
9. _____ nurse working effectively with members of the health care team
10. _____ taking a blood pressure
11. _____ caring for a dying patient
12. _____ need self-awareness and sensitivity to others to perform this skill
13. _____ bandaging a client's leg

14. What is included in the five processes of implementing?
    a.
    b.
    c.
    d.
    e.

15. Nursing activities are communicated verbally as well as in writing.
    a. True   b. False

FOCUSED STUDY TIPS

1. What are the guidelines for implementing nursing interventions?

2. What are the five components of the evaluation process?

3. What are the two components of an evaluation statement?

4. Explain the difference between quality improvement and quality assurance.

5. Why should the nurse never document in advance?

CASE STUDY

Refer to the Companion Website for the case study on "Treating a Client for Pain." Answer the questions on the Companion Website and answer the following questions regarding Mr. Raymond Sanchez.

1. *List different potential nursing diagnoses for Mr. Sanchez, give an example of subjective and objective data, and list one nursing intervention for each diagnosis.*
2. *List other comfort measures that the nurse may implement for Mr. Sanchez.*

REVIEW QUESTIONS

1. Evaluation of the client's health care while the client is still receiving care from the agency is called a:
   1. retrospective audit.
   2. audit.
   3. concurrent audit.
   4. peer review.

2. Basic nursing interventions are based on:
   1. scientific knowledge, nursing research, and evidence-based practice.
   2. creative thinking and intuition.
   3. physician's orders.
   4. client's wishes and nursing research.

3. Which of the following is the fifth and last phase of the nursing process?
   1. Evaluating
   2. Assessment
   3. Planning
   4. Implementing
   5. Diagnosing

4. The nurse documents that the goal or desired outcome was met, partially met, or not met. What part of the evaluation statement is the nurse documenting?
   1. Supporting data
   2. Collecting data
   3. Finale
   4. Conclusion

5. While implementing the plan of care for the client, the nurse should:
   1. supervise unlicensed support personnel that provide care to the client.
   2. complete every task for the client including bathing, measuring intake and output, and room cleaning services.
   3. complete a retrospective audit.
   4. supervise and direct the physician providing care.
   5. evaluate the client's reactions to the planned interventions.

6. What is meant by the nurse using interpersonal skills?
   1. These skills include problem solving, decision making, critical thinking, and creativity.
   2. These skills include all of the activities, verbal and nonverbal, that people use when interacting directly with one another.
   3. These skills include manipulating equipment, giving injections, bandaging, etc.
   4. These skills include leadership management and delegation.

7. In which of the following situations does the nurse need assistance with implementing the nursing interventions?
   1. A nurse applying Buck's traction for the fifth time
   2. A nurse who has just begun working in the hospital
   3. A nurse who turns the client in bed without the client experiencing discomfort
   4. A nurse transferring a bilateral amputee from bed to chair

8. What are two nursing phases that overlap each other in the nursing process?
   1. Assessing; diagnosing
   2. Planning; implementing
   3. Implementing; evaluation
   4. Evaluating; assessing

9. The nurse writes an evaluation statement after determining whether a nursing goal or client outcome has been met. What are the two parts in an evaluation statement?
   1. Conclusion and implementation
   2. Conclusion and supporting data
   3. Implementation and summary
   4. Implementation and data analysis

10. A quality-assurance (QA) program evaluates and promotes excellence in the health care provided to clients. Select the three components of care that are reviewed during this process from the following:
    1. structure evaluation.
    2. process evaluation.
    3. outcome evaluation.
    4. internal processes and external agency evaluations.

CHAPTER 15

DOCUMENTING AND REPORTING

CHAPTER OUTLINE

I. Ethical and Legal Considerations
  A. Ensuring Confidentiality of Computer Records
II. Purposes of Client Records
  A. Communication
  B. Planning Client Care
  C. Auditing Health Agencies
  D. Research
  E. Education
  F. Reimbursement
  G. Legal Documentation
  H. Health Care Analysis
III. Documentation Systems
  A. Source-Oriented Record
  B. Problem-Oriented Medical Record
    1. Database
    2. Problem List
    3. Plan of Care
    4. Progress Notes
  C. PIE
  D. Focus Charting
  E. Charting by Exception
  F. Computerized Documentation
  G. Case Management
IV. Documenting Nursing Activities
  A. Admission Nursing Assessment
  B. Nursing Care Plans
  C. Kardexes
  D. Flow Sheets
    1. Graphic Record
    2. Intake and Output Record
    3. Medication Administration Record
    4. Skin Assessment Record
  E. Progress Notes
  F. Nursing Discharge/Referral Summaries

MediaLink

www.prenhall.com/berman

DVD-ROM
• Audio Glossary
• NCLEX® Review
• End of Unit Concept Map Activity

Companion Website
• Additional NCLEX® Review
• Case Study: Client with Delirium Tremens
• Application Activities:
  • Establishing a Documentation System
  • HIPAA and Client Privacy
• Links to Resources

KEY TOPIC REVIEW

1. The client's record is protected legally as a private record of the client's care. Access to the client's record is limited to:
   a. Family members.
   b. Only the physician.
   c. The physician and client.
   d. Health care professionals delivering care and the client.

2. The nurse has a _____ and _____ to maintain confidentiality of the client's record.

3. Identify the purposes of client records:
   a.
   b.
   c.
   d.
   e.
   f.
   g.
   h.

4. The Joint Commission on Accreditation of Healthcare Organizations (JCAHO) requires for client record documentation to be:
   a.
   b.
   c.
   d.
   e.

5. What measures should be taken when faxing confidential health information? Is consent needed? What should be done before hitting the "send" button?

6. Students or graduates are not bound by a strict ethical code and legal responsibility to hold all information in confidence.
   a. True   b. False

7. Describe source-oriented records. What is a traditional part of source-oriented records?

8. List the advantages and disadvantages of source-oriented charting.

9. What is a problem-oriented medical record (POMR) or problem-oriented record (POR)? What are the four components of POMR?

10. List the advantages and disadvantages of POMR charting.

11. What is the SOAP format that is used in charting and progress notes? What is meant by the acronyms SOAPIE and SOAPIER?

12. Explain how charting by exception (CBE) works, and explain why some nurses are uncomfortable with this method. What are the three elements of CBE?

13. What are the advantages and disadvantages of case management?

FOCUSED STUDY TIPS

1. Explain the Security Rule of the Health Insurance Portability and Accountability Act of 1996 (HIPAA).

2. Name four suggestions for ensuring confidentiality and security of computerized records.

3. What is the PIE system of charting?

4. How does focus charting work? What are its advantages?

5. Refer to Box 15–2 in the textbook. Review the pros and cons of computer documentation. Do you agree with this information?

6. What are the requirements for documentation in a long-term care facility?

CASE STUDIES

1. *While charting, a nurse notices that she has made an error. She did not write the correct oral temperature down. It should have been 98 degrees orally instead of 101 degrees orally. Demonstrate the correct way to correct the following note:*

   12/04/06 09:10 am Pt stated "I am coughing so bad I am coughing junk up." respirations 28 breaths/minute; temp 101 degrees orally; v/s 140/76 Lt arm; sitting; pulse 96 per min.; no use of accessory muscles noted—D. . Smith, RN BSN

2. *Review the case study on the Companion Website about the client with delirium tremors. What should be included in the shift report for the next shift?*

REVIEW QUESTIONS

1. What is used to organize client data, and allows quick access for health care professionals to review information regarding the client?
   1. End-of-shift report
   2. Variance reports
   3. SOAPIER notes
   4. Kardex

2. In long-term care facilities, what are the two types of care provided?
   1. Easy
   2. Intermediate
   3. Hard
   4. Skilled
   5. Unskilled
   6. Critical

3. Which of the following clients would require more frequent documentation by the nurse?
   1. Stable, delivered OB client who is 2 days post vaginal delivery
   2. A client presenting to the emergency department with signs/symptoms of a viral respiratory problem
   3. An 86-year-old female post operative day 4 of a hip replacement
   4. A 55-year-old male admitted to the ICU after a major myocardial infarction

4. If the nurse makes an error while charting, which is the recommended method to correct the mistake?
   1. Use "correction fluid" and obliterate the error.
   2. Draw one line through the error and write "mistaken entry" above it, then sign your name or initials beside it.
   3. Draw one line through the error and write "error" above it, then sign your initials beside it.
   4. Do nothing and hope no one notices the error.

5. The client has refused to have a Foley catheter inserted after surgery. As the nurse, what would need to be charted in the client's chart?
    1. The client refused the Foley catheter. The client was educated about the need for the Foley and the consequences of refusing the treatment; client verbalized understanding of the education.
    2. The client stubbornly refused the Foley catheter insertion.
    3. The client was medicated and the Foley was inserted without difficulty.
    4. The client refused the Foley catheter.

6. Identify the three purposes of charting.
    1. To fill up the nurse's spare time
    2. To communicate care and responses to care
    3. To create a legal document
    4. To demonstrate what the nurse did every moment of the shift
    5. To provide a basis for evaluation

7. The student nurse is learning to chart effectively in the clinical setting. The student nurse can do which of the following to increase her knowledge?
    1. Chart and hope it is correct.
    2. Practice charting and hope it will improve with time.
    3. Do nothing now and learn charting after graduation.
    4. Read charts to learn from actual situations.

8. Identify the correct example of documentation recording a client situation. The nurse charts:
    1. The client was shouting "I am so mad that I am going to hit you if you come any closer."
    2. The client seems angry and moderately aggressive.
    3. The client is angry and shouting.
    4. The client stated that he was mad and wanted to hit someone.

9. During the change-of-shift report, the nurse reports that the client is having "respiratory difficulty." What should the nurse add to this report?
    1. "But she seems okay."
    2. "Her respiratory rate is up to 28 breaths/min; oral temperature is 100 degrees; heart rate is 96 beats/minute; O_2 saturation of 90%."
    3. "And I put her on 3 liters of oxygen."
    4. "I called the doctor but he didn't do anything."

10. When the nurse places a check mark or a dash in an allocated space and uses an asterisk to reflect other pertinent information that has been recorded elsewhere on the chart, this is an example of what type of documentation?
    1. Multidisciplinary charting
    2. Charting by exception
    3. Focus charting
    4. Flow-sheet charting

11. What measures can the nurse take to maintain confidentiality of the client records? (Select all that apply.)
    1. Personal passwords are not shared with anyone else.
    2. Never leave the computer unattended after logging into the system.
    3. Do not leave paperwork with the client's information in an unsecured location.
    4. Discard all unneeded computer-generated worksheets in the trash can.
    5. Know the facility's policy and procedure for correcting an entry error.
    6. Only use the client's social security number and the initials of the client.

12. Identify examples that health care professionals may use in order to communicate specific information regarding the client or their care.
    1. Change-of-shift report
    2. Discussing the client's care in the cafeteria
    3. Contacting the physician via telephone regarding new orders for medication to decrease an increased temperature
    4. Care plan conferences
    5. A laboratory report for the client

CHAPTER 16

HEALTH PROMOTION

CHAPTER OUTLINE

MediaLink

www.prenhall.com/berman

DVD-ROM
- Audio Glossary
- NCLEX® Review

Companion Website
- Additional NCLEX® Review
- Case Study: Health Promotion Program
- Care Plan Activity: Health Promotion, Health Fair, and Nursing Students
- Application Activity: Health Belief Model
- Links to Resources

KEY TOPIC REVIEW

1. List four main characteristics of homeostatic mechanisms.
2. The nurse must consider all components of health in order to ensure holistic health care. What are the components of health?
3. Maslow, a renowned needs theorist, ranks human needs on five levels. List the levels in ascending order and give an example of a need in each level.
4. What did Richard Kalish add to Maslow's hierarchy of needs, where did he add it, and why did he add it?
5. *Healthy People 2010: Understanding and Improving Health* (U.S. Department of Health and Human Services [USDHHS]) presents a comprehensive 5-year strategy for promoting health and preventing illness, disability, and premature death.
   a. True   b. False
6. List the two major goals of *Healthy People 2010* and what is reflected by those goals.
7. Health-promoting behavior is directed toward attaining positive health outcomes for the client.
   a. True   b. False
8. How do health promotion plans need to be developed to encourage clients to participate in their care?
9. To encourage a client to quit smoking, what implementations should the nurse use? Describe the nurse's behaviors while implementing the plan.
10. Which of the following should be included in a client's lifestyle assessment that would be relevant to their health care?
    1. Nutrition
    2. Physical activity
    3. Drug, alcohol, and cigarette smoking habits
    4. Spirituality
    5. Marital status

FOCUSED STUDY TIPS

1. How does understanding developmental stage theories enable the nurse to provide knowledgeable care?

2. As a nurse, what is your role in health promotion? How can you enhance health promotion actions in your community?

3. Discuss the health promotion model. Refer to the textbook, Figure 16-4.

4. When exploring the stages of change, is change always linear? Why or why not? Why is it important for nurses to understand the stages of change?

5. What is the nurse's role in health promotion? Do you believe that the nurse should be a good role model for healthy living? How would you feel if a nurse who never exercises is attempting to instruct you (a client) in the importance of exercise?

CASE STUDY

Evaluate your own risk for health concerns.

1. *What types of illnesses are apparent in your family history?*
2. *What actions could you take to prevent the development of the identified health concerns?*
3. *What types of health promotion could you utilize to increase your own good health?*
4. *Identify a site for your identified health problem for related health promotion activities.*

NCLEX® REVIEW QUESTIONS

1. A client reports that he believes he will "never kick the habit" of smoking because he has tried before and failed. Using the transtheoretical model (TTM), what stage of health behavior change is the client functioning in?
   1. Preparation stage
   2. Contemplation stage
   3. Termination stage
   4. Action stage
   5. Precontemplation stage
   6. Maintenance stage

2. Identify which of the following is the most basic type of health promotion activity. (Select all that apply.)
   1. A billboard promoting abstinence to prevent sexually transmitted diseases and unplanned pregnancies
   2. A wellness assessment program
   3. An environmental control program about pesticide uses
   4. A nurse who models healthy lifestyle behaviors
   5. A school of nursing that is holding a blood pressure fair

3. The nurse refers a new below-the-knee (BKA) amputation client to a support group for amputees. This is an example of what type of prevention?
   1. Primary
   2. Secondary
   3. Tertiary
   4. Terminal

4. The nurse is providing health education about injury and poisoning prevention to a group of young mothers at a health fair. What type of prevention is the nurse conducting?
   1. Primary prevention
   2. Secondary prevention
   3. Tertiary prevention
   4. Limited prevention

5. A client had surgery for gastrointestinal problems and required a colostomy from the surgery. What type of preventive care would this client need at this stage?
   1. Primary prevention
   2. Secondary prevention
   3. Tertiary prevention
   4. Limited prevention

6. A school nurse is teaching a group of seniors about self-examination techniques for breast and testicular cancer in their health class. What type of health care prevention is the school nurse teaching?
   1. Primary prevention
   2. Secondary prevention
   3. Tertiary prevention
   4. Limited prevention

7. Pender's health promotion model would benefit which of the following clients?
   1. An active 21-year-old client who does not smoke or drink alcohol
   2. A 50-year-old client who exercises four times a week
   3. A 32-year-old who has yearly breast exams and other routine health screenings
   4. An overweight 29-year-old who engages in risky behaviors

8. A client has complete confidence that she has learned health behaviors that will enable her to maintain her current health status by exercising three to five times a week, monitoring her dietary intake, and by no longer engaging in risky behaviors. What stage of health behavior change is this client experiencing?
   1. Maintenance
   2. Action
   3. Preparation
   4. Termination

9. The client is attending Alcoholics Anonymous (AA) meetings for support to assist in remaining sober. It is anticipated that the client will remain in this group for several years. What stage of health behavior change is this client experiencing?
   1. Maintenance
   2. Action
   3. Preparation
   4. Termination

10. Who is responsible for developing health promotion plans?
    1. Physician
    2. Family
    3. Client
    4. Nurse

CHAPTER 17

HEALTH, WELLNESS, AND ILLNESS

CHAPTER OUTLINE

MediaLink

www.prenhall.com/berman

DVD-ROM
- Audio Glossary
- NCLEX® Review

Companion Website
- Additional NCLEX® Review
- Care Plan: Health Care Promotion in a Senior Citizen Residence
- Case Study: Nonadherent Diabetic Client
- Application Activity: Multidisciplinary Care and Resources
- Links to Resources

V. Health Care Adherence
VI. Illness and Disease
    A. Illness Behaviors
       1. Stage 1 Symptom Experiences
       2. Stage 2 Assumption of the Sick Role
       3. Stage 3 Medical Care Contact

       4. Stage 4 Dependent Client Role
       5. Stage 5 Recovery or Rehabilitation
    B. Effects of Illness
       1. Impact on the Client
       2. Impact on the Family

KEY TOPIC REVIEW

1. What is the difference between illness and disease?
2. Match the theorist with the correct theory of the stages and aspects of illness.
    a. Parsons   _____ Outlines five stages of illness: symptom experience, assumption of the sick role,
    b. Suchman   medical care contact, dependent client role, and recovery or rehabilitation.
    c. Roy   _____ Describes four aspects of the sick role.
3. How is a client's usual pattern of behavior changed with illness or hospitalization?
4. Explain the internal variables in biologic, psychologic, and cognitive dimensions.
5. Select all of the factors that may influence a person's decision to improve or begin living a healthier lifestyle.
    a. A diagnosis of diabetes
    b. The physician instructs the client to lose weight
    c. A client's sister is diagnosed with lung cancer
    d. A client has reached the age of 25
6. What are three external influences on health?
7. Anspaugh, Hanrick, and Rosato (2006) proposed seven components of wellness. List the seven dimensions of wellness and give one factor within each component.
8. The causation of a disease is called its _____.
9. What are the four aspects of the sick role that Parson describes?
    a.
    b.
    c.
    d.
10. Define the following.
    a. Locus of control (LOC):
    b. Exacerbation:
    c. Health behaviors:
    d. Health beliefs:
    e. Health status:
    f. Acute illness:
    g. Remission:
    h. Risk factors:

FOCUSED STUDY TIPS

1. How are health belief and behavior models useful in nursing? What are two models used for nursing?

2. How can nurses enhance health care adherence?

3. Why do nurses have to be aware of their own personal definitions of health? How can that enhance their nursing practice?

4. Explore the various theorists that have described stages and aspects of illness. How does Parson describe the sick role?

5. The focus of *Healthy People 2010* is on health promotion. How can the nurse use the findings from *Healthy People 2010* in nursing practice?

CASE STUDY

A 52-year-old female with a family history of lung cancer requests information about smoking cessation. The client admits that she smokes one pack per day and has smoked for approximately 32 years.

1. *With the goals of* Healthy People 2010 *in mind, how can the nurse assist the client?*

NCLEX® REVIEW QUESTIONS

1. A client has severe arthritis, yet she still works 40 hours a week and takes care of her family. This is an example of which health model?
   1. Clinical model
   2. Adaptive model
   3. Role performance model
   4. Eudemonistic model

2. In this health model, illness is a condition that prevents self-actualization.
   1. Clinical model
   2. Adaptive model
   3. Role performance model
   4. Eudemonistic model

3. Osteoporosis and autoimmune diseases are examples of what type of biologic dimension that influences a person's health?
   1. Genetic makeup
   2. Gender
   3. Age
   4. Developmental levels

4. During the first years of life, infants lack physiologic and psychological maturity, so their defenses against diseases are lower. This is an example of what type of biologic dimension that influences a person's health?
   1. Genetic makeup
   2. Gender
   3. Age
   4. Developmental levels

5. The impact of illness on an individual may cause:
   1. the client to become dependent on others.
   2. the client to have role changes within the family.
   3. the client to become more outgoing and friendly.
   4. the client's self-esteem to greatly increase.

6. A nursing student is instructing a female client on healthy lifestyle choices. What are the correct examples of healthy lifestyle choices? (Select all that apply.)
   1. Tobacco use of 1 pack per day
   2. Exercising 3-4 days per week for 1 hour
   3. Regular dental checkup
   4. Seat belt use
   5. Overeating

7. A client who was grossly overweight decided to lose weight in order to feel better about himself and become healthier. What health belief model could the nurse use to assist the client?
   1. Health locus of control model
   2. Rosenstock's health belief model
   3. Becker's health belief model
   4. Pender's health belief model

8. A client reports that she has been practicing yoga for the past 2 years in order to reduce stress and increase muscle flexibility. What part of wellness is this client participating in?
   1. Physical and emotional
   2. Physical and social
   3. Social and emotional
   4. Intellectual and emotional

9. The nurse is attempting to instruct a chronic obstructive pulmonary disease client on the benefits of not smoking, yet the nurse reeks of cigarette smoke and admits that she also smokes one pack a day. What might be a factor in the client's refusal to quit smoking at this time?
   1. The client is distressed about quitting the habit of smoking.
   2. The nurse is not modeling healthy lifestyle choices.
   3. The perceived benefits of not smoking are inconclusive at this time.
   4. The client's cultural heritage demands that he smoke two packs of cigarettes per day.

10. Diabetes mellitus is an example of:
    1. acute illness.
    2. adherence.
    3. chronic illness.
    4. exacerbation.

CHAPTER 18

CULTURE AND HERITAGE

CHAPTER OUTLINE

MediaLink

www.prenhall.com/berman

DVD-ROM
- Audio Glossary
- NCLEX® Review

Companion Website
- Additional NCLEX® Review
- Care Plan Activity: Client in the ICU
- Case Study: Conveying Cultural Sensitivity
- Application Activity: Chinese Childbearing Beliefs
- Links to Resources

KEY TOPIC REVIEW

1. What is culture? How does it define health?
2. _____ are things passed down from previous generations.
3. What is the purpose of the U.S. Department of Health and Human Services (DHHS)?
4. What is a goal for the Centers for Disease Control and Prevention (CDC)?
5. What is the purpose for the National Center on Minority Health and Health Disparities (NCMHD)?
6. Describe what Racial and Ethnic Approaches to Community Health (REACH) influences in the nursing care?
7. What is one of the goals for *Healthy People 2010?*
8. How does the *National Healthcare Disparities Report* influence current nursing practice?
9. Differentiate between culturally sensitive, culturally appropriate, and culturally competent in professional nursing.
10. _____ is credited with creating the theory of culture care diversity and universality.

FOCUSED STUDY TIPS

1. What are the core practice competencies of culturally competent nursing care?

2. What does the magico-religious health belief view entail? Give an example.

3. How do scientific or biomedical health beliefs differ from holistic health beliefs?

CASE STUDIES

1. *While caring for an Asian client who became ill while visiting relatives in the United States, the nurse notices an unusual bruised circular pattern on the trunk of the client.*

   a. *If the nurse is culturally competent, what would be an appropriate comment?*
   b. *If the nurse has xenophobia, what comment might the nurse make regarding the coining or cupping that occurred?*
   c. *Give an example of an ethnocentric statement from the nurse.*
   d. *What nurse action would be considered discrimination?*

2. *A nurse is taking care of a traditional Hispanic client on a medical-surgical floor following a laporotomy appendectomy. Review Box 18–2 in the textbook for an overview of the health-related practices of different cultures.*

   a. *If the client does not return direct eye contact, is this indicative of a cultural difference or a result of a "shifty," evasive client?*
   b. *The client's family desires to spend as much time with him as possible, including staying after hours. How does the nurse handle this situation?*
   c. *The client does not want to take his preventative medication (Reglan) to prevent stress ulcers. He stated that his life and recovery status were in God's hands, and that he "had no need of pharmaceutical medications." What action should the nurse take at this time?*

NCLEX® REVIEW QUESTIONS

1. What are two driving forces for the immense need for culturally focused nursing care?
   1. Demographic changes in the United States
   2. The use of international nurses to supplement the nursing shortage in the United States
   3. The influence of immigration on health services
   4. The influence of herbal supplements being used

2. A client who has a French mother and an Italian father is described as having a _____ identification.
   1. bicultural
   2. diversity
   3. subculture
   4. acculturation
   5. assimilation

3. A client who is homosexual is described as having:
   1. biculturalism.
   2. acculturation.
   3. diversity.
   4. subculture.
   5. assimilation.

4. The involuntary process of _____ occurs when people adapt to or borrow traits from another culture.
   1. biculturalism
   2. acculturation
   3. diversity
   4. subculture
   5. assimilation

5. If a citizen of Japan permanently moves to America, then _____ may occur when that individual becomes an American citizen.
   1. biculturalism
   2. diversity
   3. assimilation
   4. subculture
   5. acculturation

6. If a nurse caring for a Chinese client orders rice for every meal without consulting the client, the nurse may be:
   1. prejudiced.
   2. discriminatory.
   3. stereotyping.
   4. racist.

7. Using the HEALTH traditions model, which of the following would be considered an example of spiritual and mental health?
   1. Avoiding persons who can cause illnesses
   2. Special foods and drinks
   3. Acupuncture
   4. Exorcism

8. Complementary and alternative medicines (CAM) are being used more frequently and are becoming more socially acceptable. What is one example of a CAM therapy?
   1. Massage
   2. Antibiotics
   3. Electric shock therapy
   4. Chicken soup

9. While caring for a Latin American client who cannot speak or understand English, the nurse recognizes that she will need a _____ in order to care for the client.
   1. family member
   2. translator
   3. representative
   4. interpreter

10. While caring for a diverse cultural population, the nurse must recognize that cultural beliefs and behaviors may lead to:
    1. stereotyping.
    2. ethnocentricity.
    3. placing of the nurse's culture to others.
    4. being confused regarding the many values and beliefs of different cultures.

11. Identify which nursing interventions would be beneficial in communication with clients that have limited knowledge of English.
    1. Use slang words, limited medical terminology, and no abbreviations.
    2. Speak slowly, in a respectful manner, and at a normal volume.
    3. Use nonverbal communication, which uses silence, touch, eye movement, facial expressions, and body posture that is acceptable to that particular culture.
    4. Ask a member of the client's family, especially a child or spouse, to act as interpreter.
    5. Address the client, not the interpreter.

12. Campinha-Bacote's model of cultural competence is based on a framework that integrates transcultural nursing, medical anthropology, and multicultural counseling. Identify 3 of the 5 constructs of this model of cultural competence.
    1. Cultural awareness
    2. Cultural appearance
    3. Cultural desires
    4. Cultural skills
    5. Cultural experiences

CHAPTER 19

COMPLEMENTARY AND ALTERNATIVE HEALING MODALITIES

CHAPTER OUTLINE

MediaLink

www.prenhall.com/berman

DVD-ROM
- Audio Glossary
- NCLEX® Review
- End of Unit Concept Map Activity

Companion Website
- Additional NCLEX® Review
- Care Plan Activity: Lyme Disease
- Case Study: Complementary Alternative Medicine
- Application Activity: Support for Alternative Therapies
- Links to Resources

KEY TOPIC REVIEW

1. _____ is the combination of mental, emotional, spiritual relationship, and environmental factors.
2. What is the focus of the American Holistic Nurses Association (AHNA)?
3. How can the nurse create a healing environment in health care?
4. Identify four methods of self-healing for nurses.
   a.
   b.
   c.
   d.
5. Identify which of the following are manual methods of healing:
   a. massage.
   b. meditation.
   c. hypnotherapy.
   d. chiropractic.
   e. hand-mediated biofield therapies.
   f. aromatherapy.
6. _____ is viewed as the force that integrates the body, mind, and spirit, and it connects everything.
7. What is the third largest independent health profession in the Western world after conventional medicine and dentistry?
8. Match the type of prayer with the correct definition.
   a. Intercessory prayer   _____ no specific outcome is requested during prayer time
   b. Nondirected prayer   _____ an informal talk with God—like talking with a good friend
   c. Ritual prayer   _____ praying person asks for a specific outcome
   d. Colloquial prayer   _____ asking God for things for oneself or others
   e. Directed prayer   _____ the use of formal prayers or rituals such as prayers from a prayer book
   f. Meditation prayer   or Jewish siddur
                               _____ contemplative prayer
9. What are the contraindications for magnetic therapy and, on principle, does this therapy work?
10. Describe chelation therapy and how it works in the body.

FOCUSED STUDY TIPS

1. Discuss the six concepts that are common to most alternative practices.

2. Describe the different mind–body therapies and the benefits of each.

3. What issues arise with animal-assisted therapies in health care? Describe the benefits of animal-assisted therapy.

4. Differentiate between conventional medicine, biomedicine, allopathic methods, and alternative or complementary medicines.

5. How are herbs used in medicine? What are some nursing guidelines for herbs used in conjunction with over-the-counter (OTC) medications?

CASE STUDY

1. *During the initial assessment interview with an elderly client, what type of questions should the nurse ask to investigate the use of complementary and alternative therapies?*

2. *The client is admitted to the hospital with uncontrolled hypertension. The client has been taking an antihypertensive medication for several years. The spouse stated that the client takes her antihypertension medication as directed, exercises, and watches her sodium intake. The client reports taking an enteric-coated aspirin daily. However, the client stated she has noted more bruising than usual lately. Refer to the "Practice Guidelines" in the textbook. What popular herbal preparation could affect bruising and cause a decrease in antihypertensive medication effectiveness?*

NCLEX® REVIEW QUESTIONS

1. Concepts that are common to most alternative practices include (select all that apply):
   1. holism.
   2. balance.
   3. spirituality.
   4. prescription medications.
   5. technology and instrumentation.

2. What is the name of the system of medicine that emphasizes client responsibility, client education, health maintenance, and disease prevention?
   1. Naturopathic medicine
   2. Nutritional medicine
   3. Homeopathic medicine
   4. Chiropractic medicine

3. Identify roles that the nurse should assess regarding alternative and complementary therapies.
   1. Recommend hydrotherapy for the older clients.
   2. Colonics for clients with Crohn's disease.
   3. Assess the use of herbs, teas, vitamins, or other natural products used in a nonjudgemental manner.
   4. Encourage the client in using alternative therapies such as acupuncture.

4. The nurse suggests to a client with osteoarthritis to participate in Pilates. What are the benefits of Pilates for this client?
   1. It will give the client an activity to perform to lessen boredom.
   2. It encourages a spiritual connection.
   3. It may improve flexibility and joint health, and relieve muscle aches.
   4. It cleanses the colon and promotes a healthy feeling.

5. A client has diabetic neuropathy in his feet and legs. He complains of a loss of sensation in his feet. What is a research-supported CAM treatment that can improve sensation in the feet, lessen pain, and improve balance?
   1. Detoxification therapies
   2. Music therapies
   3. Infrared photoenergy therapies
   4. Bioelectromagnetic therapies

6. Which of the following therapies stimulates the production of catecholamines, hormones, and endorphins? It can be used in establishing relationships, relieving tension and anxiety, and even facilitating learning.
   1. Music therapy
   2. Hypnotherapy
   3. Guided imagery therapies
   4. Humor and laughter therapy

7. The American Holistic Nurses Association and an organization called "Beyond Ordinary Healing" offer a nurses' certificate program in this CAM. A nurse is certified in which of the following after successfully passing the certification?
   1. Music therapy
   2. Hypnotherapy
   3. Guided imagery therapies
   4. Humor and laughter therapy

8. Meditation, biofeedback, and imagery use different techniques, but what do all these have in common?
   1. The process of physical resting and rhythmic breathing
   2. The process of physical activity and music therapy
   3. The process of relaxation and sleep
   4. The process of utilizing aromatherapy

9. Which of the following types of music therapy are used to induce relaxation and distract clients from pain?
   1. Rap music
   2. Opera music
   3. Piano and flute melody playing quietly
   4. Country music with yodeling

10. A client is on complete bed rest and complains of back pain from lying "in the bed all the time." What is a nursing intervention that uses a nonpharmacological method to ease the discomfort?
   1. Administering a dose of morphine for pain
   2. Assisting the client to a bedside chair
   3. Giving the client a back massage
   4. Instructing the client that the physician will see him tomorrow night
   5. Using music that contains no words
   6. Guided imagery

CHAPTER 20

CONCEPTS OF GROWTH AND DEVELOPMENT

CHAPTER OUTLINE

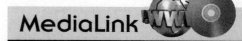

MediaLink

www.prenhall.com/berman

DVD-ROM
• Audio Glossary
• NCLEX® Review

Companion Website
• Additional NCLEX® Review
• Case Study: Treating a Six-Year-Old Client
• Care Plan Activity: Child with Developmental Problems
• Application Activity: Discharging a Young Client
• Links to Resources

KEY TOPIC REVIEW

1. What is meant by the term *growth*? What indicators of growth are used?
2. Define development.
3. List seven factors that influence growth and development.
4. What is meant by psychosocial development?
5. Sigmund Freud introduced a number of concepts about development. What are the major concepts in his theory? Define the terms used in his theory.
6. Describe social learning theory.
7. Describe Kohlberg's theory on moral development.
8. What does the behaviorist learning theory emphasize?
9. Which two theorists describe stages of spiritual development as faith? Describe their concepts in depth.
10. Define the following terms:
    a. Accommodation:

    b. Adaptation:

    c. Assimilation:

    d. Developmental task:

FOCUSED STUDY TIPS

1. What is the definition of personality? Why is it hard to define?

2. Describe Erik Erikson's stages of development.

3. What are Freud's five stages of development?

4. Describe the moral theories of Kohlberg and Gilligan.

5. Review the research note on "What Predicts Conscience in Preschoolers" in the textbook. Discuss the implications for practice.

CASE STUDY

Go to the Companion Website and click on the weblinks for this chapter. Go to the National Institute of Child Health and Human Development's website. Click on the "Health Education" tab.

1. *What topics are listed on this website?*
2. *What other information could be obtained from the site?*

NCLEX® REVIEW QUESTIONS

1. In which direction does growth and development occur from birth if it starts from the head and moves to the trunk, the legs, and the feet?
   1. Proximodistal direction
   2. Simple to complex direction
   3. Cephaproximodistal direction
   4. Cephaolocaudal direction

2. The nurse prepares to give an antibiotic injection to a toddler, age 3, who has an infection. When the toddler views the nurse with needle he begins to cry and say "no-no" while reaching for his mother. According to Piaget's phases of cognitive development, what stage/phase is the toddler experiencing?
   1. Primary circular phase
   2. Concrete operations phase
   3. Preconceptual phase
   4. Initiative thought phase

3. While caring for a 72-year-old client, the nurse perceives the client is depressed when he states that he feels like he is "falling apart now." According to Robert Peck's theory regarding adult development, what task is the client struggling with?
   1. Ego differentiation versus work-role perception
   2. Body transcendence versus body preoccupation
   3. Ego transcendence versus ego preoccupation
   4. Integrity versus despair

4. A school nurse is teaching high school students about sexually transmitted diseases and pregnancy prevention in a health education course. According to Havighurst's age periods and developmental tasks, why is this the appropriate age to introduce this discussion?
   1. Adolescents are achieving new and more mature relations with their peers and are trying to assert their independence.
   2. Adolescents are finding a congenital social group and selecting mates.
   3. Adolescents are developing a conscience, morality, and a set of values.
   4. Adolescents are establishing satisfactory affiliations with one's age group.

5. While caring for a pregnant adolescent, the client stated that she felt abortion was wrong so she decided to continue her pregnancy. What does the adolescent's comment reflect, based on the nurse's knowledge of moral theories?
   1. Morals
   2. Morality
   3. Moral behavior
   4. Moral development

6. The nurse is exploring activities that would enhance an older client's retirement per the client's request. Which theorist would explain this type of adult development?
   1. Freud
   2. Piaget
   3. Kohlberg
   4. Peck

7. According to Gould's study, which is the best example of Stage 3?
   1. A 19-year-old leaving for college
   2. A 25-year-old in the military
   3. A 30-year-old graduate student
   4. A 65-year-old retired school teacher

8. A 26-year-old female client makes the statement that she realizes that she has been selfish in her life and she needs to "do more" for her aging parents. According to Carol Gilligan's research, what stage of moral development is the client in?
   1. Stage 1—caring for oneself
   2. Stage 2—caring for others
   3. Stage 3—caring for self and others
   4. Stage 4—caring for her spouse

CHAPTER 21

PROMOTING HEALTH FROM CONCEPTION THROUGH ADOLESCENCE

CHAPTER OUTLINE

I. Conception and Prenatal Development
  A. Health Promotion
    1. Oxygen
    2. Nutrition and Fluids
    3. Rest and Activity
    4. Elimination
    5. Temperature Maintenance
    6. Safety
II. Neonates and Infants (Birth to 1 Year)
  A. Physical Development
    1. Weight
    2. Length
    3. Head and Chest Circumference
    4. Head Molding
    5. Vision
    6. Hearing
    7. Smell and Taste
    8. Touch
    9. Reflexes
    10. Motor Development
  B. Psychosocial Development
  C. Cognitive Development
  D. Moral Development
  E. Health Risks
    1. Failure to Thrive
    2. Infant Colic
    3. Crying
    4. Child Abuse
    5. Sudden Infant Death Syndrome

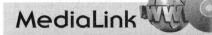

MediaLink

www.prenhall.com/berman

DVD-ROM
- Audio Glossary
- NCLEX® Review

Animations
- Adolescent Ear
- Cell Division
- Conception
- Oogenesis
- Spermatogenesis

Videos
- Drowning
- Identifying Child Abuse
- SIDS

Companion Website
- Additional NCLEX® Review
- Case Study: Motor and Social Development in Infancy
- Care Plan Activity: Teen with Lymphocytic Leukemia
- Application Activities: Safety Tips for Children Playground Bullies
- Links to Resources

    F. Health Assessment and Promotion
        1. Apgar Scoring
        2. Developmental Screening Tests
        3. Ongoing Nursing Assessments
III. Toddlers (1 to 3 years)
    A. Physical Development
        1. Weight
        2. Height
        3. Head Circumference
        4. Sensory Abilities
        5. Motor Abilities
    B. Psychosocial Development
    C. Cognitive Development
    D. Moral Development
    E. Spiritual Development
    F. Health Risks
        1. Injuries
        2. Visual Problems
        3. Dental Caries
        4. Respiratory Tract and Ear Infections
    G. Health Assessment and Promotion
IV. Preschoolers (4 and 5 years)
    A. Physical Development
        1. Weight
        2. Height
        3. Vision
        4. Hearing and Taste
        5. Motor Abilities
    B. Psychosocial Development
    C. Cognitive Development
    D. Moral Development
    E. Spiritual Development
    F. Health Risks
    G. Health Assessment and Promotion
V. School-Age Children (6 to 12 years)
    A. Physical Development
        1. Weight
        2. Height
        3. Vision
        4. Hearing and Touch
        5. Prepubertal Changes
        6. Motor Abilities
    B. Psychosocial Development
    C. Cognitive Development
    D. Moral Development
    E. Spiritual Development
    F. Health Risks
    G. Health Assessment and Promotion
VI. Adolescents (12 to 18 years)
    A. Physical Development
        1. Physical Growth
        2. Glandular Changes
        3. Sexual Characteristics
    B. Psychosocial Development
    C. Cognitive Development

     D. Moral Development
     E. Spiritual Development
     F. Health Risks
     G. Eating Disorders
     H. Health Assessment and Promotion

KEY TOPIC REVIEW

1. How long does prenatal development last?
2. _____ are the three periods of pregnancy that last about _____ months.
3. Identify the trimester and/or phases and describe what is taking place with the fetus during that time.
   a.
   b.
   c.
4. What are the five maternal factors that contribute to higher risks of low-birth-weight babies?
5. Birth weight _____ by the _____ month and _____ by the _____ month.
6. For the infant, how does cognitive development occur?
7. List milestones that toddlers develop between ages 12 months to 3 years.
8. According to Erickson, what task are preschoolers, ages 4 to 5, engaged in?
9. In the school-age period the skills learned are particularly important in relation to work later in life and the willingness to try new tasks.
   a. True
   b. False
10. Choose the major landmarks of the adolescent period.
    a. Rapid growth in height
    b. Deciduous teeth are shed
    c. Sexual maturity
    d. Increasing dependence on the family
    e. Leading causes of death are motor vehicle crashes, homicides, suicides, and other unintentional injuries

FOCUSED STUDY TIPS

1. Why is it important for the nurse to know the normal developmental tasks for each age group?

2. Identify nursing activities to assess and promote health of the fetus and the developmental milestones, noting the average time of occurrence.

3. Identify nursing activities to assess and promote health of the toddler and the developmental milestones, noting the average time of occurrence.

4. Identify nursing activities to assess and promote health of the preschooler and the developmental milestones, noting the average time of occurrence.

5. Identify nursing activities to assess and promote health of the adolescent and the developmental milestones, noting the average time of occurrence.

CASE STUDIES

1. *Go to the case study on the Companion Website on motor and social development in infancy.*

a. *What reflex disappears after 8 months of age?*
b. *If this reflex persists after 1 year and remains positive, what does that indicate?*

2. *Go to the weblinks for this chapter on the Companion Website. Choose the "World Health Organization— Health Topics" link. Click on "Adolescent Health" and then click on "Children's Environmental Health." Read the short note on this site and answer the following questions.*

   a. *Each year, how many children under the age of 5 die due to environment-related diseases?*
   b. *What are the three leading causes of death for children under the age of 5?*

NCLEX® REVIEW QUESTIONS

1. The nurse is instructing a group of pregnant women about ways to reduce the risks of birth defects. Which of the following statements indicates a need for further instruction and/or clarification?
   1. "It is okay for me to use the sauna at the health club but not the hot whirlpool bath."
   2. "I should continue taking the folic acid my physician prescribed prior to the confirmation of my pregnancy."
   3. "I need to stop smoking and try to avoid second-hand smoke."
   4. "I should stop drinking alcohol while I am pregnant."

2. A 10-year-old client has terminal cancer. What does the nurse expect to be the normal concept of death at this age?
   1. There is no concept of death at this age.
   2. Death only happens to old people.
   3. The dead can return, much like a family member returns from a trip.
   4. Death is a final and inevitable outcome of life.

3. The most common health risk occurring in today's environment for school-age children is:
   1. falls.
   2. obesity.
   3. colic.
   4. unprotected sex.

4. A woman that is approximately 5 months pregnant tells the nurse that she is beginning to feel a fluttering in her lower abodomen. She is worried that she is having a miscarriage. Based on the nurse's knowledge of prenatal development, what is the best response by the nurse?
   1. "Is your back hurting bad?"
   2. "Fetal movements may be felt around 5 months by the mother."
   3. "Fetal movements starts around 3 months and mothers may feel the movement."
   4. "Fetal movement begins at 8 months and you may be feeling that movement."

5. The Denver Developmental Screening Test (DDST-II) measures the abilities of a child compared to those of an average group of children of the same age. What are the areas of development screened? (Select all that apply.)
   1. Growth and weight charts
   2. Personal-social development
   3. Fine-motor adaptive development
   4. Language
   5. Gross motor skills
   6. Fine motor skills

6. A teenage mother questions the nurse about why her "baby's head is dented and pointed." The nurse's best response is:
   1. "His head is dented and pointy looking, almost like an eraser."
   2. "This is a normal process and the head shape will return to normal in 6 months."
   3. "The head will return to a normal shape in approximately 1 week. The baby's head is often misshapen because molding occurs during vaginal deliveries."
   4. "He looks deformed. I will get a physician to check him immediately."

7. While conducting a newborn assessment, the nurse notes that the newborn baby has a positive Babinski reflex. How does the nurse elicit the Babinski reflex?
   1. By holding the baby upright so the feet touch a flat surface—the legs move up and down as if walking
   2. By touching the side of the cheek, thus causing the baby's head to turn to the touched side
   3. By stroking the sole of the foot and observing the big toe rising and the other toes fanning out
   4. By placing an object just beneath the toes that causes the toes to curl around it

8. While working with a pediatrician, a nurse is often questioned about when to begin toilet training. What is the appropriate response by the nurse that indicates when a toddler is ready for toilet training?
   1. The toddler stands and walks well and recognizes the need for elimination.
   2. The toddler cannot delay elimination consistently.
   3. The toddler is still crawling.
   4. The toddler is 12 months or older.

9. The nurse is caring for an adolescent client. Which statement would encourage the most communication for this age group?
   1. "We need to discuss this situation with your parents."
   2. "Read this article and it will answer all of your questions."
   3. "Watch this cartoon about your problem."
   4. "You are the fifth teenager this week to have these same issues."

10. Parents of a newborn son insist that their son be circumcised on the 8th day after his birth. This is an example of a cultural religious ritual practiced by Judaism. What should the nurse do regarding the circumcision?
    1. Perform it on the second day of birth per routine orders.
    2. Notify the physician of the parents' request and obtain further orders.
    3. Take no action at this time.
    4. Inform the parents that circumcision is not allowed in the United States.

CHAPTER 22

PROMOTING HEALTH IN YOUNG AND MIDDLE-AGED ADULTS

CHAPTER OUTLINE

MediaLink

www.prenhall.com/berman

DVD-ROM
- Audio Glossary
- NCLEX® Review

Companion Website
- Additional NCLEX® Review
- Case Study: Developmental Phases of Adulthood
- Care Plan Activity: Parenting Responsibilities
- Application Activity: College Student with Manic Depression
- Links to Resources

KEY TOPIC REVIEW

1. How is adulthood categorized, and what are the age ranges?
2. What three distinct generations are included in adulthood?
3. Health risks for young adults are related to _____ and _____.
4. _____ is the state of maximal function and integration, or the state of being fully developed.
5. _____ is defined as the concern for establishing and guiding the next generation.
6. According to Havighurst, what are four developmental tasks for middle-aged adults?
7. What are two health threats that begin to affect persons in middle age?
8. Spirituality is important to young adults and is very much an out in the open public matter.
   a. True   b. False
9. Erikson's developmental task for the middle adult is _____.
10. What are three psychosocial concerns for young adults?

FOCUSED STUDY TIPS

1. Review the Research Note on "What Workforce Differences Exist Between Nursing Staff of Different Generations?" in the textbook. How did the Generations X and Y perceive themselves? In what way was that different from the Silent Generation and Baby Boomer group?

2. What are common health problems in young adults?

3. What sexually transmitted diseases (STDs) are prevalent?

4. How do you define adulthood? What are the criteria to determine this state?

5. Define the following terms: Baby Boomers, Generation X, Generation Y, intimacy, maturity.

CASE STUDY

To answer the following questions, refer to the care plan located on the Companion Website regarding Mary and Lou's situation.

1. *What health problem could Lou be at risk for, especially since Mary reported to you that he has been staying out late and arrives home with alcohol on his breath?*
2. *How can the nurse help clients and their families in dealing with this concern?*
3. *What other resources might help the couple resolve their other issues?*

NCLEX® REVIEW QUESTIONS

1. The leading causes of death for young adults are:
   1. unintentional injuries and suicides.
   2. cancer and diabetes.
   3. AIDS and STDs.
   4. SIDS and suffocation.

2. "Boomerang Kids" are young adults who have moved back into their parents' homes. What are the associated factors that influence these moves?
   1. High divorce and unemployment rates
   2. Fear of intimacy
   3. Lack of supervision
   4. The parents request that the children return

3. Which population group of young adults has a major problem with hypertension?
   1. American Indians
   2. Hispanics
   3. African Americans
   4. Anglo-Saxon males

4. While lecturing a group of young male adults, the nurse discusses the most common neoplasm in men aged 20 to 34. What type of cancer is the nurse instructing the group on?
   1. Testicular cancer
   2. Lung cancer
   3. Kidney cancer
   4. Breast cancer

5. A 47-year-old female states that she has started having periods where she is very hot and breaking out in a sweat, has insomnia, and seems to be gaining weight. What should the nurse consider as a contributory cause for the reported symptoms?
   1. Climacteric
   2. Menopause
   3. Breast cancer
   4. Loose skin

6. The nurse is caring for a 46-year-old female complaining of gaining weight. She wants to know why she has trouble losing weight now. What are leading causes of obesity in middle-aged-adults?
   1. Decreased physical and metabolic activities
   2. Increase in caloric need
   3. Lack of time to exercise
   4. Unknown at this time

7. During an admission assessment, a client reports that she is very active in civic groups and works at a local homeless soup kitchen. This is an appropriate psychosocial development task for which group?
   1. Middle adults
   2. Young adults
   3. Older adults
   4. Preschoolers

8. What comment would be indicative of a young client not meeting one of the psychosocial development tasks?
   1. "I go to my parents' house for lunch every day."
   2. "I am headed in the right direction; I am due for a promotion soon."
   3. "I never go out at night. I don't have any friends."
   4. "I never see my family."

9. If a client was born in 1963, which generation would that client be identified with?
   1. Generation X
   2. Generation Y
   3. Baby Boomer
   4. Boomerang Kid

10. A middle-aged client stated that his son and the son's child had moved back home. What may be one of the causes that promoted the son to return to his childhood home and live with his parents again?
    1. High divorce rates
    2. High wages for nondegree persons
    3. Children moving home to care for aging parents
    4. Son unable to cook and clean up after his own son

11. Identify 3 psychosocial developmental characteristics for the middle-aged adult. The middle-aged adult is:
    1. in the generatively versus stagnation phase of Erikson's stage of development.
    2. has pleasure activities as a central theme.
    3. moving from the conventional level to the postconventional level according to Kohlberg.
    4. achieving adult civic and social responsibility.
    5. adjusting to aging parents.

CHAPTER 23

PROMOTING HEALTH IN ELDERS

CHAPTER OUTLINE

MediaLink

www.prenhall.com/berman

DVD-ROM
- Audio Glossary
- NCLEX® Review
- Videos and Animations:
  - Alzheimer's Disease
  - Cardiovascular System
  - Cultural Diversity
  - Elder Mistreatment and Abuse
  - Gastrointestinal
  - Geritourinary and Renal System
  - Immune System
  - Nursing Issues and the Elderly
  - Nutrition and Aging
  - Respiratory System
  - Sleep and the Elderly
  - The Study of Aging

Companion Website
- Additional NCLEX® Review
- Case Study: Home Health and Elderly Siblings
- Care Plan Activity: Elderly Client with Nose Bleed
- Application Activity: Gerontology as a Nursing Speciality
- Links to Resources

E. Maintaining Independence and Self-Esteem
F. Facing Death and Grieving
VII. Cognitive Abilities and Aging
  A. Perception
  B. Cognitive Ability
  C. Memory
  D. Learning
VIII. Moral Reasoning
 IX. Spirituality and Aging

X. Health Problems
  A. Injuries
  B. Chronic Disabling Illness
  C. Drug Use and Misuse
  D. Alcoholism
  E. Dementia
  F. Elder Mistreatment
XI. Health Assessment and Promotion

KEY TOPIC REVIEW

1. Why are people living longer in today's world?
2. By the mid-21st century in the United States, the _____ are projected to outnumber _____ people.
3. What category of the aging population is the fastest growing of all the age groups in the country?
4. Fill in the correct data in the blanks.
   a. The young-old are _____ to _____ years old.
   b. _____ are 75 to 85 years old.
   c. Old _____ are _____ to _____ years old.
   d. Elite _____ are over _____ years old.
5. *Healthy People 2010* includes focus areas that are relevant to elders. List five topics.
   a.   d.
   b.   e.
   c.
6. Disease is a normal outcome of aging.
   a. True   b. False
7. Ageism is a term that celebrates the wondrous stage of aging that is honored throughout the world.
   a. True   b. False
8. Many elders do not consider faith, and they do not display a high level of spirituality.
   a. True   b. False
9. _____ is a term used to define the study of aging and older adults. _____ is associated with medical care of the elderly.
10. Describe gerontological nursing. How do gerontological nurses obtain certification? What degrees are needed to practice as a nurse in this field?
11. Review the Research Note "How do Elders Manage Personal Integrity During Hospitalization" in the textbook. What are some strategies that the nurse may employ to maintain the personal integrity of the elderly client?
12. What is the objective of long-term care facilities? What types of care are included in long-term care facilities?
13. Describe Alzheimer's disease (AD) and explain why specialized units are necessary for Alzheimer's patients.
14. What are the hypotheses of the wear-and-tear theory of aging?

FOCUSED STUDY TIPS

1. What are the physical changes associated with aging, and what are the rationales in the integumentary system?

2. What are the physical changes associated with aging, and what are the rationales in the gastrointestinal system?

3. What are positive health practices that can promote health and wellness for all adults?

4. What are the common biologic theories of aging? Which one do you agree with and why?

5. Review health problems associated with the older adults and list those concerns.

CASE STUDY

A retired 90-year-old widow lives alone in a rural town. Her children live in various states nearby and lead busy lives. The elderly widow insists that she is satisfied with her life. The church that she attends drives her to and from services and her friends visit her daily. Her children believe that their mother is depressed and needs medication, so they take her to a geriatric nurse practitioner.

1. *What age category of the aging population is this widow currently in?*
2. *What is the myth of aging that her children are subscribing to? What is the reality?*
3. *According to Erikson, what developmental task occurs at this phase?*

NCLEX® REVIEW QUESTIONS

1. An 84-year-old client complains of reduced visual acuity and of seeing glare around objects. On physical exam, the nurse notices less opacity. What is the term for this common vision disturbance in the elderly?
   1. Presbyopia
   2. Cataracts
   3. Glaucoma
   4. Presbycusis

2. Identify the normal findings of an elderly client's cardiovascular system.
   1. The working capacity of the heart increases with age.
   2. The heart rate at rest may increase with age.
   3. There is a slower response in the heart rate when responding to stressors.
   4. There is reduced arterial elasticity.
   5. The client may have orthostatic hypotension whenever the client lies down or stands up suddenly.

3. The client reports that she attends a senior citizen center at least three times a week. What psychosocial aging theory would explain these activities?
   1. Continuing theory
   2. Activity theory
   3. Disengagement theory
   4. Growth and developmental theory

4. A caregiver for a client with Alzheimer's disease calls and states that she has to attend a conference in another state. She requests information about what arrangements could be made for her mother's care during that time. What place could the nurse suggest?
   1. Nursing home
   2. Assisted living facility
   3. Adult day care
   4. Leave the client alone in a locked room with enough water and food

5. What types of injuries are more common in older adults than middle adults?
   1. Motor vehicle crashes
   2. Drownings
   3. Falls
   4. Homicides

6. What is the largest growing population in the United States today?
   1. Newborns
   2. Adolescents
   3. Middle-aged adults
   4. Older adults

7. Based on your knowledge of elder mistreatment, which of the following statements are true? (Select all that apply.)
   1. It may affect either sex equally.
   2. The abuse may involve physical, psychological, or emotional abuse.
   3. The elderly may be beaten and raped by family members or health care workers.
   4. Elder abuse never occurs in private settings.

8. The nurse is planning health care interventions for an older client who has a nursing diagnosis of "potential alteration in gastrointestinal functioning (constipation) related to complete bed rest/administration of pain medication/sedatives." Which of the following should be included in the interventions?
   1. Include adequate roughage and liquids in the diet.
   2. Assess risk factors for elder abuse.
   3. Obtain weight of client daily.
   4. Keep side rails up at all times.

9. The biological theory of aging, the endocrine theory, proposes that:
   1. the faster an organism lives, the quicker it dies.
   2. the organism is genetically programmed for a predetermined number of cell divisions, and then the cells die.
   3. the immune system declines with age.
   4. the hypothalamus and pituitary are responsible for changes in hormone production and response, then the organism's decline.

10. While caring for an elderly client with osteoporosis, the nurse is instructing the client and family on fall prevention measures to take at home. Which measures should the nurse include: (select all that apply)
    1. remove throw rugs.
    2. wear sturdy, rubber-soled shoes.
    3. place safety bars in the bathroom.
    4. remove all carpet and keep floors waxed.
    5. change position slowly to prevent orthostatic hypotension.

CHAPTER 24

PROMOTING FAMILY HEALTH

CHAPTER OUTLINE

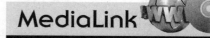

MediaLink

www.prenhall.com/berman

DVD-ROM
- Audio Glossary
- NCLEX® Review
- Video: Involving Families in NICU Settings
- End of Unit Concept Map Activity

Companion Website
- Additional NCLEX® Review
- Case Study: Home Health and an Elderly Family
- Care Plan Activity: Client in the ICU and the Family
- Application Activity: Health Care Resources
- Links to Resources

KEY TOPIC REVIEW

1. The _____ is a basic unit of society.
2. A _____ is a set of interacting, identifiable parts or components.
3. _____ _____ was introduced as a universal theory that could be applied to many fields of study.
4. What is the purpose of family assessment?
5. One of the greatest stressors on a two-couple family is _____.
6. List four potential nursing diagnoses for family assessment.
7. Of all types of households, about _____ are single-parent families, and this number continues to increase. _____ _____ of these families are headed by women and _____ _____ by men.
8. The stresses of single parenthood include _____ and _____.
9. _____ is the mechanism by which some of the output of a system is returned to the system as input.
10. The _____ _____ focuses on family structure and function. The structural component of the theory addresses the membership of the family and the relationships among family members.

FOCUSED STUDY TIPS

1. Define the following terms: nuclear family, extended family, traditional family, two-career family, single-parent family, adolescent family, foster family, blended family, intragenerational family, cohabiting family, gay and lesbian family.

2. Discuss how family communications influence families. What happens when that communication does not correctly flow among family members?

3. The incidence of family violence has increased in recent years. What factors have influenced the increase in recent years?

4. How do sociologic factors and poverty influence the different types of families?

5. Review the various theories used when dealing with family health.

CASE STUDY

A client presents to the emergency department with injuries that are suspiciously related to common patterns of physical abuse. The client reported that she "fell down several stairs while going to the basement." The client's husband is present and seems unwilling to leave the client's bedside.

1. *What would be the best interventions by the nurse in this situation?*
2. *What should the nurse be observing during the interactions between herself, the client, and the spouse?*

NCLEX®-RN REVIEW QUESTIONS

1. A nurse is reviewing data gathered from a family assessment. The single mother of two children has been treated several times for drug overdose and has a history of substance abuse. What nursing diagnoses would be appropriate for this family based on this information?
   1. Interrupted Family Process
   2. Readiness for Enhanced Family Coping
   3. Impaired Parenting
   4. Caregiver Role Strain

2. The client has a history of diabetes in her family as identified by a detailed nursing health history. This data is identified as what type of risk for health problems?
   1. Maturity factors
   2. Hereditary factors
   3. Gender or race factors
   4. Lifestyle factors

3. As a nurse instructing a client on the need for exercise, stress management, and rest, you are trying to minimize or prevent the causes of some diseases and disabilities. You are disseminating information about prevention and motivating families to make changes in which of the following areas?
   1. Maturity factors
   2. Hereditary factors
   3. Gender or race factors
   4. Lifestyle factors

4. A 6-year-old client has been living with her grandparents since her parent's divorce. Her parents are unable to care for the client because of substance abuse. What type of family unit does this client belong to?
   1. Foster family
   2. Traditional family
   3. Intragenerational family
   4. Cohabiting family

5. As the nurse, you are assessing which part of the family when you are observing the ways the family expresses affection, love, sorrow, and anger?
   1. Family structure
   2. Physical health status
   3. Interaction patterns
   4. Family roles and functions

6. If the nurse is evaluating how the family members handle stressful situations and conflicting goals, what is the nurse observing?
   1. Coping resources
   2. Family values
   3. Interaction patterns
   4. Family roles and functions

7. Identify the later symptoms seen when assessing for family violence.
   1. Depression, alcohol and substance abuse, and suicide attempts
   2. Burns, cuts, fractures, and death
   3. Alcohol and substance abuse and fractures
   4. No differentiation in the symptoms presented

8. While caring for a client who is struggling with cancer, the nurse who is committed to family-centered care will do which of the following?
   1. Ensure that the client understands the disease, treatment, and other matters related to the diagnosis of cancer.
   2. Ensure that the client and family members understand the disease, treatment, and other matters related to the diagnosis of cancer.
   3. Identify how radiation is affecting the client's skin.
   4. Ensure that the primary care provider understands how the treatment is affecting the family unit.

9. Who does the nurse evaluate when planning health care for family care?
   1. Family and community
   2. Individual and family
   3. Communities, political arenas, and families
   4. Families, individuals, and community

10. The school nurse can promote family health by presenting which of the following programs?
    1. A program describing how washing hands will reduce infection rates
    2. A program describing how truancy will influence education
    3. A program instructing students on personal hygiene
    4. A program describing head lice and how to treat it

CHAPTER 25

CARING

CHAPTER OUTLINE

MediaLink

www.prenhall.com/berman

DVD-ROM
- Audio Glossary
- NCLEX® Review

Companion Website
- Additional NCLEX® Review
- Case Study: Six C's of Caring in Nursing
- Care Plan Activity: Care of Client After Motor Vehicle Crash
- Application Activity: Watson's Theory of Human Caring
- Links to Resources

KEY TOPIC REVIEW

1. _____ means that people, relationships, and things matter and is _____ to nursing practice.
2. List what is involved with a caring practice.
3. According to Morse, Solberg, Neander, Battorff, and Johnson, what are the five viewpoints of caring as a multidimensional concept?
    a.
    b.
    c.
    d.
    e.
4. A noted philosopher, Melton Mayeroff, proposes that to care for another person is to help him grow and actualize himself.
    a. True
    b. False

For questions 5–11, match each theorist to the correct perception of "caring" in the nursing process.

5. _____ Nursing is described as a relationship in which caring is primary because it sets up the possibility of giving and receiving help.

6. _____ Caring is the moral ideal of nursing where by the end is protection, enhancement, and preservation of human dignity. The two individuals in a caring transaction are both in a process of being and becoming.

7. _____ Caring is a nurturing behavior that has been present throughout history and is critical in helping people maintain or regain health.

8. _____ Caring in nursing is contextual and is influenced by the organizational structure.

9. _____ The emphasis is on the nurse knowing self as a caring person. Caring is a lifetime process and respect for persons as caring individuals in nursing is necessary.

10. _____ A nurturing way of relating to a valued "other," toward whom one feels a personal sense of commitment and responsibility.

11. _____ Caring is the human mode of being, or the most common, authentic criterion of humanness. Caring is not unique to nursing.

a. Leininger—Theory of Cultural Care Diversity and Universality
b. Ray—Theory of Bureaucratic Caring
c. Roach—Caring, the Human Mode of Being
d. Boykin and Schoenhofer—Nursing as Caring
e. Watson—Theory of Human Care
f. Swanson—Theory of Caring
g. Benner and Wrubel—The Primacy of Caring

12. _____ is the art of nursing and is expressed by the individual nurse through creativity and style in meeting the needs of client.
13. How can an individual care for the self?
14. _____ is thinking from a critical point of view, analyzing why one acted in a certain way and assessing the results of one's actions.
15. Nursing school instructors can teach all nursing students how to care.
    a. True
    b. False

FOCUSED STUDY TIPS

1. Define the following terms used in caring: caring, caring practice, empirical knowing, ethical knowing, personal knowing.

2. What nursing theory of caring matches your own personal philosophy of caring? Why?

3. Discuss and define the six C's of caring in nursing.

4. Review the Research Note on "Believing That I Make a Difference" in the textbook. What are the nursing implications for your nursing practice?

5. Think about your encounters with various nurses in your lifetime. How does the "caring" nurse differ from others? What made you remember that caring nurse?

CASE STUDY

1. *Review the case study on "Providing Care" that is found on the Companion Website (www.prenhall.com/berman).*

   a. *What are two additional interventions to provide comfort measures?*

2. *A child who was involved in a motor vehicle crash has been admitted to your unit. The parents and a younger brother were announced dead on arrival (DOA) at the hospital.*

   a. *As a student nurse assigned to this client, which of the six C's of caring in nursing do you want to incorporate in your interventions?*
   b. *If you were using the caring processes from Swanson's theory of caring, on what five processes would you base your nursing interventions for this client?*
   c. *What type of knowing would you demonstrate if you are observing and documenting phenomena as it is occurring in this case?*

NCLEX® REVIEW QUESTIONS

1. Which theorist developed her theory of caring by the various interactions with parents at the time of pregnancy, miscarriage, and birth?
   1. Watson
   2. Miller
   3. Leininger
   4. Swanson

2. When it became apparent that the chaplain might not arrive before the death of the client, the nurse prayed with the dying client who requested a chaplain to visit. This is an example of what type of caring?
   1. Nursing presence
   2. Empowering the client
   3. Compassion from the nurse
   4. Nursing competence

3. Caring for self means taking time to nurture oneself. What are some ways that a nurse may care for herself? (Select all that apply.)
   1. A balanced diet
   2. Regular exercise
   3. Adequate rest and sleep
   4. Recreational sleep
   5. Working 60 hours per week

4. The nurse is instructing the client on ways to "self-care" for relief of stress. Identify ways in which the client can lead a healthier lifestyle and carve out enough time to care for herself. (Select all that apply.)
   1. Avoid unhealthy patterns such as replacing negative affirmations with positive affirmations.
   2. Delay exercising until stress level and job demands have lessened.
   3. Use guided imagery to promote relaxation several times a day.
   4. Begin a yoga class to unite the mind, body, and spirit.

5. The nurse demonstrates personal knowing when reflecting about the death of a client who died from having a major myocardial infarction (heart attack) by asking which of the following questions?
   1. "What were my thoughts and emotions?"
   2. "Did I act for the best?"
   3. "What additional information was needed?"
   4. "Why did I respond the way I did to the situation?"

6. A nurse quietly sits with a client who is recovering from a spontaneous abortion. This is an example of what type of caring?
   1. Knowing the client
   2. Nursing presence
   3. Empowerment
   4. Resting

7. While caring for an older client with a left-sided paralysis, the nurse strongly encourages the client to participate in her activities of daily living. What type of caring encounter is being conducted by the nurse?
   1. Knowing the client
   2. Nursing presence
   3. Empowering the client
   4. Compassion

8. The nurse repositions a bed-bound client every 2 hours. This nursing intervention is an example of what type of caring? (Select all that apply.)
   1. Competence
   2. Caring for self
   3. Spiritual care
   4. Compassionate care

9. The nurse instructs the client on mind–body therapies. Which mind–body therapy does the client practice when picturing himself lying on a beach with the sounds of the waves, the cries of the seagull, and the warmth of the sun during periods of stress?
   1. Music therapy
   2. Guided imagery
   3. Yoga
   4. Story telling

10. The postpartum nurse demonstrates caring by which of the following actions?
    1. Holding and rocking an infant so the mother can rest quietly for a few hours after being up all night
    2. Allowing the client to wait two more hours before giving pain medications
    3. Not allowing the father of the infant to visit mother and infant upon his arrival to hospital after hours
    4. Leaving the crying baby in the room with the mother for 24 hours

CHAPTER 26

COMMUNICATING

CHAPTER OUTLINE

MediaLink

www.prenhall.com/berman

DVD-ROM
- Audio Glossary
- NCLEX® Review
- Videos and Animations:
  - Communicating Effectively
  - Communication

Companion Website
- Additional NCLEX® Review
- Case Study: Facilitating Communication
- Care Plan Activity: Treating an Immigrant Family
- Application Activity: Communication Resources
- Links to Resources

3. Self-Help Groups
4. Self-Awareness/Growth Groups
5. Therapy Groups
6. Work-Related Social Support Groups

IV. Communication and the Nursing Process
V. Nursing Management
   A. Assessing
      1. Impairments to Communication
         a. Language Deficits
         b. Sensory Deficits
         c. Cognitive Impairments
         d. Structural Deficits
         e. Paralysis
      2. Style of Communication
         a. Verbal Communication
         b. Nonverbal Communication
   B. Diagnosing
   C. Planning
   D. Implementing
      1. Manipulate the Environment
      2. Provide Support
      3. Employ Measures to Enhance Communication
      4. Educate the Client and Support Persons
   E. Evaluating
      1. Client Communication
      2. Nurse Communication
VI. Communication Among Health Professionals
   A. Nurse and Physician Communication
      1. Communication Styles
      2. Assertive Communication
      3. Nonassertive Communication

KEY TOPIC REVIEW

1. Why are good communication skills essential in nursing?
2. Circle all of the following that apply to the nonverbal communication process.
   a. pace and intonation
   b. adaptability
   c. personal appearance
   d. posture
   e. clarity
   f. gestures
   g. timing and relevance
3. What are barriers to communication?
4. How can the nurse demonstrate the actions of "physical attending" when communicating?
5. Which of the following signs are components of "genuineness" in conversation? Circle all that apply.
   a. The person is spontaneous.
   b. The nurse tells the client "I know exactly how you are feeling."
   c. The client is open and nondefensive.
   d. The client states that he does not routinely practice "safe sex" while partying.
6. A nurse is caring for an 86-year-old client. During the care, the nurse needs to reposition the client; she asks the client to "please grab the side rail, Honey, while I bathe your back." What type of speech style is the nurse employing?
7. In _____ _____, the verbal and nonverbal aspects of the message match.

8. When seeking clarification during an initial health assessment, what is the best question the nurse could ask?
   a. "Would you tell me more?"
   b. "What do you mean—you smoke one pack of cigarettes a day? Are you trying to kill yourself?"
   c. "Why did you even come to the emergency room?"
   d. "I can't understand you at all. What are you saying?"
9. What is the difference between teaching groups and self-help groups? According to the Research Note on "The Effects of Disruptive Behavior" located in the textbook, what are the implications of disruptive behavior for nursing, and how would this affect your nursing practice?

FOCUSED STUDY TIPS

1. What is the difference between assertive and nonassertive communication?

2. What are the advantages and disadvantages of electronic communication? When should e-mail not be used in health care?

3. Describe personal space and proxemics. How is communication altered in accordance with the four distances?

4. What are the four phases of helping relationships?

5. How does the situational briefing model work in communication?

CASE STUDY

An 18-year-old first-year college student presents to the college's infirmary complaining of painful urination and severe back pain. She is pale, running a 101-degree oral temperature, has chills, and is teary-eyed. The client states that she has never been to a hospital or physician without her mother present. The physician orders a urine specimen to check for urinary tract infection. The client has her menstrual cycle and a "mini-catheter" is ordered. The nurse explains the procedure for the mini-catheter and the client starts crying.

1. *What could the nurse do in order to create a more positive environment for the health interview?*
2. *If the nurse shares a similar experience with the client, then what communication technique is the nurse using?*
3. *What are three therapeutic responses the nurse could employ in this situation?*
4. *Using the information from the case study, supply the following information:*
   a. *Provide a nursing diagnosis for the client.*
   b. *Identify the subjective and objective assessment information.*

NCLEX® REVIEW QUESTIONS

1. The nurse is using active listening skills, building rapport, and providing a nonjudgmental attitude and nonreactive behaviors. Based on this information, which populations is the nurse communicating with? (Select all that apply.)
   1. Infants
   2. School-age children
   3. Adolescents
   4. Toddlers

2. While assessing a postoperative client for pain, the nurse notices the client is holding the surgical site and making facial grimaces. However, the client states that she is not hurting. What part of the communication process is most important in this scenario?
   1. Sender
   2. Receiver
   3. Message
   4. Feedback

3. The nurse is administering an enema to a client with a questionable gastrointestinal blockage. The nurse is in what type of personal space for the client?
   1. Intimate
   2. Personal
   3. Social
   4. Public

4. The nurse makes direct eye contact and has a pleasant expression on her face when changing a client's colostomy bag. The nurse tells the client, "The colostomy looks good." What type of communication is the nurse demonstrating?
   1. Nonverbal communication
   2. Process recoding
   3. Congruent communication
   4. Noncongruent communication

5. The nurse is participating in a self-help group on women's health. What is one of the main functions of the nurse's role?
   1. Participate as a member of the self-help group when appropriate.
   2. Give information to the group in order to teach about women's health.
   3. Buffer the stress within the group.
   4. Lend the group an air of professionalism.

6. A client expresses anxiety about a surgical procedure. What would be the most appropriate therapeutic communication technique to use in this situation? (Select all that apply.)
   1. Using open-ended questions
   2. Probing and rejecting the comment made by the client
   3. Restating or paraphrasing the comment made by the client
   4. Offering unwarranted reassurance

7. In which of the following situations would using the therapeutic communication of "touch" be appropriate?
   1. When a family member is making inappropriate comments to the nurse, touch is appropriate.
   2. Touch is never appropriate in the nursing profession.
   3. When an upset spouse is alone and the client has just expired, touch is appropriate.
   4. When a young male client asks a young student nurse for a hug, touch is appropriate.

8. What type of behaviors is the client exhibiting if he states that he will not need assistance with any aspect of his personal care?
   1. Resistant behaviors
   2. Introductory behaviors
   3. Preinteraction behaviors
   4. Trusting behaviors

9. A primary nurse developed a contract with a newly admitted client. Which phase of the helping relationship is the nurse involved in?
   1. Preinteraction phase
   2. Introductory phase
   3. Working phase
   4. Termination phase

10. The older client asks the physician if she needs to move into an assisted living facility instead of living alone now that she is old. The physician responded by telling the client that if she were his mother, he would tell her to go into the assisted living facility because her meals would be cooked for her and she would not have to clean anything. The physician was demonstrating what type of barrier to communication?
    1. Stereotyping
    2. Being defensive
    3. Challenging
    4. Giving common advice

CHAPTER 27

TEACHING

CHAPTER OUTLINE

I. Teaching
   A. Teaching Clients and Their Families
   B. Teaching in the Community
   C. Teaching Health Personnel
II. Learning
   A. Learning Theories
      1. Behaviorism
      2. Cognitivism
      3. Humanism
   B. Using Learning Theories
   C. Factors Affecting Learning
      1. Motivation
      2. Readiness
      3. Active Involvement
      4. Relevance
      5. Feedback
      6. Nonjudgmental Support
      7. Simple to Complex
      8. Repetition
      9. Timing
     10. Environment
     11. Emotions
     12. Physiologic Events
     13. Cultural Aspects
     14. Psychomotor Ability
III. The Internet and Health Information
   A. Online Health Information
   B. Access
   C. Elders and Use of the Internet
   D. Implications
IV. Nurse as Educator

V. Nursing Management
   A. Assessing
      1. Nursing History
         a. Age
         b. Client's Understanding of Health Problem
         c. Health Beliefs and Practice
         d. Cultural Factors
         e. Economic Factors
         f. Learning Style
         g. Client Support System
      2. Physical Examination
      3. Readiness to Learn
      4. Motivation
      5. Health Literacy

MediaLink

www.prenhall.com/berman

DVD-ROM
- Audio Glossary
- NCLEX® Review

Companion Website
- Additional NCLEX® Review
- Case Study: Planning a Rural Health Education Program
- Care Plan Activity: Discharge of Client with Cardiomyopathy
- Application Activity: Overseeing a Health Fair
- Links to Resources

B. Diagnosing
    1. Learning Need as the Diagnostic Label
    2. Deficient Knowledge as the Etiology
C. Planning
    1. Determining Teaching Priorities
    2. Setting Learning Outcomes
    3. Choosing Content
    4. Selecting Teaching Strategies
    5. Organizing Learning Experiences
D. Implementing
    1. Guidelines for Teaching

2. Special Teaching Strategies
    a. Client Contracting
    b. Group Teaching
    c. Computer-Assisted Instruction (CAI)
    d. Discovery/Problem Solving
    e. Behavior Modification
3. Transcultural Teaching
E. Evaluating
    1. Evaluating Learning
    2. Evaluating Teaching
F. Documenting

KEY TOPIC REVIEW

1. Physiologic events such as a critical illness, pain, or sensory deficits inhibit learning.
    a. True   b. False

2. Motivation is generally greatest when a person recognizes a need and believes the need will be met through learning.
    a. True   b. False

3. Developmental readiness and individual readiness are other key factors associated with cognitive approaches.
    a. True   b. False

4. Active learning, such as listening to a lecture or watching a film, does not foster optimal learning.
    a. True   b. False

5. People learn best when they believe they are accepted and will not be judged.
    a. True   b. False

6. _____ is the application of the Internet and other related technologies in the health care industry to improve the access, efficiency, effectiveness, and quality of clinical and business processes utilized by health care organizations, practitioners, clients, and consumers in an effort to improve the health status of clients.

7. A high level of _____ resulting in agitation and the inability to focus or concentrate can also inhibit learning.

8. Repetition of key _____ and facts facilitates retention of newly learned material.

9. A client's learning style may be based in that client's _____ background.

10. The person who is not ready to learn is more likely to _____ the subject or situation.

11. Match the following terms with the correct definition.
    a. Teaching
    b. Learning need
    c. Imitation
    d. Motivation
    e. Modeling
    f. Learning
    g. Geragogy
    h. Pedagogy
    i. Andragogy
    j. Adherence

_____ is the term used to describe the process involved in stimulating and helping elders to learn.

_____ is a system of activities intended to produce learning.

_____ is the art and science of teaching adults.

_____ is a desire or a requirement to know something that is presently unknown to the learner.

_____ is a change in human disposition or capability that persists and that cannot be solely accounted for by growth.

_____ is a commitment or attachment to a regimen.

_____ is the discipline concerned with helping children learn.

_____ is the process by which a person learns by observing the behavior of others.

_____ means to learn is the desire to learn.

_____ is the process by which individuals copy or reproduce what they have observed.

12. _____ is the art and science of teaching adults.
    a. Pedagogy   b. Geragogy
    c. Andragogy   d. Etiology

13. _____ depicts learning as a complex cognitive activity.
    - a. Cognitivism
    - b. Humanism
    - c. Behaviorism
    - d. Colloquialism

14. The _____ domain, the "skill" domain, includes motor skills such as giving an injection.
    - a. Affective
    - b. Psychomotor
    - c. Cognitive
    - d. Thinking

15. A nurse would adhere to all of the following guidelines for teaching clients from various ethnic backgrounds EXCEPT:
    - a. Obtains teaching materials, pamphlets, and instructions in languages used by clients.
    - b. Uses visual aids, such as pictures, charts, or diagrams, to communicate meaning.
    - c. Invites and encourages questions during teaching.
    - d. Uses medical terminology or health care language, such as "taking your vital signs" or "apical pulse."

16. When a nurse is using demonstration as a teaching strategy, which major type of learning would it be?
    - a. Psychomotor
    - b. Cognitive
    - c. Affective
    - d. All types of learning

FOCUSED STUDY TIPS

1. How would a nurse know that a client is ready for patient education?

2. List the seven elements in the nursing history that provide clues to learning needs.

3. Explain computer-assisted instruction (CAI).

4. Discuss the evaluation tools for cognitive learning.

5. Describe all types of learning.

6. Identify the parts of the teaching process that should be documented in the client's chart.

7. Summarize the four physical abilities that are important for learning psychomotor skills.

8. Compare and contrast teaching and learning.

9. When is the best time and situation for a client to learn?

10. Define attitude, values, beliefs, and emotions.

11. Recall the pertinent features that a learning contract combined with behavior modification should include.

CASE STUDY

Melba is an 86-year-old client who has just been diagnosed with hypertension. Her daughter tells you her mother only completed the sixth grade and gets very anxious when learning something new because of her poor reading skills.

1. *How will you be able to determine if Melba is ready to learn?*
2. *Identify three ways you could facilitate Melba's learning.*
3. *Describe various teaching aids to help foster Melba's learning.*

NCLEX® REVIEW QUESTIONS

1. Andragogy is:
   1. the process involved in stimulating and helping elders to learn.
   2. the art and science of teaching adults.
   3. the discipline concerned with helping children learn.
   4. the commitment or attachment to a regimen.

2. Which of the following is the process by which a person learns by observing the behavior of others?
   1. Modeling
   2. Imitation
   3. Trial and error
   4. Positive reinforcement

3. Teaching a client how to self-administer insulin is in the _____ domain.
   1. Sensorimotor
   2. Psychomotor
   3. Cognitive
   4. Affective

4. In which of the following situations would the nurse be applying the humanistic theory?
   1. Encouraging the learner to establish goals and promote self-directed learning
   2. Encouraging a positive teacher–learner relationship
   3. Providing a social, emotional, and physical environment conducive to learning
   4. Selecting multisensory teaching strategies since perception is influenced by the senses

5. In teaching a client about heart disease, the client may need to know the effects of smoking before recognizing the need to stop smoking. In this situation, what factor can facilitate client learning?
   1. Readiness
   2. Active involvement
   3. Motivation
   4. Allotted time

6. Many factors inhibit learning. Which of the following is a barrier to learning?
   1. The client receives adequate support from family members.
   2. The client exhibits emotional readiness to learn.
   3. The client is experiencing an acute illness.
   4. The client is physically ready to learn.

7. Which of the following client behaviors may cause a nurse to suspect a literacy problem?
   1. The client displays a pattern of compliance.
   2. The client reads the instructions slowly.
   3. The client recognizes that he or she does not know the information.
   4. The client states a pattern of excuses for not reading the instructions.

8. Which of the following is a learning outcome for a teaching plan?
   1. The client knows the factors that affect blood sugar level.
   2. The client selects low-fat foods from a menu.
   3. Teach the client about cardiac risk factors.
   4. The client understands a low-salt diet.

9. E-health includes all of the following EXCEPT:
   1. a client making an online appointment.
   2. e-mail access between the client and health care provider.
   3. online health information.
   4. a billing statement sent to the client's home address.

10. Which of the following is NOT an element in the nursing history that provides clues to learning needs?
    1. Age
    2. Economic factors
    3. Client's support systems
    4. Social factors

CHAPTER 28

LEADING, MANAGING, AND DELEGATING

CHAPTER OUTLINE

MediaLink

www.prenhall.com/berman

DVD-ROM
- Audio Glossary
- NCLEX® Review
- End of Unit Concept Map Activity
- Videos:
  - Building and Managing Teams
  - Delegating Successfully
  - Handling Conflict
  - Initiating and Managing Change
  - Introduction to Nursing Management
  - Leading and Managing
  - Managing Stress and Time
  - Motivating and Developing Staff

Companion Website
- Additional NCLEX® Review
- Case Study: Nurse as Manager and Delegator
- Application Activity: Nursing World
- Links to Resources

KEY TOPIC REVIEW

1. A manager influences others to work together to accomplish a specific goal.
   a. True   b. False

2. The informal leader, or appointed leader, is selected by an organization and given official authority to make decisions and take action.
   a. True   b. False
3. Theories about leadership style describe traits, behaviors, motivations, and choices used by individuals to effectively influence others.
   a. True   b. False
4. An autocratic (authoritarian) leader makes decisions for the group.
   a. True   b. False
5. A leader is an employee of an organization who is given authority, power, and responsibility for planning, organizing, coordinating, and directing the work of others, and for establishing and evaluating standards.
   a. True   b. False
6. A _____ (participative, consultative) leader encourages group discussion and decision making.
7. The _____ (nondirective, permissive) leader recognizes the group's need for autonomy and self-regulation.
8. The _____ leader does not trust self or others to make decisions and instead relies on the organization's rules, policies, and procedures to direct the group's work efforts.
9. The _____ leader flexes task and relationship behaviors, considers the staff members' abilities, knows the nature of the task to be done, and is sensitive to the context or environment in which the task takes place.
10. A _____ leader is rare and is characterized by an emotional relationship with the group members.
11. Match the following terms with the correct definition.
    a. Influence
    b. First-level managers
    c. Shared leadership
    d. Upper-level (top-level) managers
    e. Shared governance
    f. Risk management
    g. Planning
    h. Transactional leader
    i. Middle-level managers
    j. Vision

    _____ has a relationship with followers based on an exchange for some resource valued by the follower.
    _____ recognizes that a professional workforce is made up of many leaders.
    _____ a method that aims to distribute decision making among a group of people.
    _____ a mental image of a possible and desirable future state.
    _____ an informal strategy used to gain the cooperation of others without exercising formal authority.
    _____ supervise a number of first-level managers and are responsible for the activities in the departments they supervise.
    _____ involves deciding what, when, where, and how to do it, by whom, and with what resources.
    _____ are organizational executives who are primarily responsible for establishing goals and developing strategic plans.
    _____ having in place a system to reduce danger to clients and staff.
    _____ are responsible for managing the work of nonmanagerial personnel and the day-to-day activities of a specific work group or groups.

12. _____ involves determining responsibilities, communicating expectations, and establishing the chain of command for authority and communication.
    a. Organizing
    b. Directing
    c. Coordinating
    d. All the above
13. _____ is defined as the legitimate right to direct the work of others.
    a. Accountability
    b. Responsibility
    c. Authority
    d. Coordinating

14. _____ is a process whereby professional links are established through which people can share ideas, knowledge, and information, offer support and direction to each other, and facilitate accomplishment of professional goals.
    a. Mentor
    b. Effectiveness
    c. Preceptor
    d. Networking

15. _____ is a measure of the resources used in the provision of nursing services.
    a. Efficiency
    b. Effectiveness
    c. Productivity
    d. Coordinating

16. _____ is the transference of responsibility and authority for an activity to a competent individual.
    a. Change
    b. Delegation
    c. Planned change
    d. Unplanned change

FOCUSED STUDY TIPS

1. Discuss the classic work of Lewin, who developed a model of change that involves three stages: unfreezing, moving, and refreezing.

2. Compare and contrast authoritarian, democratic, and laissez-faire leadership styles.

3. List several characteristics of effective leaders.

4. Describe the role of the leader/manager in planning for and implementing change.

5. List the five rights of delegation.

6. Describe the characteristics of tasks appropriate to delegate to unlicensed and licensed assistive personnel.

7. Identify the skills and competencies needed by a nurse manager.

8. Discuss the roles and functions of nurse managers.

9. Describe the four functions of management.

10. Compare and contrast the levels of management.

11. Identify characteristics of an effective leader.

12. Compare and contrast different leadership styles.

13. Differentiate formal from informal leaders.

14. Compare and contrast leadership and management.

15. Visit the following website and write a short summary of what you learned: www.nursingspectrum.com/CareerManagement/Articles/Pearls_pw2005.htm.

CASE STUDY

Nathaniel is a nursing director who influences others to work together to accomplish a specific goal. He also has initiative and the ability and confidence to innovate change, motivate, facilitate, and mentor others. He actively guides the group toward achieving group goals. He assumes that individuals are internally motivated and capable of making decisions, and he values their independence.

1. *Is Nathaniel assuming the role of a leader or manager?*
2. *Compare and contrast the role of a leader and manager.*
3. *What particular leadership style has Nathaniel developed?*

NCLEX® REVIEW QUESTIONS

1. A nurse is planning a seminar on leadership styles. Which of the following statements describes a democratic leadership style?
    1. The leader assumes a "hands-off" approach.
    2. Under this leadership style, the group may feel secure because procedures are well defined and activities are predictable.
    3. This leadership style demands that the leader have faith in the group members to accomplish the goals.
    4. This leadership style does not trust self or others to make decisions and instead relies on the organization's rules, policies, and procedures to direct the group's work efforts.

2. A nursing director who fosters creativity, risk taking, commitment, and collaboration by empowering the group to share in the organization's vision is which type of leader?
    1. Charismatic
    2. Transactional
    3. Transformational
    4. Shared

3. The organizational executives who are primarily responsible for establishing goals and developing strategic plans are considered to be:
    1. first-level managers.
    2. middle-level managers.
    3. upper-level managers.
    4. supervising managers.

4. The nursing director who has the ability and willingness to assume responsibility for one's actions and to accept the consequences of one's behavior is demonstrating what management principle?
    1. Accountability
    2. Authority
    3. Responsibility
    4. Coordinating

5. The type of change that is an intended, purposeful attempt by an individual, group, organization, or larger social system to influence its own current status is referred to as:
   1. natural.
   2. situational.
   3. unplanned.
   4. planned.

6. A nurse is planning a seminar on the comparison of leader and manager roles. Which of the following characteristics describes a leader role?
   1. Influences others toward goal setting, either formally or informally
   2. Maintains an orderly, controlled, rational, and equitable structure
   3. Relates to people according to their roles
   4. Feels rewarded when fulfilling the organizational mission or goals

7. Which of the following is NOT a characteristic of an effective leader?
   1. Uses a leadership style appropriate to the task and the members
   2. Does not involve members in all decisions
   3. Plans and organizes activities of the group
   4. Is open and encourages openness, so that real issues are confronted

8. Which of the following is considered a driving force?
   1. Low tolerance for change related to intellectual or emotional insecurity
   2. Misunderstanding of the change and its implications
   3. Perception that the change will improve the situation
   4. Lack of time or energy

9. A nurse is planning a seminar on guidelines for dealing with resistance to change. Which of the following would be an appropriate guideline for dealing with resistance to change?
   1. Clarify information and provide accurate information.
   2. Explain the positive and negative consequences of the change and how the individual or group will get the change done.
   3. Maintain a climate of trust, support, and confidence.
   4. Communicate with those who oppose the change. Get to the root of their reasons for opposition.

10. Which of the following statements is incorrect? A situational leader:
    1. flexes task and relationship behaviors.
    2. does not consider the staff members' abilities.
    3. knows the nature of the task to be done.
    4. is sensitive to the context or environment in which the task takes place.

CHAPTER 29

VITAL SIGNS

CHAPTER OUTLINE

MediaLink

www.prenhall.com/berman

DVD-ROM
- Audio Glossary
- NCLEX® Review
- Skill Checklists:
  - Assessing a Peripheral Pulse
  - Assessing an Apical-Radial Pulse
  - Assessing an Apical Pulse
  - Assessing Blood Pressure
  - Assessing Body Temperature
  - Assessing Respirations
  - Measuring Oxygen Saturation

Companion Website
- Additional NCLEX® Review
- Case Study: Assessing Vital Signs
- Care Plan Activity: Client with Pneumonia
- Application Activity: Joanna Briggs Institute
- Links to Resources

  D. Hypotension
  E. Assessing Blood Pressure
      1. Blood Pressure Sites
      2. Methods
  F. Common Errors in Assessing Blood Pressure
     Skill 29-6 Assessing Blood Pressure
  V. Oxygen Saturation
  A. Factors Affecting Oxygen Saturation Readings
     Skill 29-7 Measuring Oxygen Saturation

KEY TOPIC REVIEW

1. Core temperature reflects the balance between the heat produced and the heat lost from the body, and is measured in heat units called degrees.
   a. True   b. False
2. Surface temperature is the temperature of the skin, the subcutaneous tissue, and fat.
   a. True   b. False
3. Cardiac output is the volume of blood pumped into the arteries by the heart and equals the result of the stroke volume (SV) times the heart rate (HR) per minute.
   a. True   b. False
4. The apical pulse is a pulse located away from the heart, for example, in the foot or wrist.
   a. True   b. False
5. Body temperature is the temperature of the deep tissues of the body, such as the abdominal cavity and pelvic cavity.
   a. True   b. False
6. _____ are body temperature, pulse, respirations, and blood pressure.
7. Heat _____ is a result of excessive heat and dehydration.
8. _____ of the arteries is their ability to contract and expand.
9. A pulse _____ is any discrepancy between the two pulse rates.
10. _____ is a core body temperature below the lower limit of normal.
11. Match the following terms with the correct definition.
   a. Radiation
   b. Conduction
   c. Chemical thermogenesis
   d. Convection
   e. Pulse volume
   f. Basal metabolic rate (BMR)
   g. Tachycardia
   h. Pulse
   i. Remittent fever
   j. Heat balance

   _____ when the amount of heat produced by the body equals the amount of heat lost.
   _____ the rate of energy utilization in the body required to maintain essential activities such as breathing.
   _____ the stimulation of heat production in the body through increased cellular metabolism.
   _____ the transfer of heat from the surface of one object to the surface of another without contact between the two objects, mostly in the form of infrared rays.
   _____ the dispersion of heat by air currents.
   _____ a wide range of temperature fluctuations (more than 2°C [3.6°F]) occurs over the 24-hour period, all of which are above normal.
   _____ a wave of blood created by contraction of the left ventricle of the heart.
   _____ is an excessively fast heart rate.
   _____, also called the pulse strength or amplitude, refers to the force of blood with each beat.
   _____ the transfer of heat from one molecule to a molecule of lower temperature.

12. _____ is the act of breathing.
   a. Inhalation
   b. Exhalation
   c. Ventilation
   d. Respiration

13. _____ is the absence of breathing.
    a. Bradypnea
    b. Apnea
    c. Tachypnea
    d. Polypnea

14. _____ refers to very deep, rapid respirations.
    a. Hypoventilation
    b. Respiratory rhythm
    c. Hyperventilation
    d. Respiratory quality/character

15. _____ pressure is the pressure when the ventricles are at rest.
    a. Diastolic
    b. Arterial blood
    c. Systolic
    d. Pulse

16. _____ is a blood pressure that is persistently above normal.
    a. Hypotension
    b. Orthostatic hypotension
    c. Hypertension
    d. Pulse oximeter

FOCUSED STUDY TIPS

1. List and explain the various vital signs.

2. Identify when it is appropriate to delegate measurement of vital signs to unlicensed assistive personnel.

3. Discuss measurement of blood oxygenation using pulse oximetry.

4. Describe methods and sites used to measure blood pressure.

5. Describe five phases of Korotkoff's sounds.

6. Differentiate systolic from diastolic blood pressure.

7. Identify the components of a respiratory assessment.

8. Describe the mechanics of breathing and the mechanisms that control respirations.

9. Explain how to measure the apical pulse and the apical-radial pulse.

10. List the characteristics that should be included when assessing pulses.

11. Identify nine sites used to assess the pulse and state the reasons for their use.

12. Describe appropriate nursing care for alterations in body temperature.

13. Compare methods of measuring body temperature.

14. Identify the variations in normal body temperature, pulse, respirations, and blood pressure that occur from infancy to old age.

15. Describe factors that affect the vital signs and accurate measurement of them.

CASE STUDY

A 20-year-old client is brought in to the clinic with complaints of fever, chills, and fatigue. His vital signs upon admission are BP 120/70, P 116, RR 20, T (oral) 102.1°F. His mother reports that his temperature rises to fever level rapidly and then returns to normal within a few hours. The doctor who examines him orders blood work.

1. *What are the normal vital signs for a 20-year-old male client?*
2. *What type of fever is the client most likely experiencing?*
3. *Why has the doctor ordered blood work?*

NCLEX® REVIEW QUESTIONS

1. Conduction is:
    1. the transfer of heat from one molecule to a molecule of lower temperature.
    2. the transfer of heat from the surface of one object to the surface of another without contact between the two objects, mostly in the form of infrared rays.
    3. the continuous evaporation of moisture from the respiratory tract and from the mucosa of the mouth and from the skin.
    4. the dispersion of heat by air currents.

2. Which type of fever is a client experiencing when the body temperature alternates at regular intervals between periods of fever and periods of normal or subnormal temperatures?
    1. Intermittent
    2. Remittent
    3. Relapsing
    4. Constant

3. A client reports that he has been exercising in hot weather; he feels warm, is flushed, and is not sweating. His temperature is 106°F and he just experienced a seizure. What condition is the client most likely experiencing?
    1. Hypothermia
    2. Heat exhaustion
    3. Heatstroke
    4. Hypertension

4. The body temperature is measured in degrees on two scales: Celsius (centigrade) and Fahrenheit. When the Celsius reading is 40, the Fahrenheit reading is:
    1. 100.
    2. 101.
    3. 103.
    4. 104.

5. The posterior tibial pulse site is on the medial surface of the ankle where the posterior tibial artery passes behind the:
   1. medial malleolus.
   2. knee.
   3. inguinal ligament.
   4. wrist.

6. Which of the following can cause an erroneously low blood pressure result?
   1. Cuff wrapped too loosely or unevenly
   2. Bladder cuff too narrow
   3. Arm above level of the heart
   4. Assessing immediately after a meal or while client smokes or has pain

7. Which of the following actions by a nurse would be incorrect when taking an adult's temperature using a tympanic thermometer?
   1. Inserting the probe slowly using a circular motion until snug
   2. Pointing the probe slightly anteriorly, toward the eardrum
   3. Pulling the pinna straight back and upward
   4. Not inserting the tympanic thermometer into the client's ear when there was a presence of cerumen

8. A nurse is evaluating a nursing student's understanding of altered breathing patterns and sounds. Which of the following statements demonstrates a need for further teaching?
   1. Stertor is a snoring or sonorous respiration, usually due to a partial obstruction of the upper airway.
   2. Wheeze is a continuous, high-pitched musical squeak or whistling sound occurring on expiration and sometimes on inspiration when air moves through a narrowed or partially obstructed airway.
   3. Bubbling is a gurgling sound heard as air passes through moist secretions in the respiratory tract.
   4. Stridor is difficult and labored breathing during which the individual has a persistent, unsatisfied need for air and feels distressed obstruction.

9. A nurse is planning a seminar on secretions and coughing. Which of the following describes a condition in which there is a presence of blood in the sputum?
   1. Hemoptysis
   2. Productive cough
   3. Nonproductive cough
   4. Orthopnea

10. A nurse is evaluating a nursing student's understanding of Korotkoff's sounds. Which of the following statements demonstrates a need for further teaching?
    1. Phase 1 is the pressure level at which the first faint, clear tapping or thumping sounds are heard. These sounds gradually become more intense.
    2. Phase 2 is the period during deflation when the sounds have a muffled, whooshing, or swishing quality.
    3. Phase 4 is the time when the sounds become muffled and have a soft, blowing quality.
    4. Phase 5 is the first tapping sound heard during deflation of the cuff and is the systolic blood pressure.

HEALTH ASSESSMENT

CHAPTER OUTLINE

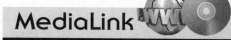

MediaLink

www.prenhall.com/berman

DVD-ROM
- Audio Glossary
- NCLEX® Review
- End of Unit Concept Map Activity
- Videos and Animations:
  - Barking Cough (14 month old with upper respiratory infection)
  - Crackles (age: 8 months; recovering from cardiac surgery
  - Continuous Murmur (caused by patent Ductus Arteriosus)
- Fast Breathing (3 month old with Bronchiolitis)
- Fixed S2 Split
- Inspiratory and Expiratory Crackles (age: 3 months with Bronchiolitis)
- Normal Heart Sound (12 year-old, heart rate is approximately 65 beats per minute)
- Normal Heart Sound (recorded from a child, heart rate is approximately 100 beats per minute)
- Normal Lung Sounds (4 month old)
- Normal Lung Sounds (4 year-old)
- Physiological S2 Split (12 year-old)
- Rhonchi (recorded from a mid right back of a 5 year-old with pneumonia)
- Stridor (16 year-old female)
- Squawks (5 year-old with pneumonia)
- Skill Checklists:
  - Assessing Appearance and Mental Status

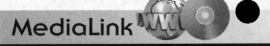

MediaLink

www.prenhall.com/berman

- Assessing the Abdomen
- Assessing the Breasts and Axillae
- Assessing the Ears and Hearing
- Assessing the Eye Structures and Visual Acuity
- Assessing the Female Genitals and Inguinal Area
- Assessing the Hair
- Assessing the Heart and Central Vessels
- Assessing the Male Genitals and Inguinal Area
- Assessing the Mouth and Oropharynx
- Assessing the Musculoskeletal System
- Assessing the Nails
- Assessing the Neck
- Assessing the Neurological System
- Assessing the Nose and Sinuses
- Assessing the Peripheral Vascular System
- Assessing the Rectum and Anus
- Assessing the Skin
- Assessing the Skull and Face
- Assessing the Thorax and Lungs

Companion Website
- Additional NCLEX® Review
- Case Study: Performing Physical Assessments
- Care Plan Activity: Client Care After Motor Vehicle Crash
- Application Activity: Physical Exam Study Guide
- Links to Resources

KEY TOPIC REVIEW

1. Inspection is the visual examination—that is, assessing by using the sense of sight.
   a. True   b. False
2. Percussion is the examination of the body using the sense of touch.
   a. True   b. False
3. The middle finger of the nondominant hand is referred to as the pleximeter.
   a. True   b. False

4. Tympany is a musical or drumlike sound produced from an air-filled stomach.
    a. True   b. False
5. Palpation is the act of striking the body surface to elicit sounds that can be heard or vibrations that can be felt.
    a. True   b. False
6. _____ (a blowing or swishing sound) is created by turbulence of blood flow due to either a narrowed arterial lumen (a common development in older people) or a condition, such as anemia or hyperthyroidism, that elevates cardiac output.
7. Any defects in or loss of the power to express oneself by speech, writing, or signs, or to comprehend spoken or written language due to disease or injury of the cerebral cortex, is called _____.
8. _____ is an automatic response of the body to a stimulus.
9. _____ is a protrusion of the intestine through the inguinal wall or canal.
10. _____ is the ability to sense whether one or two areas of the skin are being stimulated by pressure.
11. Match the following terms with the correct definitions.
    a. Hyperopia   _____ the process of listening to sounds produced within the body.
    b. Otoscope   _____ nearsightedness.
    c. Cerumen   _____ loss of elasticity of the lens and thus loss of ability to see close objects.
    d. Astigmatism   _____ an uneven curvature of the cornea that prevents horizontal and vertical
    e. Eustachian tube   rays from focusing on the retina; is a common problem that may occur
    f. Glaucoma   in conjunction with myopia and hyperopia.
    g. Miosis   _____ a disturbance in the circulation of aqueous fluid, which causes an
    h. Myopia   increase in intraocular pressure; is the most frequent cause of
    i. Auscultation   blindness in people over 40.
    j. Presbyopia   _____ constricted pupils that may indicate an inflammation of the iris or result
                                   from such drugs as morphine or pilocarpine.
                          _____ an instrument for examining the interior of the ear, especially the
                                   eardrum, consisting essentially of a magnifying lens and a light.
                          _____ a part of the middle ear that connects the middle ear to the nasopharynx.
                          _____ earwax that lubricates and protects the canal.
                          _____ farsightedness.

12. _____ is an extremely dull sound produced by very dense tissue, such as muscle or bone.
    a. Dullness
    b. Flatness
    c. Resonance
    d. Hyperresonance
13. _____ refers to the loudness or softness of a sound.
    a. Pitch
    b. Quality
    c. Duration
    d. Intensity
14. _____ is the result of inadequate circulating blood or hemoglobin and subsequent reduction in tissue oxygenation.
    a. Cyanosis
    b. Erythema
    c. Jaundice
    d. Pallor
15. _____ is the presence of excess interstitial fluid.
    a. Vitiligo
    b. Alopecia
    c. Edema
    d. Clubbing
16. _____ is what a normal head size is referred to.
    a. Exophthalmos
    b. Visual acuity
    c. Normocephalic
    d. Visual fields

FOCUSED STUDY TIPS

1. Define dullness, flatness, and resonance.

2. List the common refractive errors of the lens of the eye.

3. Explain the air-conducted transmission process.

4. Define thrill and bruit.

5. Describe common inflammatory visual problems.

6. Identify the positions that are frequently required during the physical assessment.

7. Summarize the physical health assessment.

8. Discuss variations in examination techniques appropriate for clients of different ages.

9. Describe suggested sequencing to conduct a physical health examination in an orderly fashion.

10. Identify the steps in selected examination procedures.

11. Identify expected outcomes of health assessment.

12. Explain the significance of selected physical findings.

13. Explain the four methods used in physical examination.

14. Identify the purposes of the physical examination.

15. Summarize auscultated sounds that are described according to their pitch, intensity, duration, and quality.

CASE STUDY

A nursing student is preparing for her clinical rotation at a clinic. She has been told that she will be responsible for preparing clients for physical examinations.

1. *Discuss the purposes of the physical examination.*
2. *Several positions are frequently required during the physical assessment. List client positions and provide a description of each one.*
3. *List the equipment and supplies used for a health examination.*

NCLEX® REVIEW QUESTIONS

1. A client asks the nurse "What is the purpose of a physical examination?" Which response by the nurse is NOT correct?
   1. "To obtain data at any given time about a client's functional abilities."
   2. "To obtain data that will help establish nursing diagnoses and plans of care."
   3. "To identify areas for health promotion and disease prevention."
   4. "To supplement, confirm, or refute data obtained in the nursing history."

2. Auscultation is the:
   1. visual examination—that is, assessing by using the sense of sight.
   2. examination of the body using the sense of touch.
   3. act of striking the body surface to elicit sounds that can be heard or vibrations that can be felt.
   4. process of listening to sounds produced within the body.

3. Jaundice is:
   1. the result of inadequate circulating blood or hemoglobin and subsequent reduction in tissue oxygenation.
   2. a bluish tinge and is most evident in the nail beds, lips, and buccal mucosa.
   3. a yellowish tinge, may first be evident in the sclera of the eyes and then in the mucous membranes and the skin.
   4. a redness associated with a variety of rashes.

4. Which of the following terms means nearsightedness?
   1. Myopia
   2. Hyperopia
   3. Presbyopia
   4. Astigmatism

5. A nurse is evaluating a nursing student's understanding of the air-conducted transmission process. Which of the following statements demonstrates a need for further teaching?
   1. A sound stimulus enters the external canal and reaches the tympanic membrane.
   2. The sound waves vibrate the tragus and reach the ossicles.
   3. The sound waves travel from the ossicles to the opening in the inner ear (oval window).
   4. The cochlea receives the sound vibrations.

6. A nurse is planning a seminar on the organs in the nine abdominal regions. Which of the following information is incorrect?
   1. The epigastric region includes the aorta, the pyloric end of the stomach, part of the duodenum, and the pancreas.
   2. The umbilical region includes the omentum, the mesentery, the lower part of the duodenum, and part of the jejunum and ileum.
   3. The right lumbar region includes the ascending colon, the lower half of the right kidney, and part of the duodenum and jejunum.
   4. The left lumbar region includes the stomach, the spleen, the tail of the pancreas, the splenic flexure of the colon, the upper half of the left kidney, and the suprarenal gland.

7. A nurse is evaluating a nursing student's understanding of cranial nerves. Which of the following statements demonstrates a need for further teaching? The assessment method for:
   1. cranial nerve I would be to ask the client to close his/her eyes and identify different mild aromas, such as coffee, vanilla, peanut butter, orange/lemon, or chocolate.
   2. cranial nerve IV would be to ask the client to read a Snellen-type chart.
   3. cranial nerve VI would be to assess the client's directions of gaze.
   4. cranial nerve VII would be to ask the client to smile, raise the eyebrows, frown, puff out cheeks, close eyes tightly.

8. Which adventitious breath sound is a superficial grating or creaking sound heard during inspiration and expiration?
    1. Friction rub
    2. Crackles
    3. Wheeze
    4. Gurgles

9. A nurse is preparing to complete a physical examination on a client's pelvis and vagina. The position the client is placed in for this examination is:
    1. prone.
    2. supine.
    3. lithotomy.
    4. sitting.

10. Which of the following actions is correct for the nurse assessing a client who has just had a cast applied to the lower leg?
    1. Assess tissue turgor, fluid intake and output, and vital signs.
    2. Assess peripheral perfusion of toes, capillary blanch test, pedal pulse if able, and vital signs.
    3. Assess apical pulse and compare with baseline data.
    4. Assess level of consciousness using Glasgow Coma Scale; assess pupils for reaction to light and accommodation; assess vital signs.

CHAPTER 31

ASEPSIS

CHAPTER OUTLINE

MediaLink

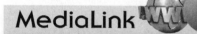

www.prenhall.com/berman

DVD-ROM
- Audio Glossary
- NCLEX® Review
- Skills Checklists:
  - Donning a Sterile Gown and Gloves (Open Method)
  - Donning and Removing Personal Protective Equipment
  - Donning and Removing Sterile Gloves (Open Method)
  - Establishing and Maintaining a Sterile Field
  - Handwashing
- Videos and Animations: Handwashing and Gloving

Companion Website
- Additional NCLEX® Review
- Case Study: Client with Mycoplasma Pneumonia
- Care Plan Activity: Client on Radiation Therapy and Medication
- Application Activity: Infection Control Today
- Links to Resources

F. Disinfecting and Sterilizing
  1. Disinfecting
  2. Sterilizing
VIII. Isolation Precautions
  A. CDC (HICPAC) Isolation Precautions (1996)
    1. Standard Precautions
    2. Transmission-Based Precautions
  B. Compromised Clients
IX. Isolation Practices
  A. Personal Protective Equipment
    1. Gloves
      Skill 31-2 Donning and Removing
      Personal Protective Equipment (Gloves,
      Gown, Mask, Eyewear)
  B. 1. Gowns
    2. Face Masks
    3. Eyewear
  C. Disposal of Soiled Equipment and Supplies
    1. Bagging
    2. Linens
    3. Laboratory Specimens
    4. Dishes

  5. Blood Pressure Equipment
  6. Thermometers
  7. Disposable Needles, Syringes, and Sharps
  D. Transporting Clients with Infections
  E. Psychosocial Needs of Isolation Clients
X. Sterile Technique
  A. Sterile Field
    Skill 31-3 Establishing and Maintaining
    a Sterile Field
  B. Sterile Gloves
    Skill 31-4 Donning and Removing Sterile
    Gloves (Open Method)
  C. Sterile Gowns
    Skill 31-5 Donning a Sterile Gown and Gloves
    (Closed Method)
XI. Infection Control for Health Care Workers
XII. Role of the Infection Control Nurse
XIII. Evaluating

KEY TOPIC REVIEW

1. A disease is an invasion of body tissue by microorganisms and their growth within that tissue.
   a. True   b. False
2. Virulence is the ability to produce disease.
   a. True   b. False
3. Pathogenicity is the ability to produce disease; thus a pathogen is a microorganism that causes disease.
   a. True   b. False
4. Surgical asepsis or sterile technique includes all practices intended to confine a specific microorganism to a specific area, limiting the number, growth, and transmission of microorganisms.
   a. True   b. False
5. Sepsis is the state of infection and can take many forms, including septic shock.
   a. True   b. False
6. If the infectious agent can be transmitted to an individual by direct or indirect contact or as an airborne infection, the resulting condition is called a _____ disease.
7. A(an) _____ pathogen causes disease only in a susceptible individual.
8. _____ is the freedom from disease-causing microorganisms.
9. _____ are by far the most common infection-causing microorganisms.
10. In medical asepsis objects are considered clean or _____.
11. Match the following terms with the correct definition.
    a. Vehicle   _____   consist primarily of nucleic acid and therefore must enter living cells
    b. Iatrogenic infections   in order to reproduce.
    c. Compromised host   _____   include yeasts and molds.
    d. Colonization   _____   live on other living organisms.
    e. Nonspecific defenses   _____   the process by which strains of microorganisms become resident
    f. Parasites   flora.
    g. Vector   _____   are the direct result of diagnostic or therapeutic procedures.
    h. Fungi   _____   a person or animal reservoir of a specific infectious agent that
    i. Carrier   usually does not manifest any clinical signs of disease.
    j. Viruses   _____   any substance that serves as an intermediate means to transport and
                                         introduces an infectious agent into a susceptible host through a
                                         suitable portal of entry.

_____ an animal or flying or crawling insect that serves as an intermediate means of transporting the infectious agent.

_____ a person at increased risk, an individual who for one or more reasons is more likely than others to acquire an infection.

_____ protect the person against all microorganisms, regardless of prior exposure.

12. _____ is limited to the specific part of the body where the microorganisms remain.
    a. Bacteremia
    b. Systemic infection
    c. Septicemia
    d. Local infection

13. _____ infections are classified as infections that are associated with the delivery of health care services in a health care facility.
    a. Acute
    b. Nosocomial
    c. Chronic
    d. Endogenous

14. _____ is a local and nonspecific defensive response of the tissues to an injurious or infectious agent.
    a. Hyperemia
    b. Leukocytes
    c. Inflammation
    d. Leukocytosis

15. _____ is the replacement of destroyed tissue cells by cells that are identical or similar in structure and function.
    a. Regeneration
    b. Antigen
    c. Immunity
    d. Antibodies

16. _____ are agents that inhibit the growth of some microorganisms.
    a. Sterilization
    b. Antiseptics
    c. Airborne precautions
    d. Disinfectants

FOCUSED STUDY TIPS

1. Discuss the relationship between hygiene, rest, activity, and nutrition in the chain of infection.

2. Discuss antimicrobial soaps and effective disinfectants.

3. Describe the steps to take in the event of a bloodborne pathogen exposure.

4. Explain aseptic practices, including hand washing; donning and removing a facemask, gown, and disposable gloves; managing equipment used for isolation clients; and maintaining a sterile field.

5. Compare and contrast category-specific, disease-specific, universal, body substance, standard, and transmission-based isolation precaution systems.

6. Identify measures that break each link in the chain of infection.

7. Identify interventions to reduce risks for infections.

8. Identify relevant nursing diagnoses and contributing factors for clients at risk for infection and for clients who have an infection.

9. Identify signs of localized and systemic infections.

10. Identify factors influencing a microorganism's capability to produce an infectious process.

11. Differentiate active from passive immunity.

12. Identify anatomic and physiologic barriers that defend the body against microorganisms.

13. Identify risks for nosocomial infections.

14. Explain the concepts of medical and surgical asepsis.

15. Visit the following website: http://en.wikipedia.org/wiki/Asepsis. Write a one-paragraph summary of what you learned.

CASE STUDY

Brent is a new nursing student. You will be his preceptor for the next 3 days. On the first day, Brent asks you the following questions:

1. *What is the difference between asepsis and sepsis, and between medical asepsis and surgical asepsis?*
2. *What four major categories of microorganisms cause infection in humans?*
3. *Explain the difference between standard precautions and transmission-based precautions.*

NCLEX® REVIEW QUESTIONS

1. Which of the following means freedom from disease-causing microorganisms?
   1. Medical asepsis
   2. Asepsis
   3. Surgical asepsis
   4. Sepsis

2. Which of the following consists primarily of nucleic acid and therefore must enter living cells in order to reproduce?
   1. Fungi   3. Viruses
   2. Bacteria   4. Parasites

3. Inflammation is a local and nonspecific defensive response of the tissues to an injurious or infectious agent. Which of the following is NOT a sign of inflammation?
   1. Pain
   2. Swelling
   3. Redness
   4. Fatigue

4. Four commonly used methods of sterilization are moist heat, gas, boiling water, and radiation. Which of the following is the most practical and inexpensive method for sterilizing in the home?
   1. Gas
   2. Moist heat
   3. Radiation
   4. Boiling water

5. A nurse is evaluating a nursing student's understanding of types of infections. Which of the following statements demonstrates a need for further teaching?
   1. A local infection is limited to the specific part of the body where the microorganisms remain.
   2. If the microorganisms spread and damage different parts of the body, it is a systemic infection.
   3. Acute infections may occur slowly, over a very long period, and may last months or years.
   4. Nosocomial infections are classified as infections that are associated with the delivery of health care services in a health care facility.

6. A nurse is planning a seminar on the chain of infection. Which of the following is NOT one of the six links?
   1. Etiologic agent
   2. Reservoir
   3. Portal of entry
   4. Mode of transmission

7. An antigen is a:
   1. host that produces antibodies in response to natural antigens (e.g., infectious microorganisms) or artificial antigens (e.g., vaccines).
   2. substance that induces a state of sensitivity or immune responsiveness (immunity).
   3. host that receives natural (e.g., from a nursing mother) or artificial (e.g., from an injection of immune serum) antibodies produced by another source.
   4. part of the body's plasma proteins.

8. The CDC recommends antimicrobial hand cleansing agents in all of the following situations EXCEPT:
   1. when there are unknown multiple nonresistant bacteria.
   2. before invasive procedures.
   3. in special care units, such as nurseries and ICUs.
   4. before caring for severely immunocompromised clients.

9. Which of the following statements about disinfectants is incorrect?
   1. A disinfectant is a chemical preparation, such as phenol or iodine compounds, used on inanimate objects.
   2. Disinfectants are frequently caustic and toxic to tissues.
   3. Disinfectants and antiseptics often have similar chemical components, but the disinfectant is a less concentrated solution.
   4. A disinfectant is an agent that destroys pathogens other than spores.

10. Which types of precautions are used for clients known or suspected to have serious illnesses transmitted by particle droplets larger than 5 microns?
    1. Airborne
    2. Droplet
    3. Contact
    4. Connection

CHAPTER 32

SAFETY

CHAPTER OUTLINE

I. Factors Affecting Safety
  A. Age and Development
  B. Lifestyle
  C. Mobility and Health Status
  D. Sensory-Perceptual Alterations
  E. Cognitive Awareness
  F. Emotional State
  G. Ability to Communicate
  H. Safety Awareness
  I. Environmental Factors
    1. Home
    2. Workplace
    3. Community
    4. Health Care Setting
    5. Bioterrorism
II. Nursing Management
  A. Assessing
    1. Nursing History and Physical Examination
      a. Risk Assessment Tools
      b. Home Hazard Appraisal
    2. National Patient Safety Goals
    3. Bioterrorism Attacks
  B. Diagnosing
  C. Planning
  D. Implementing
    1. Promoting Safety across the Life Span
      a. Newborns and Infants
      b. Toddlers
      c. Preschoolers
      d. School-Age Children
      e. Adolescents
      f. Young Adults

MediaLink

www.prenhall.com/berman

DVD-ROM
- Audio Glossary
- NCLEX® Review
- Skills Checklists
- Videos and Animation: Lead Poisoning
- Skill Checklists:
  - Applying Restraints
  - Implementing Seizure Precautions
  - Using a Bed or Chair Exit Safety Monitoring Device

Companion Website
- Additional NCLEX® Review
- Case Study: Ensuring Client Safety
- Care Plan Activity: Safety at Home
- Application Activities:
  - Disaster Nursing and the Red Cross
  - Safety in Nursing Issues
- Links to Resources

g. Middle-Aged Adults
h. Elders
i. Safety Problems across the Life Span
2. Promoting Safety in the Health Care Setting
3. Preventing Specific Hazards
   a. Scalds and Burns
   b. Fires
      i. Agency Fires
      ii. Home Fires
   c. Falls
   d. Seizures
   e. Poisoning
   f. Carbon Monoxide Poisoning
   g. Suffocation or Choking
   h. Excessive Noise

i. Electrical Hazards
j. Firearms
k. Radiation
l. Bioterrorism Attack
4. Procedure- and Equipment-Related Accidents
5. Restraining Clients
   a. Legal Implications of Restraints
   b. Selecting a Restraint
   c. Kinds of Restraints
      Skill 32-1 Using a Bed or Chair Exit Safety Monitoring Device
      Skill 32-2 Implementing Seizure Precautions
      Skill 32-3 Applying Restraints
III. Evaluating

KEY TOPIC REVIEW

1. People with impaired touch perception, hearing, taste, smell, and vision are highly susceptible to injury.
   a. True   b. False
2. Restraints are used for staff convenience or client punishment.
   a. True   b. False
3. The universal sign of distress is the victim's grasping the anterior neck and being unable to speak or cough.
   a. True   b. False
4. Generalized seizures (also called focal) involve electrical discharges from one area of the brain.
   a. True   b. False
5. People of any age can fall, but infants and elders are particularly prone to falling and causing serious injury.
   a. True   b. False
6. _____ can include chemical, biological, or nuclear weapons.
7. Suicide and _____ are two leading causes of death among teenagers.
8. A _____ is a burn from a hot liquid or vapor, such as steam.
9. _____ injury can occur from overexposure to radioactive materials used in diagnostic and therapeutic procedures.
10. _____ assessment tools are available to determine clients at risk both for specific kinds of injury, such as falls, or for the general safety of the home and health care setting.
11. Match the following terms with the correct definition.
    a. Seizure
    b. Asphyxiation
    c. Electric shock
    d. Chemical restraints
    e. Restraints
    f. Safety monitoring device
    g. Heimlich maneuver
    h. Bioterrorism
    i. Seizure precautions
    j. Carbon monoxide (CO)

    _____ is an intentional attack using weapons of viruses, bacteria, and other germs.
    _____ A bed or chair _____ has a position-sensitive switch that triggers an audio alarm when the client attempts to get out of the bed or chair.
    _____ a sudden onset of excessive electrical discharges in one or more areas of the brain.
    _____ are safety measures taken by the nurse to protect clients from injury should they have a seizure.
    _____ is an odorless, colorless, tasteless gas that is very toxic.
    _____ Suffocation, or _____, is lack of oxygen due to interrupted breathing.
    _____ The emergency response is the _____, or abdominal thrust, which can dislodge the foreign object and reestablish an airway.
    _____ are protective devices used to limit the physical activity of the client or a part of the body.

_____ occurs when a current travels through the body to the ground rather than through electric wiring, or from static electricity that builds up on the body.

_____ are medications such as neuroleptics, anxiolytics, sedatives, and psychotropic agents used to control socially disruptive behavior. The purpose of restraints is to prevent the client from injuring self or others.

12. Which of the following is NOT a type of restraint?
    a. Jacket
    b. Mitt
    c. Foot
    d. Limb

13. _____ restraints are any manual method or physical or mechanical device, material, or equipment attached to the client's body; they cannot be removed easily and they restrict the client's movement.
    a. Chemical
    b. Physical
    c. Medical
    d. Standard

14. Health care organizations are now expected to address which of the four specific phases of disaster planning?
    a. Preparedness
    b. Recovery
    c. Response
    d. Migration

15. Which of the following is NOT a basic firearm safety rule?
    a. Store the bullets in a different location from the guns.
    b. Ensure the firearm is unloaded and the action is open when handing it to someone else.
    c. Tell children never to touch a gun or stay in a friend's house where a gun is accessible.
    d. Have firearms that are regularly used inspected by a qualified gunsmith at least every 5 years.

16. Excessive noise is a health hazard that can cause hearing loss, depending on all the following EXCEPT:
    a. the overall level of noise.
    b. the frequency range of the noise.
    c. the individual family history.
    d. the duration of exposure.

FOCUSED STUDY TIPS

1. How is excessive noise a health hazard?

2. List the types of restraints.

3. Explain how to promote safety across the life span.

4. Discuss the factors affecting safety.

5. Describe the five criteria a nurse should use when selecting a restraint.

6. Identify the four sequential priorities a nurse should follow during a fire.

7. Summarize the legal implications of restraints.

8. Compare and contrast a scald and a burn.

9. Define electric shock.

10. Recall the common home hazards causing scalds.

11. Discuss risk factors and preventive measures for falls.

12. Describe alternatives to restraints.

13. Explain the home hazard appraisal.

14. Define seizure and seizure precautions.

15. Write a summary of the textbook's lead poisoning animation MediaLink found at the website www.prenhall.com/berman.

CASE STUDY

A couple just purchased a new home last week. During your assessment, the couple tells you they do not have a fire plan, fire extinguishers, carbon monoxide alarms, or working smoke alarms in their home.

1. *What preventive measures do you need to teach the couple?*
2. *Write a fire plan for the couple to follow.*
3. *Explain the three categories of fires.*

NCLEX® REVIEW QUESTIONS

1. When planning immediate injury prevention for parents of a toddler, which of the following would NOT be a focus at that time?
   1. Burns
   2. Suffocation
   3. Choking
   4. Lead poisoning

2. When evaluating a parent's understanding of safety measures for an infant, which of the following statements indicates a need for further teaching?
   1. "I will store all household chemicals in the garage."
   2. "I will make sure my infant is in his car seat before starting the car."
   3. "I will keep small crafting beads locked in the cabinet."
   4. "I will keep the trash bags in the kitchen on the bottom shelf by the sink."

3. A nurse planning a safety instruction class for parents of adolescents knows that the focus of the class should be on:
   1. teaching adolescents to sleep on a low bed.
   2. teaching adolescents about driver safety.
   3. teaching adolescents not to ingest lead paint chips.
   4. teaching adolescents not to run or ride a tricycle into the street.

4. Suicide and homicide are two leading causes of death among teenagers. When planning a workshop on adolescent suicide and homicide, the nurse knows that which of the following is NOT among the most common factors influencing the high suicide and homicide rates?
   1. Economic deprivation
   2. Stable and fulfilling friendships
   3. The availability of firearms
   4. Family breakup

5. A nurse teaching a safety class for parents identifies all of the following as main causes of death for school-age children. Which of the following is NOT one of the leading causes?
   1. Broken arms
   2. Fires
   3. Drownings
   4. Firearms

6. When planning a safety inservice program for an independent living community for older adults, the nurse will include information on which of the following as the leading cause of injury among older adults?
   1. Firearms
   2. Drownings
   3. Suicide
   4. Falls

7. Which of the following is an incorrect part of the nursing assessment before applying restraints on a client?
   1. Status of skin to which restraint is to be applied
   2. Circulatory status proximal to restraints
   3. Consideration of other protective measures that may be implemented before applying a restraint
   4. Underlying cause for assessed behavior

8. When evaluating a parent's understanding of poisoning prevention, which of the following statements indicates a need for further teaching?
   1. "We'll store toxic liquids or solids in food containers, such as soft drink bottles, peanut butter jars, or milk cartons."
   2. "We'll display the phone number of the poison control center near or on all telephones in our home so that it is available to babysitters, family, and friends."
   3. "We'll teach our children never to eat any part of an unknown plant or mushroom and not to put leaves, stems, bark, seeds, nuts, or berries from any plant into their mouths."
   4. "We'll not refer to medicine as candy or pretend false enjoyment when taking medications in front of our children."

9. A nurse establishing a client's plan of care for implementing seizure precautions should plan to include which of the following?
   1. If clients have frequent or recurrent seizures or take anticonvulsant medications, they need to wear a medical identification tag (bracelet or necklace) and carry a card delineating any medications they take.
   2. Assist the client in alerting all persons in the community about their seizure disorder.
   3. Discuss safety precautions for inside of the home only.
   4. Discuss with the client, family, and persons in the community factors that may precipitate a seizure.

10. Which of the following would NOT be a preventive measure for an older client with poor vision?
    1. Ensure eyeglasses are functional.
    2. Ensure appropriate lighting.
    3. Mark doorways only.
    4. Keep the environment tidy.

CHAPTER 33

HYGIENE

CHAPTER OUTLINE

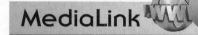

MediaLink

www.prenhall.com/berman

DVD-ROM
- Audio Glossary
- NCLEX® Review
- Skills Checklists

Companion Website
- Additional NCLEX® Review
- Case Study: Providing Basic Hygiene Care
- Care Plan Activity: Client on Radiation Therapy
- Application Activities:
  - Client with Chickenpox
  - Caring for Dentures
- Links to Resources

KEY TOPIC REVIEW

1. A dry mouth can be aggravated by poor fluid intake, heavy smoking, alcohol use, high salt intake, anxiety, and many medications.
   a. True   b. False

2. Most dentists recommend that dental hygiene should begin after the fifth tooth erupts.
   a. True   b. False

3. Fluoride toothpaste is often recommended because of its antibacterial protection.
   a. True   b. False

4. A room temperature between 20° and 23°C (68° and 74°F) is comfortable for most clients.
   a. True   b. False

5. Water used for the shampoo should be 115°F for an adult or child to be comfortable and not injure the scalp.
   a. True   b. False

6. _____ (lice) are parasitic insects that infest mammals.
7. _____ is a contagious skin infestation by the itch mite.
8. The growth of excessive body hair is called _____.
9. _____ is the fine hair on the body of the fetus, also referred to as *down* or *woolly hair*.
10. _____ is an *invisible* soft film that adheres to the enamel surface of teeth; it consists of bacteria, molecules of saliva, and remnants of epithelial cells and leukocytes.
11. Match the following terms with the correct definition.

    a. Tinea pedis
    b. Ingrown toe nail
    c. Therapeutic baths
    d. Apocrine glands
    e. Callus
    f. Fissures
    g. Tartar
    h. Hygiene
    i. Sudoriferous (sweat) glands
    j. Corn

    _____ Personal _____ is the self-care by which people attend to such functions as bathing, toileting, general body hygiene, and grooming.
    _____ are on all body surfaces except the lips and parts of the genitals.
    _____ The _____, located largely in the axillae and anogenital areas, begin to function at puberty under the influence of androgens.
    _____ are given for physical effects, such as to soothe irritated skin or to treat an area (e.g., the perineum).
    _____ A(an) _____ is a thickened portion of epidermis, a mass of keratotic material.
    _____ A(an) _____ is a keratosis caused by friction and pressure from a shoe.
    _____ (deep grooves) that frequently occur between the toes as a result of dryness and cracking of the skin.
    _____ Athlete's foot, or _____ (ringworm of the foot), is caused by a fungus.
    _____ A(an) _____, the growing inward of the nail into the soft tissues around it, most often results from improper nail trimming.
    _____ is a visible, hard deposit of plaque and dead bacteria that forms at the gum lines.

12. _____ tends to cling to clothing, so that when a client undresses, the lice may not be in evidence on the body; these lice suck blood from the person and lay their eggs on the clothing.
    a. *Pediculus corporis*
    b. *Pediculus pubis*
    c. *Pediculus capitis*
    d. Scabies
13. Dry mouth, also called _____, occurs when the supply of saliva is reduced.
    a. Xeroma
    b. Xerostomia
    c. Xerosis
    d. Xerotic
14. Dental caries occur frequently during the _____ period, often as a result of the excessive intake of sweets or a prolonged use of the bottle during naps and at bedtime.
    a. Infant
    b. Toddler
    c. School-age
    d. Newborn
15. _____ are usually conical (circular and raised).
    a. Plantar warts
    b. Calluses
    c. Corns
    d. Fissures
16. The _____ is the most widely used type because it fits snugly behind the ear. The hearing aid case, which holds the microphone, amplifier, and receiver, is attached to the earmold by a plastic tube.
    a. In-the-canal (ITC) aid
    b. Body hearing aid
    c. Behind-the-ear (BTE, or postaural) aid
    d. In-the-ear aid (ITE, or intra-aural)

FOCUSED STUDY TIPS

1. How should a proper hospital bed be made?

2. List the six different types of baths that could be given to a client.

3. Explain the factors affecting client hygiene practices.

4. Discuss the importance of brushing and combing a client's hair.

5. Describe *Pediculus capitis*, *Pediculus corporis*, and *Pediculus pubis*.

6. Identify the diseases that ticks can transmit.

7. Summarize a variety of ways to shampoo a client's hair.

8. Compare and contrast sudoriferous glands, eccrine glands, and aprocrine glands.

9. Define plaque, tartar, and gingivitis.

10. List the elements of contact lens care.

11. Discuss eyeglass care.

12. Describe general hearing aid care.

13. Explain how to insert a contact lens.

14. Define dental caries and periodontal disease.

15. Write a summary of the textbook's "Caring for Denture Application" MediaLink.

CASE STUDY

You are assigned to give a bath to an 83-year-old man who has cognitive problems.

1. *What is the proper water temperature for the client's bath?*
2. *List three reasons why a nurse would check the bath water.*
3. *Why is it important to verify the temperature of the water for this client?*

NCLEX® REVIEW QUESTIONS

1. A nurse is making the client bed. Which of the following actions should the nurse not do?
   1. Hold the soiled linen close to his or her uniform.
   2. Do not shake soiled linen in the air because shaking can disseminate secretions and excretions and the microorganisms they contain.
   3. When stripping and making a bed, conserve time and energy by stripping and making up one side as much as possible before working on the other side.
   4. Linen for one client is never (even momentarily) placed on another client's bed.

2. What is the correct bath water temperature for an adult client?
   1. 110 to 125°F
   2. 90 to 100°F
   3. 100 to 115°F
   4. 125 to 135°F

3. The parent of a toddler is cleaning the client's teeth. Which of the following statements indicates a need for further teaching?
   1. "I'll brush my child's teeth with a hard toothbrush."
   2. "I'll give a fluoride supplement daily or as recommended by the physician or dentist, unless the drinking water is fluoridated."
   3. "I'll schedule an initial dental visit for my child at about 2 or 3 years of age or as soon as all 20 primary teeth have erupted."
   4. "I'll seek professional dental attention for any problems such as discoloring of the teeth, chipping, or signs of infection such as redness and swelling."

4. During discharge planning, the nurse is teaching a client how to prevent dry skin. Which of the following statements is false?
   1. Bathe using soap or detergent only.
   2. Use bath oils, but take precautions to prevent falls caused by slippery tub surfaces.
   3. Humidify the air with a humidifier or by keeping a tub or sink full of water.
   4. Use moisturizing or emollient creams that contain lanolin, petroleum jelly, or cocoa butter to retain skin moisture.

5. When providing foot care for a client, the nurse would perform which of the following?
   1. When washing, inspect the skin of the feet for breaks or red or swollen areas.
   2. Does not cover the feet and between the toes with creams or lotions to moisten the skin.
   3. Does not check the water temperature before immersing the feet.
   4. Wash the feet every other day, and dry them well, especially between the toes.

6. A nurse is evaluating a client's understanding of nail hygiene. Which of the following statements indicates a need for further teaching?
   1. "I should have clean, short nails with smooth edges."
   2. "I should have intact cuticles."
   3. "I will avoid trimming or digging into nails at the lateral corners."
   4. "I'll cut or file around the end of the fingernail or toenail."

7. A nurse is evaluating a client's understanding of dental care. Which of the following statements indicates a need for further teaching?
   1. Brush the teeth thoroughly after meals and at bedtime.
   2. Floss the teeth daily.
   3. Avoid sweet foods and drinks between meals.
   4. Have a checkup by a dentist every year.

8. A male client is having his facial hair shaved with a razor. Which action by the student nurse is NOT correct?
   1. The student nurse holds the skin taut, particularly around creases, to prevent cutting the skin.
   2. The student nurse wears gloves in case facial nicks occur and she comes in contact with blood.
   3. The student nurse applies shaving cream or soap and water to soften the bristles and make the skin more pliable.
   4. The student nurse holds the razor so that the blade is at a 90-degree angle to the skin, and shaves in short, firm strokes in the direction of hair growth.

9. Which of the following actions is NOT appropriate for the nurse bathing a person with dementia?
   1. Move quickly and let the person know when you are going to move him or her.
   2. Use a supportive, calm approach and praise the person often.
   3. Gather everything that you will need for the bath (e.g., towels, washcloths, clothes) before approaching the person.
   4. Help the person feel in control.

10. The nurse needs to insert a hearing aid into a client's ear. Which of the following actions is NOT correct?
    1. Determine from the client if the earmold is for the left or the right ear.
    2. Gently press the earmold into the ear while rotating it forward.
    3. Inspect the earmold to identify the ear canal portion.
    4. Check that the earmold fits snugly by asking the client if it feels secure and comfortable.

CHAPTER 34

DIAGNOSTIC TESTING

CHAPTER OUTLINE

KEY TOPIC REVIEW

1. Prior to radiologic studies it is important to ask female clients if pregnancy is possible.
   a. True   b. False

2. Blood tests are one of the most commonly used diagnostic tests and can provide valuable information about the hematologic system and many other body systems.
   a. True   b. False

3. High RBC counts are indicative of anemia.
   a. True   b. False

4. The leukocyte or white blood cell (WBC) count determines the number of circulating WBCs per cubic millimeter of whole blood.
   a. True   b. False

5. Serum electrolytes are often routinely ordered for any client admitted to a hospital as a screening test for electrolyte and acid–base imbalances.
   a. True   b. False

6. Sputum and _____ culture specimens help determine the presence of disease-producing organisms.

7. A liver _____ is a short procedure, generally performed at the client's bedside, in which a sample of liver tissue is aspirated.

8. During a lumbar puncture, the physician frequently takes CSF pressure readings using a _____, a glass or plastic tube calibrated in millimeters.

9. _____ is the withdrawal of fluid that has abnormally collected (e.g., pleural cavity, abdominal cavity) or to obtain a specimen (e.g., cerebral spinal fluid).

10. _____ tests are one of the most commonly used diagnostic tests.

11. Match the following terms with the correct definitions.
    a. Phlebotomist
    b. Complete blood count (CBC)
    c. Hemoglobin
    d. Hematocrit
    e. Red blood cell (RBC) count
    f. Creatinine
    g. Serum osmolality
    h. Reagent
    i. Urine osmolality
    j. Specific gravity

    _____ The _____, a person from a laboratory who performs venipuncture, collects the blood specimen for the tests ordered by the physician.

    _____ the number of RBCs per cubic millimeter of whole blood.

    _____ the main intracellular protein of erythrocytes.

    _____ produced in relatively constant quantities by the muscles and is excreted by the kidneys.

    _____ substance used in a chemical reaction to detect a specific substance.

    _____ is a measure of the solute concentration of urine and is a more exact measurement of urine concentration than specific gravity.

    _____ an indicator of urine concentration, or the amount of solutes (metabolic wastes and electrolytes) present in the urine.

    _____ is a measure of the solute concentration of the blood.

    _____ measures the percentage of red blood cells in the total blood volume.

    _____ includes hemoglobin and hematocrit measurements, erythrocyte (RBC) count, leukocyte (WBC) count, red blood cell (RBC) indices, and a differential white cell count.

12. _____ is the mucous secretion from the lungs, bronchi, and trachea.
    a. Saliva
    b. Spit
    c. Sputum
    d. Spool

13. Which of the following is the viewing of the rectum and sigmoid colon?
    a. Proctosigmoidoscopy
    b. Anoscopy
    c. Proctoscopy
    d. Colonoscopy

14. _____ is a noninvasive test that uses ultrasound to visualize structures of the heart and evaluate left ventricular function.
    a. Angiography
    b. Echocardiogram
    c. Electrocardiography
    d. Electrocardiogram

15. _____ is a painless, noninvasive x-ray procedure that has the unique capability of distinguishing minor differences in the density of tissues.
    a. Magnetic resonance imaging
    b. Positron emission tomography
    c. Aspiration
    d. Computed tomography

16. The _____, a person from a laboratory who performs venipuncture, collects the blood specimen for the tests ordered by the physician.
    a. Venipuncturist
    b. Erotologist
    c. Phlebotomist
    d. Physician

FOCUSED STUDY TIPS

1. Discuss some of the environments that diagnostic testing occurs in.

2. Give some examples of aspiration/biopsy tests.

3. Explain some of the reasons/tests that nurses collect urine specimens for.

4. Discuss the three phases of diagnostic testing.

5. What are some of the nursing responsibilities associated with specimen collection?

6. List several blood chemistry tests that may be performed on blood serum (the liquid portion of the blood).

7. Summarize the measurement of arterial blood gases as an important diagnostic procedure.

8. Discuss what occult blood is and how it is tested for.

9. Discuss some tests performed and the purpose for timed urine specimens.

10. List some examples of visualization procedures, including indirect visualization (noninvasive) and direct visualization (invasive) techniques for visualizing body organs and system functions.

11. Discuss how to collect a stool specimen correctly.

12. What is a clean-catch or midstream voided specimen?

13. Explain what may cause inaccurate test results.

14. List and describe several of the different urine tests.

15. List some examples of aspiration/biopsy tests.

CASE STUDY

A 73-year-old female was brought into the hospital by her son. The son tells you "My mother has lost weight and has been having night sweats. She is also spitting up blood." The physician orders the client to have three sputum samples for acid-fast bacillus.

1. *Why did the physician order sputum specimens?*
2. *How will you collect the sputum specimens?*
3. *What PPE should you wear when you collect the sputum specimens?*
4. *What information should you document in the client medical record after collecting the sputum specimens?*
5. *How should the specimens be stored until they are transported to the laboratory?*

NCLEX® REVIEW QUESTIONS

1. The nurse is assessing an admitted female client's serum laboratory values. Which of the following is abnormal and should be reported immediately?
   1. Hemoglobin 13 g/dL
   2. RBC 5.1 million/mm^3
   3. Hematocrit 25%
   4. MCV 102 μm^3

2. Which serum laboratory value is abnormal and would require you to report immediately?
   1. Sodium 137 mEq/L
   2. Potassium 2.5 mEq/L
   3. Chloride 97 mEq/L
   4. Magnesium 1.9 mEq/L

3. The nurse assessing a client's serum laboratory values recognizes that the normal hematocrit level for an adult male is:
   1. 37–49%.
   2. 13–18%.
   3. 13.8–18 g/dL.
   4. 37–49 g/dL.

4. Which technique is NOT correct when collecting a urine specimen for culture and sensitivity by clean catch?
   1. Explain to the client that a urine specimen is required, give the reason, and explain the method to be used to collect it.
   2. Perform hand hygiene and observe other appropriate infection control procedures.
   3. For all female clients a circular motion should be used to clean the urinary meatus.
   4. Ensure that the specimen label is attached to the specimen cup, not the lid, and that the laboratory requisition provides the correct information.

5. Which of the following is the correct position for a client during a bone marrow biopsy?
   1. Knee-chest
   2. Prone
   3. Lithotomy
   4. Dorsal recumbent

6. Which is the correct position for a client after a lumbar puncture?
   1. Knee-chest
   2. Prone
   3. Lithotomy
   4. Dorsal recumbent

7. After a client returns from a thoracentesis, the nurse should have the client lie on the unaffected side with the head of the bed elevated _____ degrees for at least 30 minutes.
   1. 10
   2. 15
   3. 30
   4. 90

8. Which of the following situations during an abdominal paracentesis is correct?
   1. 1,500 mL is the maximum of fluid was drained at one time.
   2. The fluid was drained at several time intervals.
   3. The fluid was drained quickly.
   4. Sterile technique is not necessary.

9. The nurse is providing patient education about a fecal occult blood test. Which of the following statements is correct?
   1. "Take the sample from the center of a formed stool to ensure a uniform sample."
   2. "Use a pencil to label the specimens with your name, address, age, and date of specimen."
   3. "Urine or toilet tissue will not contaminate the specimen."
   4. "You can collect the specimens during your menstrual period."

10. The nurse needs to obtain a throat culture from a child client. Which of following techniques is NOT correct?
    1. The nurse wears sterile gloves during the procedure.
    2. The nurse wears clean gloves during the procedure.
    3. The nurse inserts the swab into the oropharynx and runs the swab along the adenoids and areas on the larynx that are reddened or contain exudate.
    4. The nurse has the client say "ugh" to relax the throat muscles and to help minimize dilation of the constrictor muscle of the larynx.

CHAPTER 35

MEDICATIONS

CHAPTER OUTLINE

MediaLink

www.prenhall.com/berman

DVD-ROM
- Audio Glossary
- NCLEX® Review
- Skills Checklists

Videos and Animations:
- Agonist and Antagonist
- Cocaine
- Drug Metabolization
- Injections
- Medical Drugs
- Pharmacology and the Elderly
- Proper Use of a Metered Dose Inhaler (MDI)
- Salmeterol
- Small Volume Nebulizer Treatment (SVN)

Companion Website
- Additional NCLEX® Review
- Case Study: Preparing Medications
- Care Plan Activity: Client on Insulin
- Application Activity: Calculating Dosages
- Links to Resources

KEY TOPIC REVIEW

1. Drugs cannot have natural (e.g., plant, mineral, and animal) sources, or they must be synthesized in the laboratory.
   a. True
   b. False
2. Drugs vary in strength and activity.
   a. True
   b. False
3. Drugs must be pure and of uniform strength if drug dosages are to be predictable in their effect.
   a. True
   b. False
4. The action of a drug in the body can be described in terms of its half-life, the time interval required for the body's elimination processes to reduce the concentration of the drug in the body by 25%.
   a. True
   b. False
5. Parenteral administration is the most common, least expensive, and most convenient route for most clients.
   a. True
   b. False
6. Medications for the _____, called ophthalmic medications, are instilled in the form of liquids or ointments.
7. A major consideration in the administration of _____ injections is the selection of a safe site located away from large blood vessels, nerves, and bone.

8. A _____ is a small glass bottle with a sealed rubber cap.

9. A needle has three discernible parts: the hub, which fits onto the syringe; the cannula, or shaft, which is attached to the hub; and the _____, which is the slanted part at the tip of the needle.

10. Syringes have three parts: the tip, which connects with the needle; the barrel, or outside part, on which the scales are printed; and the _____, which fits inside the barrel.

11. Match the following terms with the correct definition.

a. Prescription
b. Medication
c. Generic name
d. Trade name
e. Pharmacology
f. Pharmacy
g. Pharmacopoeia
h. Therapeutic effect
i. Side effect
j. Drug toxicity

_____ The written direction for the preparation and administration of a drug.

_____ A drug's name given by the drug manufacturer.

_____ The study of the effect of drugs on living organisms.

_____ A book containing a list of products used in medicine, with descriptions of the product, chemical tests for determining identity and purity, and formulas and prescriptions.

_____ A secondary effect of a drug, one that is unintended.

_____ (deleterious effects of a drug on an organism or tissue) results from overdosage, ingestion of a drug intended for external use, and buildup of the drug in the blood because of impaired metabolism or excretion (cumulative effect).

_____ The _____ of a drug, also referred to as the desired effect, is the primary effect intended, that is, the reason the drug is prescribed.

_____ The art of preparing, compounding, and dispensing drugs.

_____ Given before a drug officially becomes an approved medication.

_____ A substance administered for the diagnosis, cure, treatment, or relief of a symptom or for prevention of disease.

12. _____ is the process by which a drug changes the body (e.g., alters cell physiology).

a. Receptor
b. Pharmacodynamics
c. Agonist
d. Antagonist

13. A _____ order indicates that the medication is to be given immediately and only once.

a. prn
b. Standing
c. Single
d. Stat

14. The study of the effect of drugs on living organisms is called:

a. pharmacopoeia.
b. pharmacist.
c. pharmacy.
d. pharmacology.

15. When two different drugs increase the action of one or another drug, this effect is termed:

a. synergistic.
b. drug tolerance.
c. drug interaction.
d. cumulative effect.

16. A(an) _____ syringe comes in 2-, 2.5-, 3-, and 5-mL sizes. This syringe may have two scales marked on it: the minim and the milliliter. The milliliter scale is the one normally used; the minim scale is used for very small dosages.
    a. Insulin
    b. Tuberculin
    c. Hypodermic
    d. None of the above

FOCUSED STUDY TIPS

1. Discuss the medication ordering process.

2. List three places hospitals correctly keep controlled substances.

3. Explain how to properly handle controlled substances wasted during preparation.

4. Discuss how the client's environment can affect the action of drugs.

5. Describe how the time of administration of oral medications affects the relative speed with which they act.

6. Identify and list three factors that indicate the size and length of the needle to be used.

7. Summarize the absorption process by which a drug passes into the bloodstream.

8. Discuss the correct process of administering medications.

9. Recall that the parenteral route is defined as other than through the alimentary or respiratory tract, that is, by needle. List three routes for parenteral administration.

10. Define and discuss the types of topical applications.

11. List and describe the essential parts of a drug order.

12. List and explain three types of medication orders.

13. Recall that insertion of medications into the rectum in the form of suppositories is a frequent practice. Rectal administration is a convenient and safe method of giving certain medications. Describe how to correctly insert a rectal suppository and describe its advantages.

14. List and describe the different kinds syringes used for irrigations.

15. Visit one the following websites and write a one-paragraph summary of what you learned:

    www.rxlist.com/drugs

    www.webmd.com/drugs/index-drugs.aspx

    www.rlhleagueofnurses.org.uk/Education/Nursing_Progress/Issue8/Medication/medication.html

CASE STUDY

The physician has ordered Compazine 10 mg IM every 4 hours prn for a 37-year-old male client who is awake and alert. The client tells you that he is not currently taking any other medications or natural supplements.

1. *What are the 10 "rights" of medication administration?*
2. *The Compazine is available in an ampule. How will you properly prepare the Compazine from the ampule?*
3. *Describe the process of administering Compazine by intramuscular injection.*

NCLEX® REVIEW QUESTIONS

1. The nurse is preparing a subcutaneous injection for a client. Which of the following statements is correct?
   1. A 45-degree angle is used when 1 inch of tissue can be grasped at the site.
   2. A 90-degree angle is used when 1 inch of tissue can be grasped at the site.
   3. Generally a 3-mL syringe is used for most subcutaneous injections.
   4. A #28-gauge, 1/2-inch needle is used for adults of normal weight.

2. The nurse knows and understands that a drug that produces the same type of response as the physiologic or endogenous substance is called a/an:
   1. agonist.
   2. antagonist.
   3. receptor.
   4. biotransformation.

3. A nurse is preparing a seminar on drug misuse. Which of the following terms describes a mild form of psychological dependence, where the individual develops the habit of taking the substance and feels better after taking it, and the individual tends to continue the habit even though it may be injurious to health?
   1. Drug dependence
   2. Drug habituation
   3. Physiologic dependence
   4. Psychologic dependence

4. A client weighs 110 lbs. What is the correct kilogram amount a nurse should calculate if he or she understands how to convert pounds to kilograms?
   1. 25 kg
   2. 50 kg
   3. 75 kg
   4. 100 kg

5. Erythromycin 500 mg is ordered. It is supplied in a liquid form containing 250 mg in 5 mL. How many mL would the nurse administer?
   1. 10
   2. 20
   3. 30
   4. 40

6. The nurse is preparing a Compazine injection to be given to a client. Which of the following statements is correct?
   1. When handling a syringe, the nurse may touch the outside of the barrel and the handle of the plunger.
   2. The nurse may touch the tip of the barrel with an unsterile object.
   3. The nurse may touch the shaft of the plunger with an unsterilized object.
   4. The nurse may touch the tip of the needle with an unsterilized object.

7. A client in the emergency department is to receive a rectal suppository. Which of the following nursing actions is NOT correct for administering a rectal suppository?
   1. The client can be placed in a Sims' position.
   2. The smooth, rounded end of the rectal suppository is lubricated.
   3. After inserting the rectal suppository, press the client's buttocks together for a few minutes.
   4. Have the client remain in the left lateral position for 1 minute to help retain the suppository.

8. The nurse is performing an ear irrigation. Which nursing action is correct?
   1. The nurse explained to the client that he may experience a feeling of fullness, warmth, and, occasionally, discomfort when the fluid comes in contact with the tympanic membrane.
   2. The nurse angles the ear canal prior to inserting the tip of the syringe into the auditory meatus.
   3. The nurse pushes the solution gently downward against the bottom of the canal.
   4. The nurse places a Q-tip in the auditory meatus to absorb the excess fluid after the procedure.

9. When evaluating a client's understanding of administering a vaginal foam, which of the following statements indicates a need for further teaching?
   1. "I will gently insert the applicator into the vagina about 5 cm (2 in.)."
   2. "I will remain lying in the supine position for 2 minutes following the insertion of the vaginal foam."
   3. "I will slowly push the plunger of the applicator until the applicator is empty."
   4. "I will discard the applicator if it is a disposable type."

10. A nurse is evaluating a nursing student's transdermal patch application to a comatose client. Which of the following actions demonstrates a need for further teaching? The student:
   1. selects a clean, dry area that is free of hair.
   2. removes the patch from its protective covering.
   3. holds the patch by touching the adhesive edges.
   4. applies the patch by pressing firmly with the palm of the hand for about 10 seconds.

CHAPTER 36

SKIN INTEGRITY AND WOUND CARE

CHAPTER OUTLINE

MediaLink

www.prenhall.com/berman

DVD-ROM
- Audio Glossary
- NCLEX® Review
- Skills Checklists

Animations
- Bone Healing
- Pressure Ulcers

Companion Website
- Additional NCLEX® Review
- Case Study: Clients with Chronic Illnesses
- Care Plan Activity: Client with Pressure Ulcer
- Application Activity: Enterostomal Therapist
- Links to Resources

E. Factors Affecting Wound Healing
   1. Developmental Considerations
   2. Nutrition
   3. Lifestyle
   4. Medications
V. Nursing Management
  A. Assessing
   1. Assessment of Skin Integrity
    a. Nursing History and Physical Assessment
   2. Assessment of Wounds
    a. Untreated Wounds
    b. Treated Wounds
    c. Pressure Ulcers
    d. Laboratory Data
  Skill 36-1 Obtaining a Wound Drainage Specimen for Culture
  B. Diagnosing
  C. Planning
   1. Planning for Home Care
  D. Implementing
   1. Supporting Wound Healing
    a. Moist Wound Healing
    b. Nutrition and Fluids
    c. Preventing Infection
    d. Positioning
   2. Preventing Pressure Ulcers
    a. Providing Nutrition
    b. Maintaining Skin Hygiene
    c. Avoiding Skin Trauma
    d. Providing Supportive Devices
   3. Treating Pressure Ulcers
    a. The RYB Color Code
   4. Dressing Wounds
    a. Types of Dressings
     i. Transparent Dressings

     ii. Hydrocolloid Dressings
     iii. Securing Dressings
   5. Cleaning Wounds
    a. Wound Irrigation and Packing
  Skill 36-2 Irrigating a Wound
   6. Supporting and Immobilizing Wounds
    a. Bandages
    b. Basic Turns for Roller Bandages
     i. Circular Turns
     ii. Spiral Turns
     iii. Spiral Reverse Turns
     iv. Recurrent Turns
     v. Figure-Eight Turns
    c. Binders
     i. Triangular Arm Sling
     ii. Straight Abdominal Binder
     iii. Securing Peritoneal Dressings
   7. Heat and Cold Applications
    a. Local Effects of Heat
    b. Local Effects of Cold
    c. Systemic Effects of Heat and Cold
    d. Thermal Tolerance
    e. Adaptation of Thermal Receptors
    f. Rebound Phenomenon
   8. Applying Heat and Cold
    a. Hot Water Bag
    b. Aquathermia Pad
    c. Hot and Cold Packs
    d. Electric Pads
    e. Ice Bags, Ice Gloves, and Ice Collars
    f. Compresses
    g. Soak
    h. Sitz Bath
    i. Cooling Sponge Bath
  E. Evaluating

KEY TOPIC REVIEW

1. The skin is the largest organ in the body and serves a variety of important functions in maintaining health and protecting the individual from injury.
  a. True
  b. False
2. Hypoproteinemia is an abnormally high protein content in the blood.
  a. True
  b. False
3. Wound beds that are too dry or disturbed too often fail to heal.
  a. True
  b. False
4. Because an inadequate intake of calories, protein, vitamins, and iron is believed to be a risk factor for pressure ulcer development, nutritional supplements should not be considered for nutritionally compromised clients.
  a. True
  b. False

5. Any at-risk client confined to bed, even when a special support mattress is used, should be repositioned at least every 2 hours, depending on the client's need, to allow another body surface to bear the weight.
   a. True
   b. False

6. The appearance of the skin and skin integrity are influenced by internal factors such as genetics, age, and the underlying _____ of the individual as well as external factors such as activity.

7. Moisture from incontinence promotes skin _____ (tissue softened by prolonged wetting or soaking) and makes the epidermis more easily eroded and susceptible to injury.

8. Wound _____ involves the removal of debris (i.e., foreign materials, excess slough, necrotic tissue, bacteria, and other microorganisms).

9. Using _____ syringes instead of bulb syringes to irrigate a wound reduces the risk of aspirating drainage and provides safe, effective pressure.

10. The _____ is the largest organ in the body and serves a variety of important functions in maintaining health and protecting the individual from injury.

11. Match the following terms with the correct definitions.
    a. Regeneration
    b. Hemostasis
    c. Exudate
    d. Bandage
    e. Ischemia
    f. Irrigation (lavage)
    g. Pressure ulcer
    h. Collagen
    i. Friction
    j. Immobility

    _____ is a force acting parallel to the skin surface.
    _____ refers to a reduction in the amount and control of movement a person has.
    _____ is renewal of tissues.
    _____ is the cessation of bleeding that results from vasoconstriction of the larger blood vessels in the affected area, retraction (drawing back) of injured blood vessels, the deposition of fibrin (connective tissue), and the formation of blood clots in the area.
    _____ a whitish protein substance that adds tensile strength to the wound.
    _____ a material, such as fluid and cells, that has escaped from blood vessels during the inflammatory process and is deposited in tissue or on tissue surfaces.
    _____ the washing or flushing out of an area.
    _____ a strip of cloth used to wrap some part of the body.
    _____ any lesion caused by unrelieved pressure (a compressing downward force on a body area) that results in damage to underlying tissue, as defined by the U.S. Public Health Service's Panel for the Prediction and Prevention of Pressure Ulcers in Adults.
    _____ is a deficiency in the blood supply to the tissue.

12. The _____ phase, the second phase in healing, extends from day 3 or 4 to about day 21 postinjury.
    a. Maturation
    b. Proliferative
    c. Inflammatory
    d. Remodeling

13. _____ is a process in which extra blood floods to the area to compensate for the preceding period of impeded blood flow.
    a. Vasodilation
    b. Friction
    c. Shearing force
    d. Immobility

14. If the wound does not close by epithelialization, the area becomes covered with dried plasma proteins and dead cells. This is called _____.
    a. keloid
    b. eschar
    c. exudate
    d. suppuration

15. The risk of hemorrhage is greatest during the first _____ hours after surgery.
    a. 48
    b. 72
    c. 96
    d. 120

16. _____ is the partial or total rupturing of a sutured wound.
    a. Evisceration
    b. Debridement
    c. Dehiscence
    d. Protein

FOCUSED STUDY TIPS

1. Describe the phases of healing.

2. List the four recognized stages of pressure ulcers related to observable tissue damage.

3. Discuss some of the chronic illnesses and their treatments and how they can affect skin integrity.

4. Discuss some of the factors contributing to the formation of pressure ulcers.

5. The aging process brings about several changes in the skin and its supporting structures, making the older person more prone to impaired skin integrity. Describe some of these changes.

6. List the three phases that wound healing can be broken down into.

7. Discuss the four different ways debridement may be achieved.

8. Compare and contrast the proper procedures for untreated wounds versus treated wounds.

9. List some of the purposes for which wound dressings would be applied.

10. Discuss gauze packing using the wet-to-moist technique.

11. Discuss some of the items that may cause hemorrhage from a wound.

12. Describe what the nurse notes when a pressure ulcer is present.

13. Discuss some of the different types of dressings.

14. List the type of heat and cold applications.

15. Discuss basic turns for roller bandages.

CASE STUDY

The client is a 17-year-old high school senior who sustained a left ankle injury during a soccer game 1 hour ago. The physician has ordered an ice pack to be applied to the injured area for 20 minutes.

1. *Explain the local effects of cold.*
2. *Explain the systemic effects of cold.*
3. *List some indications for applying ice to the injured ankle.*
4. *Summarize the guidelines a nurse should follow for all local cold applications.*

NCLEX® REVIEW QUESTIONS

1. The nurse is assessing a wound and notes that the exudate is purulent. What would you expect the exudate to look like?
   1. The exudate is thick with the presence of pus and is yellow in color.
   2. The exudate is clear and appears blood-tinged.
   3. The exudate is red to pink and watery.
   4. The exudate is bright red and bloody.

2. During discharge planning, the nurse is teaching a client how to apply an electric heat pad to his back. Which of the following statements is false?
   1. "I will not insert any sharp objects (e.g., pins) into the electric heating pad because the pin could damage a wire and cause an electric shock."
   2. "I will ensure that my back is dry unless there is a waterproof cover on the electric heating pad because electricity in the presence of water can cause a shock."
   3. "I do not need to use an electric heating pad with a preset heating switch."
   4. "I will not lie on top of the electric heating pad because the heat will not dissipate, and I may be burned."

3. Which of the following actions taken by a client self-administering a hot water bottle to his back indicates to the nurse the need for further teaching?
   1. The client fills the bag two-thirds full with water.
   2. After filling the bag with water the client dries the bag and holds it upside down to test it for leakage.
   3. The client expels the remaining air out of the bag before securing the top.
   4. The client fills the bag with water at a temperature of 135°F.

4. The nurse is assessing a student nurse's knowledge of bandages. Which of the following statements from the student nurse indicates a need for further teaching?
   1. "Bandages can be used to support a wound."
   2. "Bandages can be used to immobilize a wound."
   3. "Bandages can be used to apply pressure to a wound."
   4. "Bandages must be firm and tight."

5. A nurse is planning a seminar on dressing wounds. Which of following is NOT correct information about the purpose of dressing wounds? Dressings are applied to:
   1. potect the wound from mechanical injury.
   2. prevent hemorrhage.
   3. prevent thermal insulation.
   4. protect the wound from microbial contamination.

6. During a discharge teaching session with a client, which statement by the client indicates a need for further teaching?
   1. "Transparent dressings act as temporary skin."
   2. "Transparent dressings are nonporous, nonabsorbent, and self-adhesive."
   3. "Transparent dressings cannot be placed over a joint without disrupting mobility."
   4. "Transparent dressings adhere only to the skin area around the wound and not to the wound itself because they keep the wound moist."

7. The nurse is caring for a client who has a wound covered with thick necrotic tissue, or eschar, and it requires debridement. What color would this wound most likely be?
   1. Red
   2. Yellow
   3. Black
   4. Blue

8. Any at-risk client confined to bed, even when a special support mattress is used, should be repositioned at least every 2 hours, depending on the client's need, to allow another body surface to bear the weight. The nurse should NOT place the client in which position?
   1. Prone
   2. Knee-chest
   3. Supine
   4. Sims'

9. The nurse knows albumin is an important indicator of nutritional status. The nurse understands that a value below _____ g/dL indicates poor nutrition and may increase the risk of poor healing and infection.
   1. 3.4
   2. 3.6
   3. 3.8
   4. 3.9

10. The nurse is preparing to obtain a wound drainage specimen for culture from a client. Which of the following is part of the preparation?
    1. Check the progress notes to determine if the specimen is to be collected for an aerobic (growing only in the presence of oxygen) culture.
    2. Check the medical orders to determine if the specimen is to be collected for an anaerobic (growing only in the absence of oxygen) culture.
    3. Administer an analgesic 90 minutes before the procedure if the client is complaining of pain at the wound site.
    4. Administer an analgesic 5 minutes before the procedure if the client is complaining of pain at the wound site.

CHAPTER 37

PERIOPERATIVE NURSING

CHAPTER OUTLINE

MediaLink

www.prenhall.com/berman

DVD-ROM
- Audio Glossary
- NCLEX® Review
- Skills Checklist
- End of Unit Concept Map Activity

Video
- Preoperative and Postoperative Care

Companion Website
- Additional NCLEX® Review
- Case Study: Clients Having Surgical Procedures
- Care Plan Activity: Coronary Artery Bypass Procedure
- Application Activities:
  - Developing Operative Care Policies
  - Preadmission Testing
- Links to Resources

Skill 37-2 Applying Antiemboli Stockings
 m. Sequential Compression Devices
 E. Evaluating
IV. Intraoperative Phase
 A. Types of Anesthesia
V. Nursing Management
 A. Assessing
 B. Diagnosing
 C. Planning
 D. Implementing
  1. Surgical Skin Preparation
  2. Positioning
 E. Evaluating
 F. Documentation
VI. Postoperative Phase
 A. Immediate Postanesthetic Phase
 B. Preparing for Ongoing Care of the
  Postoperative Client
VII. Nursing Management
 A. Assessing
 B. Diagnosing
 C. Planning
  1. Planning for Home Care
 D. Implementing

1. Pain Management
2. Positioning
3. Deep-Breathing and Coughing Exercises
4. Leg Exercises
5. Moving and Ambulation
6. Hydration
7. Diet
8. Urinary Elimination
9. Suction
Skill 37-3 Managing Gastrointestinal Suction
10. Wound Care
 a. Surgical Dressings
 b. Wound Drains and Suction
Skill 37-4 Cleaning a Sutured Wound and
Applying a Sterile Dressing
11. Sutures
12. Home Care Teaching
 a. Maintaining Comfort
 b. Promoting Healing
 c. Restoring Wellness
 d. Community Agencies and Other
  Sources of Help
 e. Referrals
E. Evaluating

KEY TOPIC REVIEW

1. The intraoperative phase begins when the decision to have surgery is made and ends when the client is transferred to the operating table.
 a. True
 b. False
2. An embolus is a blood clot that has moved.
 a. True
 b. False
3. Adequate nutrition is not necessarily required for normal tissue repair.
 a. True
 b. False
4. Prior to any surgical procedure, informed consent is required from the client or legal guardian.
 a. True
 b. False
5. Surgery is least risky when the client's general health is good.
 a. True
 b. False
6. Pale, cyanotic, cool, and moist skin may be a sign of _____ problems.
7. A _____ is a thread used to sew body tissues together.
8. Conscious _____ refers to minimal depression of the level of consciousness in which the client retains the ability to maintain a patent airway and respond appropriately to commands.
9. Thrombus is a stationary _____ adhered to the wall of a vessel.
10. A _____-wound drainage system consists of a drain connected to either an electric suction or a portable drainage suction.

11. Match the following terms with the correct definition.
    a. Preoperative phase
    b. Intraoperative phase
    c. Postoperative phase
    d. Regional anesthesia
    e. Local anesthesia
    f. Tissue perfusion
    g. Intravenous block (Bier block)
    h. Epidural (peridural) anesthesia
    i. Nerve block
    j. Topical (surface) anesthesia

    _____ begins with the admission of the client to the postanesthesia area and ends when healing is complete.

    _____ a technique in which the anesthetic agent is injected into and around a nerve or small nerve group that supplies sensation to a small area of the body.

    _____ used most often for procedures involving the arm, wrist, and hand.

    _____ an injection of an anesthetic agent into the epidural space, the area inside the spinal column but outside the dura mater.

    _____ the passage of blood through the vessels.

    _____ begins when the decision to have surgery is made and ends when the client is transferred to the operating table.

    _____ (infiltration) is injected into a specific area and is used for minor surgical procedures such as suturing a small wound or performing a biopsy.

    _____ is applied directly to the skin and mucous membranes, open skin surfaces, wounds, and burns.

    _____ the temporary interruption of the transmission of nerve impulses to and from a specific area or region of the body.

    _____ begins when the client is transferred to the operating table and ends when the client is admitted to the postanesthesia care unit (PACU), also called the postanesthetic room or recovery room.

12. _____ anesthesia is the loss of all sensation and consciousness.
    a. Regional
    b. Local
    c. Topical
    d. General

13. Which of the following routine preoperative tests is given to evaluate fluid and electrolyte status?
    a. Complete blood count (CBC)
    b. Blood grouping and cross-matching
    c. Serum electrolytes
    d. Fasting blood glucose

14. Which of the following routine preoperative tests is given to evaluate liver function?
    a. Blood urea nitrogen (BUN) and creatinine
    b. ALT, AST, LDH, and bilirubin
    c. Serum albumin and total protein
    d. Urinalysis

15. Which of the following routine preoperative tests is given to evaluate respiratory status and heart size?
    a. Chest x-ray
    b. Electrocardiogram
    c. Pregnancy test
    d. Complete blood count (CBC)

16. The _____ phase begins with the admission of the client to the postanesthesia area and ends when healing is complete.
    a. Intraoperative
    b. Preoperative
    c. Postoperative
    d. None of the above

FOCUSED STUDY TIPS

1. Discuss some of the risks involved with surgery.

2. List some factors affecting the degree of risk involved in a surgical procedure.

3. Explain the three different types/classifications of anesthesia.

4. What is preoperative consent?

5. Describe how to properly give a physical assessment.

6. Identify three commonly used preoperative medications and their uses.

7. List some of the different types of antiemboli stockings and what they are used for.

8. Compare and contrast elective surgery and emergency surgery.

9. State the overall goal during the preoperative period.

10. Discuss the fluid and nutrition requirements before surgery.

11. Discuss elimination requirements before surgery.

12. Describe how to properly prepare for ongoing care of the postoperative client.

13. Discuss proper client hygiene before a surgery.

14. The Joint Commission on Accreditation of Healthcare Organizations (JCAHO) established, effective July 2004, the Universal Protocol for Preventing Wrong Site, Wrong Procedure, Wrong Person Surgery. List the three steps involved in this protocol.

15. Compare and contrast major surgery and minor surgery.

CASE STUDY

A 58-year-old client has been admitted for abdominal surgery. After you have taken his vital signs he asks, "What is the difference between a major surgery and a minor surgery?" He then states "I have a lot of hair on my belly. Will I have that hair shaved off before the surgery?"

1. *Define major surgery and minor surgery.*
2. *Give two examples of major surgery and two examples of minor surgery.*
3. *Why would you need to remove the hair on the client's abdomen before surgery?*

NCLEX® REVIEW QUESTIONS

1. Surgery is a unique experience of a planned physical alteration encompassing three phases. Which phase begins when the client is transferred to the operating table and ends when the client is admitted to the postanesthesia care unit (PACU)?
   1. Preoperative
   2. Intraoperative
   3. Postoperative
   4. Perioperative

2. The regular use of certain medications can increase surgical risk. Which of the following would NOT increase surgical risk as much as the others?
   1. Anticoagulants
   2. Tranquilizers
   3. Diuretics
   4. Antibiotics

3. Which of the following is NOT a correct action to reduce the risk of postoperative wound infection?
   1. Clean the surgical site only.
   2. Always remove hair from the surgical site.
   3. Document surgical skin preparation in the client's record.
   4. Only prepare the surgical site with an antimicrobial agent.

4. Which of the following actions is appropriate for the nurse removing skin sutures?
   1. The nurse puts on exam gloves.
   2. The nurse removes the skin sutures without an order.
   3. The nurse grasps the suture at the knot with a pair of clamps.
   4. The nurse cuts the suture as close to the skin as possible.

5. During discharge planning, the nurse is teaching the client how to maintain comfort, promote healing, and restore wellness. Which of the following actions is NOT correct?
   1. Instruct the client to use pain medications as ordered, not allowing pain to become severe before taking the prescribed dose.
   2. Teach the client to avoid using alcohol or other central nervous system depressants while taking narcotic analgesics.
   3. Instruct the client to report promptly to the primary care practitioner any decreased redness, swelling, pain, or discharge from the incision or drain sites.
   4. Emphasize the importance of adequate rest for healing and immune function.

6. The spouse of a client is preparing to apply a sterile dressing. Which of the following indicates a need for further teaching? The spouse:
   1. puts on sterile gloves.
   2. places the bulk of the dressing along the edges of the wound.
   3. secures the dressing with tape or ties.
   4. applies the sterile dressings one at a time over the drain and the incision.

7. A nurse is evaluating a client's understanding of performing deep-breathing exercises. Which of the following statements indicates a need for further teaching?
   1. "I will hold my breath for 6 to 8 seconds."
   2. "I will exhale slowly through the mouth."
   3. "I will always be in a sitting position."
   4. "I will inhale slowly and evenly through the nose until the greatest chest expansion is achieved."

8. When irrigating a gastrointestinal tube for a client, which of the following would NOT be appropriate? The nurse:
   1. attaches the syringe to the nasogastric tube.
   2. aspirates the solution harshly.
   3. draws up 90 mL of irrigating solution into the syringe.
   4. quickly injects the solution.

9. A nurse is evaluating a nursing student who is applying antiemboli stockings to a client. Which of the following actions demonstrates a need for further teaching?
   1. Assists the client to a sitting position in bed
   2. Reaches inside the stocking from the top and, grasping the heel, turns the upper portion of the stocking inside out so the foot portion is inside the stocking leg
   3. Has the client to point his or her toes, then positions the stocking on the client's foot
   4. Eases the stocking over the toes, taking care to place the toe and heel portions of the stocking appropriately

10. A nurse is planning a seminar on potential postoperative problems. Which of the following describes a condition in which alveoli collapse and are not ventilated?
    1. Thrombophlebitis
    2. Pulmonary embolism
    3. Pneumonia
    4. Atelectasis

CHAPTER 38

SENSORY PERCEPTION

CHAPTER OUTLINE

MediaLink

www.prenhall.com/berman

DVD-ROM
- Audio Glossary
- NCLEX® Review
- Skills Review
- Animation: Reflex Arc

Companion Website
- Additional NCLEX® Review
- Case Study: Clients with Altered Sensory Perception
- Care Plan Activity: The Confused and Agitated Client
- Application Activity: Client with Second-Degree Burns
- Links to Resources

KEY TOPIC REVIEW

1. Sensory reception is the process of receiving stimuli or data.
    a. True
    b. False
2. Visceral refers to the ability to perceive and understand an object through touch by its size, shape, and texture.
    a. True
    b. False
3. Glaucoma is a group of diseases of the eye caused by increased intraocular pressure that can lead to optic nerve damage and eventual vision loss.
    a. True
    b. False
4. Confusion can occur in clients of all ages, but it is most commonly seen in older people.
    a. True
    b. False
5. Sensory overload is generally thought of as a decrease in or lack of meaningful stimuli.
    a. True
    b. False
6. For an individual to be aware of the surroundings, four aspects of the sensory process must be present: a stimulus, a receptor, impulse conduction, and _____.
7. During times of increased _____, people may find their senses already overloaded and thus seek to decrease sensory stimulation.
8. An individual's _____ often determines the amount of stimulation that a person considers usual or "normal."
9. Gaining the _____ of a client with a hearing impairment is an essential first step toward effective communication.
10. Sensory _____ can prevent the brain from ignoring or responding to specific stimuli.
11. Match the following terms with the correct definitions.
    a. Sensory reception
    b. Gustatory
    c. Visceral
    d. Sensory perception
    e. Awareness
    f. Stereognosis
    g. Kinesthetic
    h. Olfactory
    i. Tactile
    j. Sensoristasis

    _____ smell.
    _____ the ability to perceive and understand an object through touch by its size, shape, and texture.
    _____ the ability to perceive environmental stimuli and body reactions and to respond appropriately through thought and action.
    _____ term used to describe when a person is in optimal arousal.
    _____ involves the conscious organization and translation of the data or stimuli into meaningful information.
    _____ refers to any large organ within the body.
    _____ awareness of the position and movement of body parts.
    _____ touch.
    _____ taste.
    _____ the process of receiving stimuli or data.

12. Approximately 40 to 45% of people over age 65 and more than _____ % over the age of 70 have a hearing impairment.
    a. 53
    b. 63
    c. 73
    d. 83
13. Which of the following states of awareness would be best described as extreme drowsiness but will respond to stimuli?
    a. Confused
    b. Somnolent
    c. Semicomatose
    d. Coma

14. All of the following would be correctly categorized as an affective change EXCEPT:
    a. hallucinations.
    b. rapid mood swings.
    c. depression.
    d. anxiety.
15. Which of the following states of awareness would be best described as: reduced awareness, easily bewildered; poor memory, misinterprets stimuli; impaired judgment?
    a. Full consciousness
    b. Disoriented
    c. Confused
    d. Somnolent
16. Age-related macular degeneration (ARMD) is the leading cause of vision impairment in adults _____ and older.
    a. 55
    b. 65
    c. 75
    d. 85

FOCUSED STUDY TIPS

1. Explain how the client's environment can affect the senses.

2. Discuss some of the techniques used to help prevent sensory deprivation.

3. Discuss sensory deprivation.

4. Describe some of the tasks nurses need to perform in a health care setting for clients with visual impairments.

5. Explain how physical assessment determines whether the senses are impaired.

6. Discuss the importance of communication, particularly with clients who have sensory deficits.

7. Explain some of the sensory aids that are available for clients who have visual and hearing deficits.

8. Discuss sensory overload.

9. Describe some of the techniques used to help prevent sensory overload.

10. Discuss some of the techniques used in promoting healthy sensory function.

11. List the four aspects of the sensory process that must be present for an individual to be aware of the surroundings.

12. Explain some of the techniques used when one sense is lost to promote the use of the other senses.

13. Discuss some considerations for clients with impaired tactile senses.

14. Discuss some considerations for clients with impaired olfactory senses.

15. Describe some of the tasks nurses need to perform in a health care setting for clients with hearing impairments.

CASE STUDY

An 87-year-old client was admitted to your floor yesterday. During report you are told that she has visual and hearing impairments.

1. *What actions should you take to help with her visual impairment?*
2. *What actions should you take to help with her hearing impairments?*
3. *How can environmental stimuli be adjusted for this client?*

NCLEX® REVIEW QUESTIONS

1. A nurse is evaluating a nursing student who is assisting a client who has a visual deficit. Which of the following actions demonstrates a need for further teaching? The student nurse:
   1. Announced her presence when entering the client's room and identified herself by name.
   2. Speaks in louder voice than necessary.
   3. Speaks in a warm and pleasant tone of voice.
   4. Always explains what she is about to do before touching the client.

2. A nurse planning a seminar on delirium and dementia plans to explain the characteristics differentiating the two. Which of the following describes an alertness that fluctuates—that is, the client may be alert and oriented during the day but becomes confused and disoriented at night?
   1. Dementia
   2. Delirium
   3. Hallucinations
   4. Delusions

3. During discharge planning, the nurse is teaching the client how to prevent sensory disturbances. Which of the following actions is correct?
   1. Wear protective eye goggles when using power tools, riding motorcycles, spraying chemicals, and so on.
   2. Wear ear protectors when working in an environment with low noise levels.
   3. When wearing sunglasses it's ok to look directly into the sun.
   4. Have health examinations every 5 to 10 years.

4. Which of the following actions is NOT appropriate for the nurse who is promoting a therapeutic environment for a client with acute confusion?
   1. "Good morning, Mr. Richards. I am Betty Brown. I will be your nurse today."
   2. "Today is December 5, and it is 8:00 in the morning."
   3. "Where are you?"
   4. "I'm going to turn on the radio while you read the newspaper, and I'll leave the window open for you."

5. The spouse of a client is preparing sensory aids for the visual and hearing deficits of her husband. Which of the following indicates a need for further teaching? The spouse:
   1. Gets a phone dialer with large numbers.
   2. Gets reading material with cursive print.
   3. Gets amplified telephones.
   4. Gets a magnifying glass.

6. The nurse is providing care to an unconscious client. Which of the following actions by the nurse is correct?
   1. Provides nose care
   2. Performs range-of-motion exercises
   3. Provides a lot of environmental stimuli
   4. Informs client of the care that is being provided

7. Stereognosis is:
   1. The process of receiving stimuli or data.
   2. The ability to perceive and understand an object through touch by its size, shape, and texture.
   3. The conscious organization and translation of the data or stimuli into meaningful information.
   4. The term used to describe when a person is in optimal arousal.

8. When planning interventions to prevent sensory deprivation, which of the following would NOT be included in the client's plan of care?
   1. Encourage the client to use eyeglasses and hearing aids only when interacting with someone.
   2. Address the client by name and touch the client while speaking if this is not culturally offensive.
   3. Provide a telephone, radio and/or TV, clock, and calendar.
   4. Encourage the use of self-stimulation techniques such as singing, humming, whistling, or reciting.

9. Which of the following questions by the nurse assesses the gustatory sensory reception?
   1. "When did you last visit an eye doctor?"
   2. "Do you experience any dizziness or vertigo?"
   3. "Have you experienced any changes in taste?"
   4. "Can you distinguish foods by their odors and tell when something is burning?"

10. The nurse is assessing for sensory function. Using a Snellen chart or other reading material such as a newspaper, and visual fields, assesses which of the following?
    1. Hearing acuity
    2. Visual acuity
    3. Olfactory senses
    4. Tactile senses

CHAPTER 39

SELF-CONCEPT

CHAPTER OUTLINE

MediaLink

www.prenhall.com/berman

DVD-ROM
- Audio Glossary
- NCLEX® Review

Companion Website
- Additional NCLEX® Review
- Case Study: Refusal to Accept a Medical Diagnosis
- Care Plan Activity: Client Who Lost His Job
- Application Activity: A Change in Attitude
- Links to Resources

KEY TOPIC REVIEW

1. Self-concept is one's mental image of oneself.
   a. True
   b. False
2. A patient's attitude to a newly acquired disability is rarely the determining factor in successful rehabilitation.
   a. True
   b. False
3. Individuals who grow up in families whose members value each other are likely to feel good about themselves.
   a. True
   b. False
4. The weavings that form the patterns in one's life are experiences, knowledge, and dreams.
   a. True
   b. False
5. Self-awareness refers to the relationship between one's perception of himself or herself and others' perceptions of him or her.
   a. True
   b. False
6. A _____ self-concept is essential to a person's physical and psychological well-being.
7. Self-esteem is derived from _____ and others.
8. _____ self-esteem is how much one approves of a certain part of oneself.
9. Nursing interventions to promote a positive self-concept include helping a client to identify areas of _____.
10. A person's self-perception can differ from the person's perception of how others see them and from the _____ self, that is, how the person would like to be.
11. Match the following terms with the correct definitions.
    a. Ideal self
    b. Body image
    c. Role mastery
    d. Role development
    e. Global self-esteem
    f. Role ambiguity
    g. Self-awareness
    h. Role performance
    i. Role
    j. Personal identity

    _____ occurs when expectations are unclear, and people do not know what to do or how to do it and are unable to predict the reactions of others to their behavior.
    _____ involves socialization into a particular role.
    _____ means that the person's behaviors meet social expectations.
    _____ relates what a person in a particular role does to the behaviors expected of that role.
    _____ a set of expectations about how the person occupying one position behaves.
    _____ the image of physical self—how a person perceives the size, appearance, and functioning of the body and its parts.
    _____ the conscious sense of individuality and uniqueness that is continually evolving throughout life.
    _____ how we should be or would prefer to be.
    _____ refers to the relationship between one's perception of himself or herself and others' perceptions of him or her.
    _____ how much one likes one's self as a whole.

12. Which of the following would NOT be considered a stress that affects self-concept?
    a. Loss of body parts
    b. Lack of positive feedback from significant others
    c. Abusive relationship
    d. Loss of financial security
13. Which of the following is NOT one of Erikson's stages of psychosocial development?
    a. Infancy: trust vs. mistrust
    b. Toddlerhood: autonomy vs. shame and doubt
    c. Early childhood: initiative vs. guilt
    d. Early adulthood: segregation vs. separation

14. _____ is one's judgment of one's own worth, that is, how that person's standards and performances compare to others and to one's ideal self.
    a. Self-esteem
    b. Self-knowledge
    c. Self-expectation
    d. Self-concept
15. All of the following would be considered an identity stressor EXCEPT:
    a. Change in physical appearance
    b. Inability to achieve goals
    c. Sexuality concerns
    d. Ambiguous or conflicting role expectations
16. Which one of the following is NOT one of the four dimensions of self-concept?
    a. Self-knowledge
    b. Social evaluation
    c. Self-expectation
    d. Self-evaluation

FOCUSED STUDY TIPS

1. List some strategies nurses can employ to reinforce strengths.

2. Discuss the stage of development as a factor that can affect self-concept.

3. Discuss the concept of body image, including how and when it develops.

4. List some of the guidelines for conducting a psychosocial assessment.

5. Discuss family and culture and how they can affect self-concept.

6. Define and discuss personal identity.

7. Discuss the formation of self-concept according to Erickson.

8. List three of the NANDA nursing diagnostic labels relating specifically to the domain of self-perception and the classes of self-concept, self-esteem, and body image.

9. Discuss stressors as a factor that can affect self-concept.

10. People are thought to base their self-concept on how they perceive and evaluate themselves in several areas. List some of these areas.

11. Discuss resources and how they can affect self-concept.

12. Discuss illness and how it can affect self-concept.

13. Give some examples of questions a nurse can ask to determine a client's self-esteem.

14. List some nursing techniques that may help clients analyze the problem and enhance the self-concept.

CASE STUDY

You are working in a psychiatric facility. One of the clients you are caring for is elderly. The client told you she has low self-esteem.

1. *What nursing techniques may help clients analyze the problem and enhance self-concept?*
2. *List five stressors that affect self-concept.*
3. *During your assessment, what questions should you ask the client?*

NCLEX® REVIEW QUESTIONS

1. When planning interventions to reinforce a client's strengths, which of the following would NOT be included in the client's plan of care?
   1. Stress self-negation rather than positive thinking.
   2. Notice and verbally reinforce client strengths.
   3. Provide honest, positive feedback.
   4. Encourage the setting of attainable goals.

2. The nurse is conducting a psychosocial assessment. Which of the following actions by the nurse is correct?
   1. Create a quiet, private environment.
   2. Do not limit interruptions.
   3. Sporadic eye contact.
   4. Sit above the eye level of the client.

3. A nurse is planning a seminar on conducting a psychosocial assessment. Which of the following guidelines is appropriate for conducting a psychosocial assessment?
   1. Indicate acceptance of the client by not criticizing, frowning, or demonstrating shock.
   2. Ask close-ended questions.
   3. Maximize the writing of detailed notes during the interview.
   4. Ask more personal questions than what are actually needed.

4. A nurse is evaluating a nursing student who is asking a client questions to determine the client's self-esteem. Which of the following statements demonstrates a need for further teaching?
   1. "Are you satisfied with your life?"
   2. "How do you feel about yourself?"
   3. "Are you accomplishing what you want?"
   4. "What are your responsibilities in the family?"

5. During discharge planning, the nurse is teaching the client how to enhance her son's self-esteem. Which of the following actions is correct?
   1. Give him opportunities to "practice" who he is.
   2. Do not allow him to explore and experiment with the world around him.
   3. Do not allow him to express himself as a unique individual.
   4. Encourage him to stay connected with all memories.

6. Which of the following questions is NOT appropriate for the nurse assessing body image?
    1. Is there any part of your body you would like to change?
    2. What are your relationships like with your other relatives?
    3. Are you comfortable discussing your surgery?
    4. How do you feel about your appearance?

7. Ideal self is:
    1. the collective beliefs and images one holds about oneself.
    2. how a person perceives the size, appearance, and functioning of the body and its parts.
    3. the individual's perception of how one should behave based on certain personal standards, aspirations, goals, and values.
    4. one's mental image of oneself.

8. According to Erikson's stages of psychosocial development, the middle adulthood stage is:
    1. identity vs. role confusion.
    2. intimacy vs. isolation.
    3. integrity vs. despair.
    4. generativity vs. stagnation.

9. When a client feels or is made to feel inadequate or unsuited to a role, he or she is experiencing which of the following?
    1. Role conflict
    2. Role strain
    3. Role ambiguity
    4. Role development

10. Which of the following is considered to be a stressor affecting self-concept?
    1. Change or loss of job or other significant role
    2. Financial security
    3. Stable relationship
    4. Realistic expectations

CHAPTER 40

SEXUALITY

CHAPTER OUTLINE

MediaLink

www.prenhall.com/berman

DVD-ROM
- Audio Glossary
- NCLEX® Review
- Animations:
  - Oogenesis and Spermatogenesis
  - Spermatogenesis
- Videos:
  - Gender Identity

Companion Website
- Additional NCLEX® Review
- Case Study: Client in a Motor Vehicle Crash
- Care Plan Activity: Client with a Mastectomy
- Application Activities:
  - Society for Human Sexuality
  - Campus Health Promotion
- Links to Resources

    D. Implementing
        1. Providing Sexual Health Teaching
           a. Sex Education
           b. Teaching Self-Examination
           c. Responsible Sexual Behavior
               i. STI Prevention
              ii. Preventing Unwanted Pregnancies
        2. Counseling for Altered Sexual Function
           a. Permission Giving
           b. Limited Information
           c. Specific Suggestions
           d. Intensive Therapy
        3. Dealing with Inappropriate Sexual Behavior
    E. Evaluating

KEY TOPIC REVIEW

1. The development of sexuality begins with conception and ends with puberty.
    a. True
    b. False
2. The ability of the human body to experience a sexual response is present before birth.
    a. True
    b. False
3. Although it is difficult to apply statistical data on large populations to local populations, it is generally accepted that sexual experimentation is currently occurring at ages older than in previous decades.
    a. True
    b. False
4. Sexually transmitted infections (STIs) are the most common bacterial infections among adolescents.
    a. True
    b. False
5. Older women remain capable of multiple orgasms and may, in fact, experience an increase in sexual desire after menopause.
    a. True
    b. False
6. Sexual health includes both freedoms and _____.
7. Current practice dictates the use of a _____ in both forms of intercourse to prevent the transmission of disease.
8. The sexual response cycle starts in the _____.
9. Sexual _____ refers to the physiologic responses and subjective sense of excitement experienced during sexual activity.
10. The term commonly applied in the past to women who did not experience orgasm, _____, implied that the woman was totally incapable of responding sexually.
11. Match the following terms with the correct definition.
    a. Sexual self-concept   _____ painful menstruation.
    b. Gender-role behavior   _____ how one values oneself as a sexual being.
    c. Masturbation   _____ one's self-image as a female or male.
    d. Sexual aversion disorder   _____ the outward expression of a person's sense of
    e. Orgasmic phase   maleness or femaleness as well as the expression of
    f. Resolution phase   what is perceived as gender-appropriate behavior.
    g. Dysmenorrhea   _____, or flexibility in gender roles, is the belief that most
    h. Sexual orientation   characteristics and behaviors are human qualities that
    i. Androgyny   should not be limited to one specific gender or the other.
    j. Gender identity   _____ one's attraction to people of the same sex, other sex, or both sexes.
                                       _____ the ongoing love affair that each of us has with ourselves throughout our lifetime.

_____ the involuntary climax of sexual tension, accompanied by physiologic and psychologic release.

_____ the period of return to the unaroused state; may last 10 to 15 minutes after orgasm, or longer if there is no orgasm.

_____ a severe distaste for sexual activity or the thought of sexual activity, which then leads to a phobic avoidance of sex.

12. _____ the involuntary spasm of the outer one-third of the vaginal muscles, making penetration of the vagina painful and sometimes impossible.
    a. Vestibulitis
    b. Vaginismus
    c. Vulvodynia
    d. Dyspareunia

13. Testicular cancer occurs in more than _____ American men each year.
    a. 2,000
    b. 4,000
    c. 6,000
    d. 8,000

14. _____ is oral stimulation of the penis by licking and sucking.
    a. Masturbation
    b. Fellatio
    c. Genital intercourse
    d. Intersex

15. Which of the following is NOT one of the five critical components of sexual health?
    a. Freedoms and responsibilities
    b. Gender role behavior
    c. Mental image
    d. Body image

16. The _____ defined sexual health in 1975 as "the integration of the somatic, emotional, intellectual, and social aspects of sexual being, in ways that are positively enriching and that enhance personality, communication, and love."
    a. NAFTA
    b. World Trade Organization
    c. OPEC
    d. World Health Organization

FOCUSED STUDY TIPS

1. Discuss how older adults (elders) may define sexuality.

2. List some of the common sexual messages children get from their families.

3. Discuss how family influences a person's sexuality.

4. Discuss the desire phase of the sexual response cycle.

5. What are some of the health factors that can interfere with people's expression of sexuality?

6. Discuss how culture influences a person's sexuality.

7. Identify the forms of male and female sexual dysfunction.

8. Discuss the orgasmic phase of the sexual response cycle.

9. What is rapid ejaculation?

10. Summarize how religion influences a person's sexuality.

11. Explain sexual pain disorders.

12. Describe physiologic changes in males and females during the sexual response cycle.

13. Discuss some of the problems with sexual satisfaction.

14. Discuss the resolution phase of the sexual response cycle.

15. Describe how to correctly perform a breast self-examination and explain its importance.

CASE STUDY

A 21-year-old man is in the clinic today to get an employment physical. The physician has asked you to provide the client with education about testicular cancer and STIs. After you are done providing this education, the client makes a sexual advance toward you.

1. *Explain how to provide client teaching for testicular self-examination.*
2. *Explain how to prevent the transmission of STIs and HIV.*
3. *Summarize the nursing strategies to deal with the client's inappropriate sexual behavior.*

NCLEX® REVIEW QUESTIONS

1. During discharge planning, the nurse is teaching the client how to prevent transmission of STIs and HIV. Which of the following actions is correct?
   1. Use condoms in monogamous relationships only.
   2. Follow safe sex practices only during intercourse.
   3. Report to a health care facility for examination only when there are signs of an STI.
   4. When an STI is diagnosed, notify all partners and encourage them to seek treatment.

2. A nurse is evaluating a client's understanding of performing breast self-examination. Which of the following statements indicates a need for further teaching?
   1. Use the finger pads (tips) of the three middle fingers (held together) on your left hand to feel for lumps.
   2. Press the breast tissue against the chest wall firmly enough to know how your breast feels. A ridge of firm tissue in the lower curve of each breast is abnormal.
   3. Use small circular motions systematically all the way around the breast as many times as necessary until the entire breast is covered.
   4. Look for any change in size or shape; lumps or thickenings; any rashes or other skin irritations; dimpled or puckered skin; any discharge or change in the nipples.

3. A nurse is evaluating a nursing student who is discussing nursing strategies for inappropriate sexual behavior from a client. Which of the following actions demonstrates a need for further teaching?
   1. "I will communicate that the behavior is not acceptable."
   2. "I will identify the client behaviors that are acceptable."
   3. "I will set firm limits with the client."
   4. "I will not report the incident to my nursing instructor, charge nurse, or clinical nurse specialist."

4. A nurse is planning a seminar on methods of contraception. Which of the following is NOT a correct method of contraception?
   1. Chemical barriers including vaginal diaphragm, cervical cap, and condom
   2. Abstinence
   3. Surgical sterilization: tubal ligation and vasectomy
   4. Intrauterine devices (IUDs)

5. The nurse is providing education to a client about effects of medications on sexual function. Which of the following statements by the nurse is correct?
   1. "Antipsychotics increase sexual desire."
   2. "Diuretics decrease vaginal lubrication."
   3. "Narcotics increase sexual desire and response."
   4. "Barbiturates in small amounts increase sexual desire."

6. The spouse of a client is verbalizing understanding of common conceptions of sex. Which of the following indicates a need for further teaching? The spouse states:
   1. "sexual ability is not lost due to age."
   2. "there is no evidence that sexual activity weakens a person."
   3. "chronic alcoholism is associated with erectile dysfunction."
   4. "alcohol is a sexual stimulant."

7. The orgasmic phase is:
   1. the response cycle that starts in the brain, with conscious sexual desires.
   2. the involuntary climax of sexual tension, accompanied by physiologic and psychologic release.
   3. the period of return to the unaroused state, may last 10 to 15 minutes after orgasm, or longer if there is no orgasm.
   4. an increase of tension in muscles; may increase until released by orgasm, or it may also simply fade away.

8. Body image is:
   1. a central part of the sense of self, and is constantly changing.
   2. one's self-image as a female or male.
   3. the outward expression of a person's sense of maleness or femaleness as well as the expression of what is perceived as gender-appropriate behavior.
   4. the belief that most characteristics and behaviors are human qualities that should not be limited to one specific gender or the other.

9. The nurse who is evaluating a sexual health class recognizes that further teaching is necessary when which of the following statements is made by a participant?
   1. "*Rapid ejaculation* is one of the most common sexual dysfunctions among men."
   2. "*Preorgasmic* women have experienced an orgasm."
   3. "Vulvodynia is constant, unremitting burning that is localized to the vulva with an acute onset."
   4. "Vestibulitis causes severe pain only on touch or attempted vaginal entry."

10. One technique nurses can use to help clients with altered sexual function is the _____ model.
    1. PLISSIT
    2. PLIISIT
    3. PLLISSIT
    4. PLISIT

SPIRITUALITY

CHAPTER OUTLINE

MediaLink

www.prenhall.com/berman

DVD-ROM
- Audio Glossary
- NCLEX® Review
- Video: Emotional, Social, and Spiritual Needs

Companion Website
- Additional NCLEX® Review
- Case Study: Supporting a Client's Spiritual Practices
- Care Plan Activity: Care of a Paralyzed Client
- Application Activities:
  - Researching Atheism
  - Spirituality, Health, and Holistic Nursing
- Links to Resources

KEY TOPIC REVIEW

1. Faith generally involves a belief in a relationship with some higher power, creative force, divine being, or infinite source of energy.
   a. True
   b. False

2. A holy day is a day set aside for special religious observance.
   a. True
   b. False

3. Prayer is human communication with divine and spiritual entities.
   a. True
   b. False

4. Meditation is the act of focusing one's thoughts or engaging in self-reflection or contemplation.
   a. True
   b. False

5. Transcendence is defined by Coward as the capacity to reach out beyond oneself, to extend oneself beyond personal concerns and to take on broader life perspectives, activities, and purposes.
   a. True
   b. False

6. Religious law may dictate how food is prepared; for example, many Jewish people require _____ food, which is food prepared according to Jewish law.

7. _____, which is defined as being present, being there, or just being with a client, is a term that identifies one of the competencies incorporated by expert nurses.

8. In the _____ phase, the nurse identifies interventions to help the client achieve the overall goal of maintaining or restoring spiritual well-being so that spiritual strength, serenity, and satisfaction are realized.

9. _____ symbols include jewelry, medals, amulets, icons, totems, or body ornamentation (e.g., tattoos) that carry religious or spiritual significance.

10. Clients facing imminent death may seek _____ from others as well as from God.

11. Match the following terms with the correct definitions.
    a. Spiritual distress
    b. Religion
    c. Atheist
    d. Polytheism
    e. Spirituality
    f. Faith
    g. Hope
    h. Monotheism
    i. Agnostic
    j. Spiritual health/well-being

    _____ to believe in or be committed to something or someone.
    _____ a concept that incorporates spirituality.
    _____ the belief in more than one god.
    _____ the belief in the existence of one God.
    _____ one without belief in a God.
    _____ a person who doubts the existence of God or a supreme being or believes the existence of God has not been proved.
    _____ an organized system of beliefs and practices.
    _____ a challenge to the spiritual well-being or to the belief system that provides strength, hope, and meaning to life.
    _____ is manifested by a feeling of being "generally alive, purposeful, and fulfilled."
    _____ refers to that part of being human that seeks meaningfulness through intra-, inter-, and transpersonal connection.

12. Which of the following is NOT one of the aspects of spirituality?
    a. Meaning
    b. Value
    c. Connection
    d. Religion

13. _____ will most likely not have insurance coverage and rely on the religious community for support.
    a. Amish, Mennonites
    b. Buddhists
    c. Christian Scientists
    d. Hindus

14. _____ avoid alcohol, caffeine, and smoking. They prefer to wear temple undergarments. Arrange for priestly blessing if requested.
    a. Jehovah's Witnesses
    b. Jews
    c. Latter-Day Saints/Mormons
    d. Muslims
15. According to Vardey, organized religions offer all of the following EXCEPT:
    a. a sense of community bound by common beliefs.
    b. a place of aversion.
    c. the collective study of scripture.
    d. the performance of ritual.
16. Spiritual _____ refers to a challenge to the spiritual well-being or to the belief system that provides strength, hope, and meaning to life.
    a. Duress
    b. Interest
    c. Guidance
    d. Distress

FOCUSED STUDY TIPS

1. Describe nursing interventions to support clients' spiritual beliefs and religious practices.

2. Identify the desired outcomes for evaluating the client's spiritual health.

3. List some of the factors associated with spiritual distress and the manifestations of that stress.

4. Discuss the influence of spiritual and religious beliefs about diet on health care.

5. What are some of the ways people nurture or enhance their spirituality?

6. Describe the spiritual development of the individual across the life span.

7. Discuss the influence of spiritual and religious beliefs about birth and death on health care.

8. Explain the concept of forgiveness.

9. Describe the influence of spiritual and religious beliefs about prayer and meditation on health care.

10. Discuss the concept of hope.

11. Describe the concept of spirituality.

12. List some of the characteristics of spiritual health.

13. Discuss the influence of spiritual and religious beliefs about dress on health care.

14. Briefly explain some of the varying religious beliefs related to birth.

15. One acronym that can help the nurse ask appropriate questions is FICA. What does the acronym FICA stand for?

CASE STUDY

A 37-year-old male client has been admitted to the hospital with terminal cancer. His condition is rapidly deteriorating. He has been living at home with his mother and father for the past 6 months. He is expressing fear and anger about his condition and states that he does not believe he will be alive much longer.

1. *The client asks you to pray with him. Explain the guidelines you should follow.*
2. *Summarize the practice guidelines you should follow to support the client's religious practices.*
3. *Give some examples of spiritual needs that would be related to others.*

NCLEX® REVIEW QUESTIONS

1. It is important for nurses to understand health-related information about specific religions. Which religion avoids unnecessary treatments on the Sabbath (Sabbath begins Friday sundown, ends Saturday sundown)?
   1. Buddhism
   2. Jehovah's Witness
   3. Latter-Day Saints (LDS or Mormon)
   4. Seventh-Day Adventist

2. Religion is:
   1. an organized system of beliefs and practices. It offers a way of spiritual expression that provides guidance for believers in responding to life's questions and challenges.
   2. a challenge to the spiritual well-being or to the belief system that provides strength, hope, and meaning to life.
   3. manifested by a feeling of being "generally alive, purposeful, and fulfilled."
   4. part of being human that seeks meaningfulness through intra-, inter-, and transpersonal connection.

3. A client tells you he is an atheist. You know this to mean:
   1. he is a person who doubts the existence of God or a supreme being or believes the existence of God has not been proved.
   2. he is a person without a belief in a God.
   3. he is a person who believes in the existence of one God.
   4. he is a person who believes in more than one god.

4. A client's religion may have rules about which foods and beverages are allowed and which are prohibited. Clients of which religion do not eat shellfish or pork?
   1. Buddhism
   2. Orthodox Jew
   3. Hindu
   4. Mormon

5. A nurse is evaluating a nursing student's understanding of presencing. Which of the following statements demonstrates a need for further teaching? A distinguishing feature of presencing is:
   1. "giving of self in the present moment."
   2. "being there in a way that is meaningful to yourself."
   3. "listening, with full awareness of the privilege of doing so."
   4. "being available with all of the self."

6. The nurse who is evaluating a supporting religious practices class recognizes that further teaching is necessary when which of the following statements is made by a participant?
   1. "Create a trusting relationship with the client so that any religious concerns or practices can be openly discussed and addressed."
   2. "If unsure of client religious needs, ask how nurses can assist in having these needs met."
   3. "Always discuss personal spiritual beliefs with a client."
   4. "Acquaint yourself with the religions, spiritual practices, and cultures of the area in which you are working."

7. A nurse is evaluating a nursing student who is just about to pray with a client. Which of the following actions demonstrates a need for further teaching? The student nurse tells the nurse:
   1. "clients' preferences for prayer reflect their personalities."
   2. "before praying, assess what clients would like for you to pray."
   3. "prayer may be the springboard to further discussion or catharsis."
   4. "prayers should never be personalized."

8. A nurse caring for a Muslim client recognizes that the client practices prayer _____ times a day and that the Muslim client may need assistance to maintain this commitment.
   1. Three
   2. Four
   3. Five
   4. Six

9. When a nurse is planning in relation to a client's spiritual needs, plans should NOT be designed to do which of the following?
   1. Help the client fulfill religious obligations
   2. Help the client draw on and use inner resources more effectively to meet the present situation
   3. Help the client find meaning in existence and the present situation
   4. Promote a sense of hopelessness

10. A nurse is planning a seminar on spiritual needs. Which of the following is NOT an example of spiritual needs related to the self?
    1. Need for meaning and purpose
    2. Need to express creativity
    3. Need for hope
    4. Need to cope with loss of loved ones

CHAPTER 42

STRESS AND COPING

CHAPTER OUTLINE

MediaLink

www.prenhall.com/berman

DVD-ROM
- Audio Glossary
- NCLEX® Review
- Animation: Reuptake

Companion Website
- Additional NCLEX® Review
- Case Study: Becoming Parents
- Care Plan Activity: Client Going Through a Divorce
- Application Activities:
  - Resources for Stress Management
  - School Nursing Care of Teenagers
- Links to Resources

KEY TOPIC REVIEW

1. A stressor is a condition in which the person experiences changes in the normal balanced state.
   a. True
   b. False
2. In stimulus-based stress models, stress is defined as a stimulus, a life event, or a set of circumstances that arouses physiologic and/or psychologic reactions that may increase the individual's vulnerability to illness.
   a. True
   b. False
3. Problem solving involves thinking through the threatening situation, using specific steps to arrive at a solution.
   a. True
   b. False
4. Structuring (discipline) is assuming a manner and facial expression that convey a sense of being in control or in charge.
   a. True
   b. False
5. Self-control is the arrangement or manipulation of a situation so that threatening events do not occur.
   a. True
   b. False
6. _____ is consciously and willfully putting a thought or feeling out of mind: "I won't deal with that today. I'll do it tomorrow."
7. _____, or daydreaming, is likened to make-believe.
8. _____ may be described as dealing with change—successfully or unsuccessfully.
9. Crisis _____ is a short-term helping process of assisting clients to work through a crisis to its resolution and restore their precrisis level of functioning.
10. A coping _____ (coping mechanism) is a natural or learned way of responding to a changing environment or specific problem or situation.
11. Match the following terms with the correct definition.
    a. Shock phase
    b. Stage of resistance
    c. Anger
    d. Stressor
    e. Ego defense mechanisms
    f. Depression
    g. Local adaptation syndrome
    h. Anxiety
    i. Countershock phase
    j. Fear

    _____ unconscious psychologic adaptive mechanisms or, according to Sigmund Freud (1946), mental mechanisms that develop as the personality attempts to defend itself, establish compromises among conflicting impulses, and calm inner tensions.

    _____ an extreme feeling of sadness, despair, dejection, lack of worth, or emptiness; affects millions of Americans a year.

    _____ an emotional state consisting of a subjective feeling of animosity or strong displeasure.

    _____ an emotion or feeling of apprehension aroused by impending or seeming danger, pain, or other perceived threat.

    _____ a state of mental uneasiness, apprehension, dread, or foreboding or a feeling of helplessness related to an impending or anticipated unidentified threat to self or significant relationships.

    _____ when the body's adaptation takes place.

    _____ the changes produced in the body during the shock phase are reversed.

    _____ the stressor may be perceived consciously or unconsciously by the person.

    _____ one organ or a part of the body reacts alone.

    _____ any event or stimulus that causes an individual to experience stress.

12. _____ focuses on solving immediate problems and involves individuals, groups, or families.
    a. Crisis intervention
    b. Caregiver burden
    c. Crisis counseling
    d. Burnout

13. All of the following are common psychologic indicators of stress EXCEPT:
    a. Anxiety
    b. Fear
    c. Anger
    d. Happiness

14. _____ is resorting to an earlier, more comfortable level of functioning that is characteristically less demanding and responsible.
    a. Reaction formation
    b. Projection
    c. Minimization
    d. Regression

15. _____ is displacement of energy associated with more primitive sexual or aggressive drives into socially acceptable activities.
    a. Sublimation
    b. Substitution
    c. Undoing
    d. Repression

16. Which of the following is NOT a cognitive indicator or thinking response to stress?
    a. Structuring
    b. Suppression
    c. Anxiety
    d. Problem solving

FOCUSED STUDY TIPS

1. Compare and contrast anxiety and fear.

2. List and define 10 defense mechanisms.

3. Explain burnout.

4. Summarize ways to mediate anger.

5. Recall the concepts and sources of stress.

6. Define general adaptation syndrome (GAS) and local adaptation syndrome (LAS).

7. Describe interventions to help clients minimize and manage stress.

8. Identify nursing diagnoses related to stress.

9. Identify essential aspects of assessing a client's stress and coping patterns.

10. Discuss types of coping and coping strategies.

11. Identify behaviors related to specific ego defense mechanisms.

12. Differentiate four levels of anxiety.

13. Identify physiologic, psychologic, and cognitive indicators of stress.

14. Describe the three stages of Selye's general adaptation syndrome.

15. Differentiate the concepts of stress as a stimulus, as a response, and as a transaction.

CASE STUDY

A 37-year-old client has an inability to relax, concentrate, and focus. She also complains of headache, dizziness, and nausea. The physician has asked for you to provide the client with information about anxiety.

1. *What level of anxiety is the client most likely experiencing?*
2. *Describe various methods you could teach the client to minimize stress and anxiety.*
3. *Explain the difference between anxiety and fear.*

NCLEX® REVIEW QUESTIONS

1. A client comes into the clinic with tremors and pitch changes in her voice. She also has facial twitches and shakiness. Her respiratory and heart rates are slightly elevated. At the end of her assessment she tells you "I feel like I have butterflies in my stomach." Which level of anxiety is this client experiencing?
   1. Mild
   2. Moderate
   3. Severe
   4. Panic

2. The spouse of a client is discussing the difference between anxiety and fear. Which of the following statements indicates a need for further teaching?
   1. "The source of anxiety is identifiable and the source of fear may not be identifiable."
   2. "Anxiety is related to the future, that is, to an anticipated event. Fear is related to the present."
   3. "Anxiety is vague, whereas fear is definite."
   4. "Anxiety is the result of psychologic or emotional conflict; fear is the result of a discrete physical or psychologic entity."

3. Which of the following is an appropriate strategy for dealing with a client's anger?
   1. Try to understand the meaning of the client's anger.
   2. Do not let clients talk about their anger until you are ready.
   3. After the interaction is completed, never process your feelings and your responses to the client with your colleagues.
   4. Listen to the client, and act just like the client.

4. Which of the following techniques prevents burnout for nurses?
   1. Avoid collegial support groups.
   2. Do not get involved in constructive change efforts.
   3. Learn to say no.
   4. Exercise when you can to direct energy inward.

5. At which developmental stage would a client experience marriage, leaving home, managing a home, getting started in an occupation, continuing one's education, and having children?
   1. Adolescent
   2. Young adult
   3. Middle adult
   4. Older adult

6. Which of the following is an example of the defense mechanism of displacement?
   1. A husband and wife are fighting, and the husband becomes so angry he hits a door instead of his wife.
   2. A woman, though told her father has metastatic cancer, continues to plan a family reunion 18 months in advance.
   3. A mother is told her child must repeat a grade in school, and she blames this on the teacher's poor instruction.
   4. A woman wants to marry a man exactly like her dead father and settles for someone who looks a little bit like him.

7. A nurse is taking care of an adult client when he throws a temper tantrum because he does not get his own way. Which defense mechanism is the adult client displaying?
   1. Repression
   2. Regression
   3. Reaction formation
   4. Rationalization

8. A nurse is planning a seminar on minimizing stress and anxiety. Which of the following statements is NOT correct?
   1. Provide an atmosphere of warmth and trust; convey a sense of caring and empathy.
   2. Listen attentively; try to understand the client's perspective on the situation.
   3. Control the environment to minimize additional stressors, such as by reducing noise, limiting the number of persons in the room, and providing care by the same nurse as much as possible.
   4. Communicate in long, detailed sentences.

9. During discharge planning, the nurse is teaching the client common characteristics of crises. Which of the following statements is NOT correct?
   1. The person is not aware of a warning signal and does not "see it coming."
   2. The crisis is often experienced as ultimately life threatening, whether this perception is realistic or not.
   3. Communication with significant others is often increased.
   4. There will not be a perceived or real displacement from familiar surroundings or loved ones.

10. A nurse is evaluating a nursing student's understanding of the clinical manifestations of stress. Which of the following statements by the nursing student demonstrates a need for further teaching?
    1. "Pupils constrict to decrease visual perception when serious threats to the body arise."
    2. "Sweat production (diaphoresis) increases to control elevated body heat due to increased metabolism."
    3. "Heart rate and cardiac output increase to transport nutrients and by-products of metabolism more efficiently."
    4. "Skin is pallid because of constriction of peripheral blood vessels, an effect of norepinephrine."

CHAPTER 43

LOSS, GRIEVING, AND DEATH

CHAPTER OUTLINE

MediaLink

www.prenhall.com/berman

DVD-ROM
- Audio Glossary
- NCLEX® Review
- End of Unit Concept Map Activity
- Video: Terminally Ill Patients

Companion Website
- Additional NCLEX® Review
- Case Study: Helping a Family Accept a Terminal Illness
- Care Plan Activity: Client with an Arm Amputation
- Application Activities:
  - Dealing with a Pet Loss
  - Care of a Grieving Parent
- Links to Resources

KEY TOPIC REVIEW

1. Everyone experiences loss, grieving, and death at some time.
   a. True
   b. False
2. Actual loss is experienced before the loss actually occurs.
   a. True
   b. False
3. Higher brain death occurs when the higher brain center, the cerebral cortex, is irreversibly destroyed.
   a. True
   b. False
4. In closed awareness, the client is not made aware of impending death.
   a. True
   b. False
5. With mutual pretense, the client, family, and health personnel know that the prognosis is terminal but do not talk about it and make an effort not to raise the subject.
   a. True
   b. False
6. Rigor _____ is the stiffening of the body that occurs about 2 to 4 hours after death.
7. _____ mortis is the gradual decrease of the body's temperature after death.
8. A _____ is a person trained in care of the dead.
9. A _____ is a large piece of plastic or cotton material used to enclose a body after death.
10. _____ occurs when the person perceives no solutions to a problem.
11. Match the following terms with the correct definition.
    a. Grief
    b. Bereavement
    c. Mourning
    d. Loss
    e. Open awareness
    f. End-of-life care
    g. Hospice
    h. Palliative care
    i. Anticipatory grief
    j. Perceived loss

    _____ an actual or potential situation in which something that is valued is changed or no longer available.

    _____ experienced by one person but cannot be verified by others.

    _____ the total response to the emotional experience related to loss.

    _____ the subjective response experienced by the surviving loved ones after the death of a person with whom they have shared a significant relationship.

    _____ the behavioral process through which grief is eventually resolved or altered; it is often influenced by culture, spiritual beliefs, and custom.

    _____ is experienced in advance of the event, such as the wife who grieves before her ailing husband dies.

    _____ the client and others know about the impending death and feel comfortable discussing it, even though it is difficult.

    _____ is care that focuses on support and care of the dying person and family, with the goal of facilitating a peaceful and dignified death.

    _____ is an approach that improves the quality of life of patients and their families facing the problems associated with life-threatening illness, through the prevention and relief of suffering by means of early identification and impeccable assessment and treatment of pain and other problems—physical, psychosocial, and spiritual.

    _____ the care provided in the final weeks before death.

12. Someone who conducts rituals of mourning (e.g., funeral) is said to be in which of the following of Engel's stages of grieving?
    a. Shock and disbelief
    b. Developing awareness
    c. Restitution
    d. Resolving the loss

13. More than _____ nurses in the United States are nationally certified in hospice and palliative care.
    a. 9,000
    b. 14,000
    c. 19,000
    d. 24,000

14. A(an)_____ is a large piece of plastic or cotton material used to enclose a body after death.
    a. Undertaker
    b. Hospice
    c. Mortician
    d. Shroud

15. Which of the following age groups has the following beliefs/attitudes about the concept of death?
    ■ Understands death as the inevitable end of life.
    ■ Begins to understand own mortality, expressed as interest in afterlife or as fear of death.
    a. Infancy to 5 years
    b. 5 to 9 years
    c. 9 to 12 years
    d. 12 to 18 years

16. Someone who is displaying the behavioral response of separation anxiety would be in which of the following of Sander's phases of bereavement?
    a. Shock
    b. Awareness of loss
    c. Conservation/withdrawal
    d. Healing: the turning point

FOCUSED STUDY TIPS

1. Discuss the dying person's bill of rights.

2. Describe the types and sources of losses.

3. Discuss selected frameworks for identifying stages of grieving.

4. Identify clinical symptoms of grief.

5. Discuss factors affecting a grief response.

6. Identify measures that facilitate the grieving process.

7. List clinical signs of impending and actual death.

8. Describe helping clients die with dignity.

9. Describe nursing measures for care of the body after death.

10. Describe the role of the nurse in working with families or caregivers of dying clients.

11. Define grief, bereavement, and mourning.

12. List the factors influencing the loss and grief responses.

13. Discuss various responses to dying and death.

14. Explain the steps in postmortem care.

15. Visit the Companion Website (www.prenhall.com/berman) and look at the Case Study about helping a family accept a terminal illness. Write a summary of what you learned from this Case Study.

CASE STUDY

You are visiting with a 22-year-old male client. During the assessment phase you discover he had to put his dog to sleep due to a terminal illness yesterday. The client raised this dog from a puppy and it was his first dog.

1. *Which type of loss is the client experiencing?*
2. *Explain grief, bereavement, and mourning.*
3. *List four appropriate questions to ask during the assessment.*

NCLEX® REVIEW QUESTIONS

1. Bereavement is:
    1. the total response to the emotional experience related to loss.
    2. the subjective response experienced by the surviving loved ones after the death of a person with whom they have shared a significant relationship.
    3. the behavioral process through which grief is eventually resolved or altered; it is often influenced by culture, spiritual beliefs, and custom.
    4. an actual or potential situation in which something that is valued is changed or no longer available.

2. A nurse's client just past away. The nurse understands that rigor mortis is the stiffening of the body that occurs about _____ hours after death.
    1. 2 to 4
    2. 5 to 7
    3. 8 to 10
    4. 11 to 13

3. A nurse is taking care of a client who just lost her husband to stomach cancer. The client is refusing to believe that loss is happening. Which of Kübler-Ross's stages of grieving is the client experiencing?
    1. Denial
    2. Anger
    3. Bargaining
    4. Depression

4. A nursing student has a client who just lost her brother to suicide. The client accepts the situation intellectually, but denies it emotionally. Which of Engel's stages of grieving is the client experiencing?
    1. Shock and disbelief
    2. Developing awareness
    3. Restitution
    4. Resolving the loss

5. Which of the following is a correct description of Sander's conservation/withdrawal phase of bereavement? During this phase:
    1. the bereaved move from distress about living without their loved one to learning to live more independently.
    2. the survivors feel a need to be alone to conserve and replenish both physical and emotional energy.
    3. friends and family resume normal activities. The bereaved experience the full significance of their loss.
    4. the survivors are left with feelings of confusion, unreality, and disbelief that the loss has occurred.

6. A nurse is evaluating a nursing student who is caring for a dying client's physiological needs. Which of the following actions demonstrates a need for further teaching?
    1. For a unconscious client with an airway clearance problem the nursing student places him in a Fowler's position.
    2. The client is diaphoretic the nursing student gives the client frequent baths and changes the linen.
    3. The nursing student regularly changes client's position.
    4. The nursing student provides the client with skin care in response to incontinence of urine or feces.

7. A nurse is planning a seminar on the dying person's bill of rights. Which of the following statements is NOT part of the dying person's bill of rights?
    1. I have the right to express my feelings and emotions about my approaching death in my own way.
    2. I have the right to expect continuing medical and nursing attention even though cure goals must be changed to comfort goals.
    3. I have the right to be free from pain.
    4. I have the right to die alone.

8. The nurse is providing care to an unconscious client who is dying. Which of the following is not a clinical manifestation of impending clinical death?
    1. Difficulty swallowing and gradual loss of the gag reflex
    2. Mottling and cyanosis of the extremities
    3. Rapid, shallow, irregular, or abnormally slow respirations
    4. Faster and weaker pulse

9. At what age does a client believe his or her own death can be avoided?
    1. Infancy to 5 years
    2. 5 to 9 years
    3. 9 to 12 years
    4. 12 to 18 years

10. Which of the following actions is NOT appropriate for the nurse providing postmortem care?
    1. One pillow is placed under the head and shoulders to prevent blood from discoloring the face by settling in it.
    2. The eyelids are closed and held in place for a few seconds so they remain closed.
    3. Dentures are always removed and placed with the client's personal belongings.
    4. All jewelry is removed, except a wedding band in some instances, which is taped to the finger.

CHAPTER 44

ACTIVITY AND EXERCISE

CHAPTER OUTLINE

I. Normal Movement
   A. Alignment and Posture
   B. Joint Mobility
   C. Balance
   D. Coordinated Movement
II. Exercise
   A. Types of Exercise
   B. Benefits of Exercise
      1. Musculoskeletal System
      2. Cardiovascular System
      3. Respiratory System
      4. Gastrointestinal System
      5. Metabolic/Endocrine System
      6. Urinary System
      7. Immune System
      8. Psychoneurologic System
      9. Cognitive Function
      10. Spiritual Health
III. Factors Affecting Body Alignment
    and Activity
    A. Growth and Development
    B. Nutrition
    C. Personal Values and Attitudes
    D. External Factors
    E. Prescribed Limitations
IV. Effects of Immobility
    A. Musculoskeletal System
    B. Cardiovascular System
    C. Respiratory System
    D. Metabolic System
    E. Urinary System
    F. Gastrointestinal System
    G. Integumentary System
    H. Psychoneurologic
       System

V. Nursing Management
   A. Assessing
      1. Nursing History
      2. Physical Examination
         a. Body Alignment
         b. Gait
         c. Appearance and Movement of Joints
         d. Capabilities and Limitations for Movement
         e. Muscle Mass and Strength

f. Activity Tolerance
g. Problems Related to Immobility
B. Diagnosing
C. Planning
1. Planning for Home Care
D. Implementing
1. Using Body Mechanics
a. Lifting
b. Pulling and Pushing
c. Pivoting
2. Preventing Back Injury
3. Positioning Clients
a. Fowler's Position
b. Orthopneic Position
c. Dorsal Recumbent Position
d. Prone Position
e. Lateral Position
f. Sims' Position
4. Moving and Turning Clients in Bed
Skill 44-1 Moving a Client Up in Bed
Skill 44-2 Turning a Client to the Lateral or
Prone Position in Bed
Skill 44-3 Logrolling a Client
Skill 44-4 Assisting the Client to Sit on the
Side of the Bed (Dangling)
5. Transferring Clients
Skill 44-5 Transferring Between Bed
and Chair

Skill 44-6 Transferring Between Bed and
Stretcher
6. Using a Hydraulic Lift
7. Providing ROM Exercises
8. Ambulating Clients
a. Preambulatory Exercises
b. Assisting Clients to Ambulate
Skill 44-7 Assisting the Client to
Ambulate
9. Using Mechanical Aids for Walking
a. Canes
b. Walkers
c. Crutches
i. Measuring Clients for Crutches
ii. Crutch Gaits
iii. Crutch Stance (Tripod Position)
iv. Four-Point Alternate Gait
v. Three-Point Gait
vi. Two-Point Alternate Gait
vii. Swing-To Gait
viii. Swing-Through Gait
ix. Getting into a Chair
x. Getting out of a Chair
xi. Going Up Stairs
xii. Going Down Stairs
E. Evaluating

KEY TOPIC REVIEW

1. An activity-exercise pattern refers to a person's routine of exercise, activity, leisure, and recreation.
    a. True
    b. False
2. A person maintains balance as long as the line of gravity (an imaginary horizontal line drawn through the body's center of gravity) passes through the center of gravity.
    a. True
    b. False
3. The base of support is the foundation on which the body rests.
    a. True
    b. False
4. The range of motion (ROM) of a joint is the maximum movement that is possible for that joint.
    a. True
    b. False
5. Proprioception is the term used to describe awareness of posture, movement, and changes in equilibrium and the knowledge of position, weight, and resistance of objects in relation to the body.
    a. True
    b. False
6. _____ is commonly seen in the arm muscles of a tennis player, the leg muscles of a skater, and the arm and hand muscles of a carpenter.
7. _____ is a condition in which the bones become brittle and fragile due to calcium depletion.
8. Unused muscles _____ (decrease in size), losing most of their strength and normal function.
9. When the muscle fibers are not able to shorten and lengthen, eventually a _____ (permanent shortening of the muscle) forms, limiting joint mobility.

10. Without movement, the collagen (connective) tissues at the joint become _____ (permanently immobile).

11. Match the following terms with the correct definition.

    a. Physical activity
    b. Exercise
    c. Isotonic (dynamic) exercises
    d. Aerobic exercise
    e. Mobility
    f. Anaerobic exercise
    g. Isokinetic (resistive) exercises
    h. Osteoporosis
    i. Ventilation
    j. Isometric (static or setting) exercises

    _____ the ability to move freely, easily, rhythmically, and purposefully in the environment; is an essential part of living.

    _____ bodily movement produced by skeletal muscle contraction that increases energy expenditure.

    _____ a type of physical activity defined as a planned, structured, and repetitive bodily movement performed to improve or maintain one or more components of physical fitness.

    _____ are those in which the muscle shortens to produce muscle contraction and active movement.

    _____ are those in which there is muscle contraction without moving the joint (muscle length does not change).

    _____ involve muscle contraction or tension against resistance; thus, they can be either isotonic or isometric.

    _____ activity during which the amount of oxygen taken in the body is greater than that used to perform the activity.

    _____ involves activity in which the muscles cannot draw out enough oxygen from the bloodstream, and anaerobic pathways are used to provide additional energy for a short time.

    _____ air circulating into and out of the lungs.

    _____ a condition in which the bones become brittle and fragile due to calcium depletion.

12. The Diabetes Prevention Program, a large 3-year study, showed that even a modest 5% decrease in body weight (about 10 pounds in most participants) achieved through exercise and dietary modification reduced the risk of diabetes by _____%.

    a. 28
    b. 38
    c. 48
    d. 58

13. Which of the following means having too much muscle tone?

    a. Meningitis
    b. Paresis
    c. Flaccid
    d. Spastic

14. _____ refers to holding the breath and straining against a closed glottis.

    a. Valsalva maneuver
    b. Orthostatic hypotension
    c. Stasis
    d. Venous vasodilation

15. Which of the following is NOT one of the three factors that collectively predispose a client to the formation of a thrombophlebitis (a clot that is loosely attached to an inflamed vein wall)?

    a. Increased oil in the diet
    b. Impaired venous return to the heart
    c. Hypercoagulability of the blood
    d. Injury to a vessel wall

16. _____ refers to the sum of all the physical and chemical processes by which living substance is formed and maintained and by which energy is made available for use by the body.
    a. Metabolism
    b. Catabolism
    c. Anabolism
    d. Anorexia

FOCUSED STUDY TIPS

1. Discuss how the U.S. Department of Health and Human Services defines exercise and physical activity.

2. Describe the effects of exercise on cognitive function.

3. List some of the factors that affect an individual's body alignment, mobility, and daily activity level.

4. Define and discuss the term *body mechanics*.

5. Describe the three different ways the intensity of exercise can be measured.

6. Discuss the importance of the musculoskeletal system.

7. Describe how to use safe practices when positioning, moving, lifting, and ambulating clients.

8. Describe a variety of movement interventions and therapies to improve physical health, mobility, strength, balance, mood, and cognition.

9. Develop nursing diagnoses and outcomes related to activity, exercise, and mobility problems.

10. Discuss the activity-exercise pattern, alignment, mobility capabilities and limitations, activity tolerance, and potential problems related to immobility.

11. Identify factors influencing a person's body alignment and activity.

12. Compare the effects of exercise and immobility on body systems.

13. Differentiate isotonic, isometric, isokinetic, aerobic, and anaerobic exercise.

14. Describe four basic elements of normal movement.

15. List some of the factors that increase the potential for lower back injuries.

CASE STUDY

A 43-year-old male client who has two children is recovering from a back injury and is receiving care from a home health nurse. A major aspect of discharge planning involves instructional needs of the client and family.

1. *Provide the client and his family education about the following topics:*
   - *Maintaining musculoskeletal function*
   - *Preventing injury*
   - *Managing energy to prevent fatigue*
   - *Preventing back injuries*

NCLEX® REVIEW QUESTIONS

1. A nurse is planning a seminar on preventing back injuries. Which of the following statements is correct?
   1. When sitting for a period of time, periodically move legs and hips, and flex one hip and knee and rest your foot on an object if possible.
   2. When sitting, keep your knees slightly lower than your hips.
   3. Use a hard mattress and firm pillow that provide good body support at natural body curvatures.
   4. Exercise regularly to maintain overall physical condition and regulate weight; include exercises that strengthen the pelvic, abdominal, and spinal muscles.

2. During discharge planning, the nurse is evaluating the client's understanding of wheelchair safety. Which of the following statements indicates a need for further teaching?
   1. Always lock the brakes on both wheels of the wheelchair when the client transfers in or out of it.
   2. Lower the footplates before transferring the client into the wheelchair.
   3. Lower the footplates after the transfer, and place the client's feet on them.
   4. Ensure the client is positioned well back in the seat of the wheelchair.

3. A nurse is evaluating a nursing student's understanding of stretcher safety. Which of the following statements demonstrates a need for further teaching?
   1. Never leave a client unattended on a stretcher unless the wheels are locked and the side rails are raised on both sides and/or the safety straps are securely fastened across the client.
   2. Always push a stretcher from the end where the client's head is positioned. This position protects the client's head in the event of a collision.
   3. Maneuver the stretcher when entering the elevator so that the client's feet go in first.
   4. Fasten safety straps across the client on a stretcher, and raise the side rails.

4. Which of the following actions is appropriate for the nurse performing active ROM exercises?
   1. Perform each ROM exercise as taught to the point of slight resistance, but not beyond, and never to the point of discomfort.
   2. Perform the movements systematically, using a different sequence during each session.
   3. Perform each exercise five times.
   4. Perform each series of exercises three times daily.

5. During discharge planning, the nurse is teaching the client how to control postural hypotension. Which of the following statements is correct?
   1. Bend down all the way to the floor and stand up quickly after stooping.
   2. Wear elastic stockings day and night to inhibit venous pooling in the legs.
   3. Use a rocking chair to improve circulation in the lower extremities.
   4. Get out of a hot bath very quickly, because high temperatures can lead to venous pooling.

6. Isotonic (dynamic) exercises:
    1. are those in which there is muscle contraction without moving the joint (muscle length does not change).
    2. involve muscle contraction or tension against resistance; thus, they can be either isotonic or isometric.
    3. are activities during which the amount of oxygen taken in the body is greater than that used to perform the activity.
    4. are those in which the muscle shortens to produce muscle contraction and active movement.

7. A nurse is evaluating a nursing student's understanding of positioning clients. Which of the following statements indicates a need for further teaching?
    1. Positioning a client in good body alignment and changing the position regularly (every 3 hours) and systematically are essential aspects of nursing practice.
    2. Any position, correct or incorrect, can be detrimental if maintained for a prolonged period.
    3. For all clients, it is important to assess the skin and provide skin care before and after a position change.
    4. Frequent change of position helps to prevent muscle discomfort, undue pressure resulting in pressure ulcers, damage to superficial nerves and blood vessels, and contractures.

8. Fowler's position is a bed position:
    1. in which the head and trunk are raised 45 to 90 degrees.
    2. in which the client's head and shoulders are slightly elevated on a small pillow.
    3. in which the client lies on the abdomen with the head turned to one side.
    4. in which the person lies on one side of the body. Flexing the top hip and knee and placing this leg in front of the body creates a wider, triangular base of support and achieves greater stability.

9. General guidelines for transfer techniques include all of the following EXCEPT:
    1. obtain essential equipment before starting (e.g., transfer belt, wheelchair), and check its function.
    2. always support or hold equipment rather than the client to ensure safety and dignity.
    3. remove obstacles from the area used for the transfer.
    4. explain the transfer to the nursing personnel who are helping; specify who will give directions (one person needs to be in charge).

10. Which of the following actions is appropriate for the nurse assisting a client with crutches?
    1. The client lies in a prone position and the nurse measures from the anterior fold of the axilla to the heel of the foot and adds 2.5 cm (1 in.).
    2. The client stands erect and positions the crutch. The nurse makes sure the shoulder rest of the crutch is at least three finger widths, that is, 2.5 to 5 cm (1 to 2 in.), below the axilla.
    3. The client stands upright and supports the body weight by the axilla.
    4. The nurse measures the angle of elbow flexion. It should be about 10 degrees.

CHAPTER 45

SLEEP

CHAPTER OUTLINE

MediaLink

www.prenhall.com/berman

DVD-ROM
- Audio Glossary
- NCLEX® Review
- Video: Sleep and the Elderly

Companion Website
- Additional NCLEX® Review
- Case Study: Client with Difficulty Falling Asleep
- Care Plan Activity: Client with a Sleep Disorder
- Application Activity: Diagnosing Sleep Apnea
- Links to Resources

KEY TOPIC REVIEW

1. Somnology is the study of sleep.
   a. True
   b. False
2. Stage I is the deepest stage of sleep.
   a. True
   b. False
3. Most dreams take place during REM sleep, but usually will not be remembered unless the person arouses briefly at the end of the REM period.
   a. True
   b. False
4. Sleep apnea is characterized by frequent short breathing pauses during sleep.
   a. True
   b. False
5. Sleep hypnotics is a term referring to interventions used to promote sleep.
   a. True
   b. False
6. _____ has come to be considered an altered state of consciousness in which the individual's perception of and reaction to the environment are decreased.
7. Biological _____ exist in plants, animals, and humans.
8. During adolescence, boys begin to experience nocturnal emissions (orgasm and emission of semen during sleep), known as "_____," several times each month.
9. _____ is described as the inability to fall asleep, remain asleep, or awaken feeling rested.
10. _____ is a disorder of excessive daytime sleepiness caused by the lack of the chemical hypocretin in the area of the central nervous system that regulates sleep.
11. Match the following terms with the correct definition.
    a. Sundown syndrome
    b. Insomnia
    c. Cognitive therapy
    d. Sleep quality
    e. Narcolepsy
    f. Hypersomnia
    g. Quantity of sleep
    h. Stimulus control
    i. Sleep architecture
    j. Somnology

    _____ the study of sleep

    _____ refers to the basic organization of normal sleep.

    _____ a pattern of symptoms (e.g., agitation, anxious, aggressive, and sometimes delusional) that occur in the late afternoon.

    _____ is a subjective characteristic and is often determined by whether or not a person wakes up feeling energetic or not.

    _____ is the total time the individual sleeps.

    _____ is the most common sleep complaint in America.

    _____ learning to develop positive thoughts and beliefs about sleep.

    _____ creating a sleep environment that promotes sleep.

    _____ refers to conditions where the affected individual obtains sufficient sleep at night but still cannot stay awake during the day.

    _____ a disorder of excessive daytime sleepiness caused by the lack of the chemical hypocretin in the area of the central nervous system that regulates sleep.

12. Newborns sleep _____ hours a day, on an irregular schedule with periods of 1 to 3 hours spent awake.
    a. 10 to 12
    b. 12 to 14
    c. 14 to 16
    d. 16 to 18

13. Most healthy adults need _____ hours of sleep a night.
    a. 7 to 9
    b. 9 to 11
    c. 11 to 13
    d. 13 to 15
14. Stress is considered by most sleep experts to be the number _____ cause of short-term sleeping difficulties.
    a. one
    b. two
    c. three
    d. four
15. Which of the following medications has the largest half-life (i.e., 47–100 hours)?
    a. Chloral hydrate (Noctec)
    b. Flurazepam (Dalmane)
    c. Lorazepam (Ativan)
    d. Zolpidem (Ambien)
16. Approximately _____ million Americans have a chronic disorder of sleep and wakefulness that hinders daily functioning and adversely affects health.
    a. 10 to 30
    b. 30 to 50
    c. 50 to 70
    d. 70 to 90

FOCUSED STUDY TIPS

1. Identify factors that affect normal sleep.

2. Describe variations in sleep patterns throughout the life span.

3. Identify the characteristics of the sleep states of NREM and REM sleep.

4. Explain the functions and the physiology of sleep.

5. Discuss the following three types of sleep apnea: obstructive apnea, central apnea, and mixed apnea.

6. Identify items included in and the purpose of a sleep diary.

7. Summarize the major goal for clients with sleep disturbances.

8. Discuss the importance of bedtime rituals.

9. List several of the factors that can affect sleep.

10. Discuss several techniques for reducing environmental distractions in hospitals.

11. Discuss three nursing responsibilities to help clients sleep.

12. List seven drugs that may disrupt REM sleep, delay onset of sleep, or decrease sleep time.

13. Describe common sleep disorders.

14. Identify the components of a sleep pattern assessment.

15. Describe interventions that promote normal sleep.

CASE STUDY

A 21-year-old client came into the clinic today complaining of difficulty sleeping. The client is a part-time college student and he also works 40 to 50 hours per week at an automotive body shop. He is not taking any prescription medications and has an occasional alcoholic beverage at special events.

1. *Explain the two types of sleep.*
2. *Describe factors that affect sleep.*
3. *Explain the information that should be included in a sleep diary.*

NCLEX® REVIEW QUESTIONS

1. During discharge planning, the nurse is teaching the client how to maintain a sleep diary. Which of the following statements is correct?
   1. Document the activities you perform 5 to 6 hours before going to bed.
   2. Document the consumption of caffeinated beverages and alcohol and amounts of those beverages.
   3. Do not list the bedtime rituals before bed.
   4. List only the prescribed medications taken during the day.

2. A nurse is evaluating a client's understanding of comfort measures that are essential to help fall asleep and stay asleep. Which of the following statements indicates a need for further teaching?
   1. "I should wear loose-fitting nightwear."
   2. "I will void before bedtime."
   3. "I will perform hygienic routines prior to bedtime."
   4. "When I'm in pain, I will take the prescribed analgesics 3 hour before I go to sleep."

3. A nurse is evaluating a nursing student's understanding of medications. Which of the following statements indicates a need for further teaching?
   1. "Antianxiety medications decrease levels of arousal by facilitating the action of neurons in the CNS that suppress responsiveness to stimulation."
   2. "Sleep medications vary in their onset and duration of action and will impair waking function as long as they are chemically active."
   3. "Sleep medications affect NREM sleep more than REM sleep."
   4. "Initial doses of medications should be low and increases added gradually, depending on the client's response."

4. Hypersomnia is:
   1. a condition where the affected individual obtains sufficient sleep at night but still cannot stay awake during the day.
   2. a disorder of excessive daytime sleepiness caused by the lack of the chemical hypocretin in the area of the central nervous system that regulates sleep.
   3. characterized by frequent short breathing pauses during sleep.
   4. a behavior that may interfere with sleep and/or occurs during sleep.

5. NREM (slow-wave) sleep consists of four stages. Which stage of sleep lasts only about 10 to 15 minutes, the eyes are generally still, the heart and respiratory rates decrease slightly, and body temperature falls?
   1. Stage I
   2. Stage II
   3. Stage III
   4. Stage IV

6. A nurse is evaluating a nursing student who is discussing physiologic changes during NREM sleep. Which of the following actions demonstrates a need for further teaching?
   1. Arterial blood pressure falls.
   2. Pulse rate decreases.
   3. Peripheral blood vessels constrict.
   4. Cardiac output decreases.

7. When planning interventions to reduce environmental distractions in hospitals, which of the following would NOT be included in the client's plan of care?
   1. Lower the ring tone of nearby telephones.
   2. Discontinue use of the paging system after a certain hour or reduce its volume.
   3. Keep required staff conversations at low levels; conduct nursing reports or other discussions in a separate area away from client rooms.
   4. Perform noisy activities only during the day, never during sleeping hours.

8. A nurse is planning a seminar on promoting sleep. Which of the following is correct information?
   1. Establish a regular bedtime and wake-up time for all days of the week to enhance biological rhythm.
   2. Deal with office work or family problems before bedtime.
   3. Get adequate exercise during the day to reduce stress, but avoid excessive physical exertion 1 hour before bedtime.
   4. Establish a regular, relaxing bedtime routine before sleep such as reading, listening to soft music, or taking a cool shower.

9. When planning interventions to promote sleep, which of the following would be included in the client's plan of care?
   1. Create a sleep-conducive environment that is dark, quiet, comfortable, and cool.
   2. Give analgesics 3 hours before bedtime to relieve aches and pains.
   3. If a bedtime snack is necessary, give only high-carbohydrate snacks or a milk drink.
   4. Avoid giving the client heavy meals 4 to 5 hours before bedtime.

10. A nurse is evaluating a client's understanding of her child's night terrors. Which of the following statements indicates a need for further teaching?
    1. Night terrors are usually seen in children 3 to 6 years of age.
    2. Children usually cannot be wakened during night terrors, but should be protected from injury, helped back to bed, and soothed back to sleep.
    3. Children do not remember the night terror the next day, and there is no indication of a neurological or emotional problem.
    4. Night terrors are partial awakenings from non-REM, stage I or II sleep.

CHAPTER 46

PAIN MANAGEMENT

CHAPTER OUTLINE

MediaLink

www.prenhall.com/berman

DVD-ROM
- Audio Glossary
- NCLEX® Review
- Skill Checklist
- Video: Pain Management
- Animations:
  - Morphine
  - Naproxen

Companion Website
- Additional NCLEX® Review
- Case Study: Client with Stomach Cancer
- Care Plan Activity: Treating Chronic Back Pain
- Application Activities:
  - The Mayday Pain Project
  - Resources for Arthritis
- Links to Resources

2. Key Strategies in Pain Management
   a. Acknowledging and Accepting Client's Pain
   b. Assisting Support Persons
   c. Reducing Misconceptions about Pain
   d. Reducing Fear and Anxiety
   e. Preventing Pain
3. Pharmacologic Pain Management
   a. World Health Organization (WHO) Three-Step Approach
   b. Nonopioids/NSAIDs
   c. Opioids
      i. Weak or Mixed Opioid Analgesics
      ii. Strong Opioid Analgesics
      iii. Opioid Side Effects
   d. Equianalgesic Dosing
   e. Coanalgesics
4. Administration of Placebos
5. Routes for Opiate Delivery
   a. Oral
   b. Nasal
   c. Transdermal
   d. Rectal
   e. Subcutaneous
   f. Intramuscular
   g. Intravenous
   h. Intraspinal
   i. Continuous Local Anesthetics
6. Patient-Controlled Analgesia
7. Nonpharmacologic Pain Management
   a. Physical Interventions
   b. Cutaneous Stimulation
      i. Massage
         Skill 46-1 Providing a Back Massage
      ii. Heat and Cold Applications
      iii. Acupressure
      iv. Contralateral Stimulation
   c. Immobilization/Bracing
   d. Transcutaneous Electrical Nerve Stimulation
   e. Cognitive-Behavioral Interventions
      i. Distraction
      ii. Eliciting the Relaxation Response
      iii. Repatterning Unhelpful Thinking
      iv. Facilitating Coping
      v. Selected Spiritual Interventions
8. Nonpharmacologic Invasive Therapies

E. Evaluating

KEY TOPIC REVIEW

1. Central neuropathic pain occurs occasionally when abnormal connections between pain fibers and the sympathetic nervous system perpetuate problems with both the pain and sympathetically controlled functions
   a. True
   b. False
2. Pain tolerance is the least amount of stimuli that is needed for a person to feel a sensation he or she labels as pain.
   a. True
   b. False
3. Pain management is the alleviation of pain or a reduction in pain to a level of comfort that is acceptable to the client.
   a. True
   b. False
4. Preemptive analgesia is the administration of analgesics prior to an invasive or operative procedure in order to treat pain before it occurs.
   a. True
   b. False
5. Pain threshhold is the maximum amount of painful stimuli that a person is willing to withstand without seeking avoidance of the pain or relief.
   a. True
   b. False
6. A full agonist _____ includes morphine (e.g., Kadian, MSContin), oxycodone (e.g. Percocet, OxyContin), and hydromorphine (e.g., Dilaudid, Palladone).
7. Partial agonists have a _____ effect in contrast to a full agonist.
8. _____ refers to the relative potency of various opioid analgesics compared to a standard dose of parenteral mophine.
9. _____ is "any medication or procedure, including surgery that produces an effect in a client because of its implicit or explicit intent and not because of its specific physical or chemical properties."

10. _____ drug therapy is advantageous in that it delivers a relatively stable plasma drug level and is noninvasive.

11. Match the following terms with the correct definition.

    a. Chronic pain
    b. Mild pain
    c. Physiological pain
    d. Peripheral neuropathic pain
    e. Neuropathic pain
    f. Referred pain
    g. Somatic pain
    h. Visceral pain
    i. Moderate pain
    j. Acute pain

    _____ appear to arise in different areas.
    _____ pain arising from organs or hollow viscera.
    _____ when pain lasts only through the expected recovery period.
    _____ prolonged, usually recurring or persisting over 6 months or longer, and interferes with functioning.
    _____ pain in the 1 to 3 range.
    _____ experienced when an intact, properly functioning nervous system sends signals that tissues are damaged, requiring attention and proper care.
    _____ originates in the skin, muscles, bone, or connective tissue.
    _____ experienced by people who have damaged or malfunctioning nerves.
    _____ follow damage and/or sensitization of peripheral nerves.
    _____ pain in the 4 to 6 range.

12. A _____ block is a chemical interruption of a nerve pathway, effected by injecting a local anesthetic into the nerve.

    a. Nerve
    b. Anesthetic
    c. Chemical
    d. Pathway

13. A _____ obliterates pain and temperature sensation below the level of the spinothalamic portion of the anterolateral tract severed, and is usually done for pain in the legs and trunk.

    a. Rhizotomy
    b. Neurectomy
    c. Sympathectomy
    d. Cordotomy

14. Which of the following is NOT a type of pain stimuli?

    a. Mechanical
    b. Thermal
    c. Electrical
    d. Chemical

15. Which of the following terms is described as a painful sensation felt from a part of the body that has been amputated?

    a. Nociceptive pain
    b. Phantom pain
    c. Neuropathic pain
    d. Sensitization

16. All of the following are reasons clients may be reluctant to report pain EXCEPT:

    a. Unwillingness to trouble staff who are perceived as busy.
    b. Don't want to be labeled as a "complainer" or "bad" patient.
    c. Concern that use of drugs now will render the drug inefficient later in life.
    d. Belief that others will think they are strong if they express pain.

FOCUSED STUDY TIPS

1. List the four physiologic processes that are involved in nociception.

2. What is the "fifth vital sign"?

3. Describe the World Health Organization's ladder step approach developed for cancer pain control.

4. Describe pharmacologic interventions for pain.

5. Compare and contrast barriers to effective pain management.

6. Identify examples of nursing diagnoses for clients with pain.

7. Identify subjective and objective data to collect and analyze when assessing pain.

8. Describe the gate control theory and its application to nursing care.

9. Describe how the contribution of physical, mental, spiritual, and social aspects of pain contribute to concepts such as pain tolerance, suffering, and pain behavior.

10. Describe the four processes involved in nociception and how pain interventions can work during each process.

11. Discriminate between physiological and neuropathic pain categories.

12. Give an example of rational polypharmacy as described by the American Pain Society.

13. Differentiate between tolerance, dependence, and addiction.

14. Identify risks and benefits of various analgesic delivery routes and analgesic delivery technologies.

15. Describe nonpharmacologic pain control interventions.

16. List three nonpharmacological interventions, each directed at the body, the mind, the spirit, and social interactions.

CASE STUDY

A 43-year-old client is complaining of abdominal pain. He locates his pain in the epigastric region. On a 0 to 10 scale, he rates his pain as an 8. He describes the pain as "constant throbbing."

1. *As the fifth vital sign, pain should be screened for every time vital signs are evaluated. Define pain.*
2. *Identify the two major components of a pain assessment.*
3. *Explain the pain intensity scale.*

NCLEX® REVIEW QUESTIONS

1. Which of the following statements about pain is TRUE?
   1. Pain is a sign, not a symptom.
   2. Pain presents only physiologic dangers to health and recovery.
   3. Severe pain is viewed as an emergency situation deserving attention and prompt professional treatment.
   4. Pain is a low-priority problem.

2. When pain lasts only through the expected recovery period, it is described as:
   1. chronic pain.
   2. acute pain.
   3. referred pain.
   4. visceral pain.

3. Pain tolerance is:
   1. the least amount of stimuli that is needed for a person to feel a sensation labeled as pain.
   2. the maximum amount of painful stimuli that a person is willing to withstand without seeking avoidance of the pain or relief.
   3. an unpleasant abnormal sensation.
   4. a situation in which nonpainful stimuli (e.g., contact with linen, water, or wind) produce pain.

4. A client who describes her pain as 3 on a scale of 0 to 10 is having:
   1. mild pain.
   2. moderate pain.
   3. severe pain.
   4. intense pain.

5. The nurse is evaluating a client's understanding of acute pain and chronic pain. The nurse recognizes that further teaching is necessary when which of the following statements is made by the client?
   1. Acute pain increases a client's pulse rate.
   2. With chronic pain the client appears depressed and withdrawn.
   3. With chronic pain the client exhibits behavior indicative of pain: crying, rubbing area, and holding area.
   4. Acute pain increases a client's respiratory rate.

6. Which of the following would be a misconception of pain?
   1. The person who experiences the pain is the only authority about its existence and nature.
   2. Pain is a subjective experience, and the intensity and duration of pain vary considerably among individuals.
   3. Even with severe pain, periods of physiologic and behavioral adaptation can occur.
   4. The amount of tissue damage is directly related to the amount of pain.

7. Which of the following statements about nonopioids is TRUE?
   1. Nonopioids alone are often sufficient to relieve severe pain, but they are an important part in the total analgesic plan.
   2. A nonopioid should not be given at the same time as an opioid.
   3. Side effects from long-term use of NSAIDs are considerably less severe and life threatening than the side effects from daily doses of oral morphine or other opioids.
   4. Giving a dose of nonopioid at the same time as a dose of opioid poses no more danger than giving the doses at different times.

8. A nurse is planning a seminar on COLDERR, which is a mnemonic for pain assessment. Which of the following statements is NOT correct?
   1. *Character* describes the sensation of the pain (e.g., sharp, aching, burning).
   2. *Location* is where the pain hurts (all locations).
   3. *Onset* is when the pain started and how it has changed.
   4. *Relief* means a pattern of shooting/spreading/location of pain away from its origin.

9. A nurse is evaluating a nursing student's understanding of transcultural differences in responses to pain. Which of the following actions demonstrates a need for further teaching?
   1. The African American culture believes pain and suffering is a part of life and is to be endured.
   2. The Mexican American culture believes that enduring pain is a sign of strength.
   3. The Asian American culture tends to be loud and outspoken in expressions of pain.
   4. Native Americans are quiet, less expressive verbally and nonverbally, and may tolerate a high level of pain.

10. The nurse evaluating a practice guideline for a client-with-pain at a seminar, recognizes that further teaching is necessary when which of the following statements is made by a participant?
    1. A trusting relationship promotes expression of the client's thoughts and feelings and enhances effectiveness of planned pain therapies.
    2. Consider the client's ability and willingness to participate actively in pain relief measures.
    3. Provide measures to relieve pain before it becomes severe.
    4. Maintain a biased attitude about what may relieve the pain.

CHAPTER 47

NUTRITION

CHAPTER OUTLINE

MediaLink

www.prenhall.com/berman

DVD-ROM
- Audio Glossary
- NCLEX® Review
- Skills Checklists
- Videos:
  - Anorexia
  - Bulimia
  - Eating Disorders
- Animations:
  - Carbohydrates
  - Lipids
  - Inserting a Nasogastric Tube
- Labeling Activities:
  - A & P Review
  - Cellular Metabolism
  - Organic Compounds

Companion Website
- Additional NCLEX® Review
- Case Study: Client with PEG Tube
- Care Plan Activity: Client Experiencing Loss of Appetite
- Application Activity: Vegetarian Nutrition
- Links to Resources

K. Alcohol Consumption
L. Advertising
M. Psychologic Factors
V. Nutritional Variations throughout the Life Cycle
   A. Neonate to 1 year
   B. Toddler
   C. Preschooler
   D. School-Age Child
   E. Adolescent
   F. Young Adult
   G. Middle-Aged Adult
   H. Elders
VI. Standards for a Healthy Diet
   A. Dietary Guidelines
     for Americans
     1. The Food Guide Pyramid
   B. Recommended Dietary Intake
   C. Vegetarian Diets
VII. Altered Nutrition
VIII. Nursing Management
   A. Assessing
     1. Nutritional Screening
     2. Nursing History
     3. Physical Examination
     4. Calculating Percentage
       of Weight Loss
     5. Dietary History
     6. Anthropometric Measurements
     7. Laboratory Data
       a. Serum Proteins

       b. Urinary Tests
       c. Total Lymphocyte Count
   B. Diagnosing
   C. Planning
     1. Planning for Home Care
   D. Implementing
     1. Assisting with Special Diets
       a. Clear Liquid Diet
       b. Full Liquid Diet
       c. Soft Diet
       d. Diet as Tolerated
       e. Modification for Disease
       f. Dysphagia
     2. Stimulating the Appetite
     3. Assisting Clients with Meals
     4. Special Community Nutritional Services
     5. Enteral Nutrition
       a. Enteral Access Devices
         Skill 47-1 Inserting a Nasogastric Tube
         Skill 47-2 Removing a Nasogastric Tube
       b. Testing Feeding Tube Placement
       c. Enteral Feedings
         Skill 47-3 Administering a Tube
         Feeding
         Skill 47-4 Administering a Gastrostomy
         or Jejunostomy Tube Feeding
     6. Managing Clogged Feeding Tubes
     7. Parenteral Nutrition
   E. Evaluating

KEY TOPIC REVIEW

1. Foods differ greatly in their nutritive value (the nutrient content of a specified amount of food), and no single food provides all essential nutrients.
   a. True
   b. False
2. The body's most basic nutrient need is water.
   a. True
   b. False
3. Micronutrients—vitamins and minerals—are those required in small amounts (e.g., milligrams or micrograms) to metabolize the energy-providing nutrients.
   a. True
   b. False
4. Sugars, the most complex of all carbohydrates, are fat soluble and are produced naturally by both plants and animals.
   a. True
   b. False
5. Of the three monosaccharides (glucose, fructose, and galactose), fructose is by far the most abundant simple sugar.
   a. True
   b. False
6. _____ is the sum of all the interactions between an organism and the food it consumes. In other words, nutrition is what a person eats and how the body uses it.

7. _____ are organic and inorganic substances found in foods that are required for body functioning.
8. _____ are the insoluble, nonsweet forms of carbohydrate.
9. _____, a complex carbohydrate derived from plants, supplies roughage, or bulk, to the diet.
10. _____ are biologic catalysts that speed up chemical reactions.
11. Match the following terms to the correct definition.
   a. Complete proteins
   b. Incomplete proteins
   c. Amino acids
   d. Oils
   e. Monounsaturated fatty acids
   f. Nonessential amino acids
   g. Fats
   h. Fatty acids
   i. Lipids
   j. Essential amino acids

   _____ are organic molecules made up primarily of carbon, hydrogen, oxygen, and nitrogen, which combine to form proteins.
   _____ are those that cannot be manufactured in the body and must be supplied as part of the protein ingested in the diet.
   _____ are those that the body can manufacture.
   _____ contain all of the essential amino acids plus many nonessential ones.
   _____ lack one or more essential amino acids (most commonly lysine, methionine, or tryptophan) and are usually derived from vegetables.
   _____ are organic substances that are greasy and insoluble in water but soluble in alcohol or ether.
   _____ lipids that are solid at room temperature.
   _____ lipids that are liquid at room temperature.
   _____ made up of carbon chains and hydrogen; are the basic structural units of most lipids.
   _____ fatty acids with one double bond.

12. Which of the following is NOT one of the three major functions of nutrients?
   a. Providing energy for body processes and movement
   b. Providing structural material for body tissues
   c. Regulating body processes
   d. Supplemental nutrients function to replace natural nutrients found in food
13. All of the following are considered macronutrients EXCEPT:
   a. Vitamins and minerals.
   b. Carbohydrates.
   c. Fats.
   d. Protein.
14. Every cell in the body contains some protein, and about _____ of body solids are proteins.
   a. one-eighth
   b. one-fourth
   c. one-half
   d. three-quarters
15. _____ have three fatty acids and account for more than 90% of the lipids in food and in the body.
   a. Triglycerides
   b. Cholesterol
   c. Glycerides
   d. Minerals
16. Carbohydrates are composed of all of the following elements EXCEPT:
   a. nitrogen.
   b. carbon.
   c. hydrogen.
   d. oxygen.

FOCUSED STUDY TIPS

1. Discuss energy balance in terms of energy intake and energy output.

2. List several of the factors affecting nutrition.

3. Discuss some of the psychological factors that can affect nutrition.

4. Describe how to correctly assist with special diets (e.g., clear liquid, full liquid, soft, diet as tolerated, and modification for disease).

5. Describe the term *body mass index* and give an example of how it is calculated.

6. Discuss nursing interventions to treat clients with nutritional problems.

7. Describe nursing interventions to promote optimal nutrition.

8. Identify risk factors for and clinical signs of malnutrition.

9. Discuss essential components and purposes of nutritional screening and nutritional assessment.

10. Identify developmental nutritional considerations.

11. Identify factors influencing nutrition.

12. Discuss body weight and body mass standards.

13. Explain essential aspects of energy balance.

14. Describe normal digestion, absorption, and metabolism of carbohydrates, proteins, and lipids.

15. Identify essential nutrients and their dietary sources.

CASE STUDIES

A 37-year-old African American client is experiencing loss of appetite.

1. *Explain the combinations of plant proteins that provide complete proteins.*
2. *Identify ways this client can improve his appetite.*
3. *Describe variations in nutritional practices and preferences among the client's culture.*

NCLEX® REVIEW QUESTIONS

1. Which of the following is NOT a macronutrient?
   1. Carbohydrates
   2. Fats
   3. Proteins
   4. Vitamins

2. A nurse is evaluating a nursing student's understanding of nutrition. Which of the following statements demonstrates a need for further teaching?
   1. Starches are the insoluble, nonsweet forms of carbohydrate.
   2. Most sugars are produced naturally by plants, especially fruits, sugar cane, and sugar beets.
   3. Fiber, a complex carbohydrate derived from plants, supplies roughage, or bulk, to the diet.
   4. Fiber is present in the inner layer of grains, bran, and in the skin, seeds, and pulp of many vegetables and fruits.

3. The spouse of a client is learning about nutrition. Which of the following statements indicates a need for further teaching?
   1. Essential amino acids are those that cannot be manufactured in the body and must be supplied as part of the protein ingested in the diet.
   2. The essential amino acids are alanine, aspartic acid, cystine, glutamic acid, glycine, hydroxyproline, proline, serine, and tyrosine.
   3. Nonessential amino acids are those that the body can manufacture.
   4. Most animal proteins, including meats, poultry, fish, dairy products, and eggs, are complete proteins.

4. During discharge planning, the nurse is teaching the client about lipids. Which of the following statements is NOT correct?
   1. Lipids are inorganic substances that are greasy and soluble in water but soluble in alcohol or ether.
   2. In common use, the terms *fats* and *lipids* are used interchangeably.
   3. Fats are lipids that are liquid at room temperature.
   4. Oils are lipids that are solid at room temperature.

5. The nurse is calculating a client's BMI. The client's height is 1.5 m and his weight is 70 kg. Which of the following calculations is the correct BMI?
   1. 31.11
   2. 46.67
   3. 0.02
   4. 36.16

6. Which of the following suggestions will not help parents meet the child's nutritional needs and promote effective parent–child interactions?
   1. Make mealtime a pleasant time by avoiding tensions at the table and discussions of bad behavior.
   2. Routinely use sweet desserts after dinners.
   3. Schedule meals, sleep, and snack times that will allow for optimum appetite and behavior.
   4. Offer a variety of simple, attractive foods in small portions.

7. A food diary is a:
   1. recall of all the food and beverages the client consumes during a typical 24-hour period when at home.
   2. detailed record of measured amounts (portion sizes) of all food and fluids a client consumes during a specified period, usually 3 to 7 days.
   3. comprehensive, time-consuming assessment of a client's food intake that involves an extensive interview by a nutritionist or dietitian.
   4. checklist that indicates how often general food groups or specific foods are eaten.

8. A nurse is evaluating a nursing student's understanding of special diets. Which of the following statements demonstrates a need for further teaching?
   1. A clear liquid diet is limited to water, tea, coffee, clear broths, ginger ale, or other carbonated beverages, strained and clear juices, and plain gelatin.
   2. A full liquid diet contains only liquids or foods that turn to liquid at body temperature, such as ice cream.
   3. A soft diet is easily chewed and digested.
   4. Note that the word "clear" in clear diet means "colorless."

9. Enteral feedings can be given intermittently or continuously. Intermittent feedings are the administration of _____ mL of enteral formula several times per day.
   1. 50 to 100
   2. 100 to 200
   3. 300 to 500
   4. 600 to 700

10. When planning interventions to improve a client's appetite, which of the following would be included in the client's plan of care?
    1. Unpleasant or uncomfortable treatments can be performed before or after a meal.
    2. Provide unfamiliar food to try.
    3. Encourage or provide oral hygiene after mealtime.
    4. Provide a tidy, clean environment that is free of unpleasant sights and odors.

CHAPTER 48

URINARY ELIMINATION

CHAPTER OUTLINE

MediaLink

www.prenhall.com/berman

DVD-ROM
- Audio Glossary
- NCLEX® Review
- Skills Checklists
- Animations:
  - Female Catheterization
  - Kidney

Companion Website
- Additional NCLEX® Review
- Case Study: Intermittent Self-Catheterization
- Care Plan Activity: Client with Urinary Retention Catheter
- Application Activity: Urinary Incontinence
- Links to Resources

2. Physical Assessment
3. Assessing Urine
   a. Measuring Urinary Output
   b. Measuring Residual Urine
4. Diagnostic Tests
B. Diagnosing
C. Planning
   1. Planning for Home Care
D. Implementing
   1. Maintaining Normal Urinary Elimination
      a. Promoting Fluid Intake
      b. Maintaining Normal Voiding Habits
      c. Assisting with Toileting
   2. Preventing Urinary Tract Infections
   3. Managing Urinary Incontinence
      a. Continence (Bladder) Training
      b. Pelvic Muscle Exercises
      c. Maintaining Skin Integrity
      d. Applying External Urinary
         Drainage Devices
         Skill 48-1 Applying an External
         Catheter

4. Managing Urinary Retention
5. Urinary Catheterization
   Skill 48-2 Performing Urethral Urinary
   Catheterization
6. Nursing Interventions for Clients with
   Retention Catheters
   a. Fluids
   b. Dietary Measures
   c. Perineal Care
   d. Changing the Catheter and Tubing
   e. Removing Indwelling Catheters
7. Clean Intermittent Self-Catheterization
8. Urinary Irrigations
   Skill 48-3 Performing Bladder
   Irrigation
9. Suprapubic Catheter Care
10. Urinary Diversions
    a. Incontinent
    b. Continent
E. Evaluating

KEY TOPIC REVIEW

1. The most common urinary diversion is the ileal conduit or ileal loop.
   a. True
   b. False
2. Urinary tract infections (UTIs) are the most common infection in children.
   a. True
   b. False
3. The paired kidneys are situated on either side of the spinal column, behind the peritoneal cavity.
   a. True
   b. False
4. The urinary bladder (vesicle) is a hollow, muscular organ that serves as a reservoir for urine and as the organ of excretion.
   a. True
   b. False
5. The urethra serves only as a passageway for the elimination of urine.
   a. True
   b. False
6. _____ increase urine formation by preventing the reabsorption of water and electrolytes from the tubules of the kidney into the bloodstream.
7. Clients who have a _____ bladder (weak, soft, and lax bladder muscles) may use manual pressure on the bladder to promote bladder emptying.
8. _____ is a flushing or washing-out with a specified solution.
9. _____ diverts urine from the kidney to a stoma.
10. A _____ may be formed when the bladder is left intact but voiding through the urethra is not possible (e.g., due to an obstruction or a neurogenic bladder).

11. Match the following terms with the correct definition.
    a. Anuria
    b. Polyuria (diuresis)
    c. Nocturnal enuresis
    d. Residual urine
    e. Bladder training
    f. Creatinine clearance
    g. Dysuria
    h. Habit training
    i. Oliguria
    j. Nocturia

    _____ bed-wetting.

    _____ the production of abnormally large amounts of urine by the kidneys, often several liters more than the client's usual daily output.

    _____ low urine output.

    _____ refers to a lack of urine production.

    _____ voiding two or more times at night.

    _____ voiding that is either painful or difficult.

    _____ urine remaining in the bladder following the voiding.

    _____ a test that uses 24-hour urine and serum creatinine levels to determine the glomerular filtration rate, a sensitive indicator of renal function.

    _____ requires that the client postpone voiding, resist or inhibit the sensation of urgency, and void according to a timetable rather than according to the urge to void.

    _____ referred to as timed voiding or scheduled toileting, attempts to keep clients dry by having them void at regular intervals.

12. Normal bladder capacity is between _____ mL of urine.
    a. 300 and 600
    b. 600 and 900
    c. 900 and 1200
    d. 1200 and 1500

13. An infant may urinate as often as _____ times a day.
    a. 5
    b. 10
    c. 15
    d. 20

14. About _____% of all 6-year-olds experience difficulty controlling the bladder.
    a. 10
    b. 20
    c. 30
    d. 40

15. Although people's patterns of urination are highly individual, most people void about _____ times a day.
    a. 3 to 4
    b. 5 to 6
    c. 7 to 8
    d. 9 to 10

16. All of the following refer to the process of emptying the urinary bladder EXCEPT:
    a. Micturition.
    b. Voiding.
    c. Urination.
    d. Elimination.

FOCUSED STUDY TIPS

1. Discuss several practice guidelines to prevent catheter-associated urinary infections.

2. What are the accuracy and clinical benefits with using a bladder scanner?

3. List and discuss several factors that influence urinary elimination.

4. Problems of urinary elimination also may become the etiology for other problems experienced by the client. Discuss several of these other problems.

5. Describe and list several different types of urinary catheters available.

6. List several medications that may cause urinary retention.

7. Explain the care of clients with retention catheters or urinary diversions.

8. Discuss ways to prevent urinary infection.

9. Develop nursing diagnoses, desired outcomes, and interventions related to urinary elimination.

10. Identify normal and abnormal characteristics and constituents of urine.

11. Describe nursing assessment of urinary function including subjective and objective data.

12. Identify common causes of selected urinary problems.

13. Identify factors that influence urinary elimination.

14. Describe the process of urination, from urine formation through micturition.

15. Visit the following website: www.webmd.com/hw/lab_tests/hw6580.asp and write a short summary of what you learned.

CASE STUDY

A 68-year-old client has been experiencing urinary elimination problems. He has given you a urine specimen and asks how to maintain normal urinary elimination.

1. *List the steps a nurse must follow to measure fluid output.*
2. *Identify various goals for clients with urinary elimination problems.*
3. *Explain how this client can maintain normal urinary elimination.*

NCLEX® REVIEW QUESTIONS

1. Oliguria is:
   1. low urine output.
   2. the production of abnormally large amounts of urine by the kidneys, often several liters more than the client's usual daily output.
   3. excessive fluid intake.
   4. a lack of urine production.

2. Urinary frequency is:
   1. voiding two or more times at night.
   2. voiding at frequent intervals, that is, more than four to six times per day.
   3. the sudden strong desire to void.
   4. voiding that is either painful or difficult.

3. During discharge planning, the nurse is teaching the client ways to prevent a recurrence of a UTI. Which of the following actions is correct?
   1. Drink six 6-ounce glasses of water per day to flush bacteria out of the urinary system.
   2. Wear nylon rather than cotton underclothes.
   3. Girls and women should always wipe the perineal area from back to front following urination or defecation in order to prevent introduction of gastrointestinal bacteria into the urethra.
   4. Avoid tight-fitting pants or other clothing that creates irritation to the urethra and prevents ventilation of the perineal area.

4. A nurse is evaluating a client's understanding of intermittent self-catheterization. Which of the following statements indicates a need for further teaching? Intermittent self-catheterization:
   1. reduces incidence of urinary tract infection.
   2. enables the client to retain independence and gain control of the bladder.
   3. allows normal sexual relations without incontinence.
   4. protects the lower urinary tract from reflux.

5. Which of the following is an abnormal color or clarity of urine?
   1. Straw
   2. Amber
   3. Dark amber
   4. Transparent

6. A nurse is testing urine for specific gravity. Which of the following would be considered a normal result range?
   1. 0.100–0.999
   2. 1.000–1.050
   3. 1.010–1.025
   4. 1.050–1.100

7. The nurse is performing urethral urinary catheterization on a male client. Which of the following actions by the nurse is correct?
   1. Lubricates the catheter 1 to 2 inches
   2. Picks up a cleansing ball with the forceps in the nondominant hand and wipes from the top of the meatus in a circular motion around the glans
   3. Grasps the catheter firmly 2 to 3 inches from the tip; asks the client to take a slow deep breath and inserts the catheter as the client exhales
   4. Puts on examination gloves

8. A nurse evaluating a facilitating and promoting urinary elimination class recognizes that further teaching is necessary when which of the following statements is made by a participant?
   1. Advise the client and family to install grab bars and elevated toilet seats as needed.
   2. Teach the client to empty the bladder completely at each voiding.
   3. Emphasize the importance of drinking five to six 8-ounce glasses of water daily.
   4. Suggest clothing that is easily removed for toileting, such as elastic-waist pants or pants with Velcro closures.

9. During discharge planning, the nurse is teaching the client how to perform pelvic muscle exercises (Kegels). Which of the following actions is correct?
   1. Initially perform each contraction 10 times, five times daily. Gradually increase the count to a full 10 seconds for both contraction and relaxation.
   2. To control episodes of stress incontinence, perform a pelvic muscle contraction only after activities that increase intra-abdominal pressure, such as coughing, laughing, sneezing, or lifting.
   3. Develop a schedule that will help remind you to do these exercises, for example, before getting out of bed in the morning.
   4. Contract your pelvic muscles whereby you pull your rectum, urethra, and vagina up inside, and hold for a count of 1 to 2 seconds. Then relax the same muscles for a count of 1 to 2 seconds.

10. A nurse is evaluating a client's understanding of preventing catheter-associated urinary infections. Which of the following statements indicates a need for further teaching?
   1. Maintain a sterile closed-drainage system.
   2. Always disconnect the catheter and drainage tubing.
   3. Provide routine perineal hygiene, including cleansing with soap and water after defecation.
   4. Prevent contamination of the catheter with feces.

CHAPTER 49

FECAL ELIMINATION

CHAPTER OUTLINE

MediaLink

www.prenhall.com/berman

DVD-ROM
- Audio Glossary
- NCLEX® Review
- Skills Checklists
- Animations:
  - Enema
- Labeling Activity:
  - Intestinal Wall

Companion Website
- Additional NCLEX® Review
- Case Study: Client After Abdominal Surgery
- Care Plan Activity: Client Who Had a Stroke
- Application Activities:
  - The United Ostomy Association
  - Wound Ostomy Nurse
- Links to Resources

c. Nutrition and Fluids
   i. For Constipation
   ii. For Diarrhea
   iii. For Flatulence
d. Exercise
e. Positioning
2. Teaching about Medications
   a. Cathartics and Laxatives
   b. Antidiarrheal Medications
   c. Antiflatulent Medications
3. Decreasing Flatulence
4. Administering Enemas
   a. Cleansing Enemas
   b. Carminative Enema

c. Retention Enema
d. Return-Flow Enema
   Skill 49-1 Administering an Enema
5. Digital Removal of
   a Fecal Impaction
6. Bowel Training Programs
7. Fecal Incontinence Pouch
8. Ostomy Management
   a. Stoma and Skin Care
   Skill 49-2 Changing a Bowel Diversion
   Ostomy Appliance
   b. Colostomy Irrigation
E. Evaluating

KEY TOPIC REVIEW

1. Elimination of the waste products of digestion from the body is essential to health.
   a. True
   b. False
2. The small intestine extends from the ileocecal (ileocolic) valve, which lies between the large and small intestines, to the anus.
   a. True
   b. False
3. Normal feces are made of about 25% water and 75% solid materials.
   a. True
   b. False
4. Constipation is the most common bowel-management problem in the elder population.
   a. True
   b. False
5. The colon (large intestine) in the adult is generally about 125 to 150 cm (50 to 60 in.) long.
   a. True
   b. False
6. _____ is the presence of excessive flatus in the intestines and leads to stretching and inflation of the intestines (intestinal distention).
7. _____ is an opening for the gastrointestinal, urinary, or respiratory tract onto the skin.
8. Clients restricted to bed may need to use a _____, a receptacle for urine and feces.
9. An _____ is a solution introduced into the rectum and large intestine.
10. _____ are drugs that induce defecation.
11. Match the following terms with the correct definition.
   a. Hemorrhoids
   b. Laxatives
   c. Bowel/fecal incontinence
   d. Constipation
   e. Diarrhea
   f. Defecation
   g. Fecal impaction
   h. Ingestion
   i. Gastrocolic reflex
   j. Chyme

   _____ the act of taking food.
   _____ waste products leaving the stomach through the small intestine and then passing through the ileocecal valve.
   _____ a condition that can occur when the veins become distended, as can occur with repeated pressure.
   _____ the expulsion of feces from the anus and rectum.
   _____ increased peristalsis of the colon after food has entered the stomach.
   _____ medications that stimulate bowel activity and so assist fecal elimination.
   _____ fewer than three bowel movements per week.

_____ a mass or collection of hardened feces in the folds of the rectum.

_____ the passage of liquid feces and an increased frequency of defecation.

_____ the loss of voluntary ability to control fecal and gaseous discharges through the anal sphincter.

12. The contents of the colon normally represent foods ingested over the previous _____ days.
    a. 2
    b. 3
    c. 4
    d. 5

13. All of the following may be causes and factors that contribute to constipation EXCEPT:
    a. lack of privacy.
    b. daily routines.
    c. insufficient fiber intake.
    d. insufficient fluid intake.

14. The rate of fecal incontinence among elders living in the community has been reported to be 4% to 17% compared to 2% in the general community population and _____ % in elderly nursing home residents.
    a. 4 to 20
    b. 20 to 54
    c. 54 to 84
    d. 84 to 96

15. All of the following are thought to contribute to constipation EXCEPT:
    a. overuse of laxatives.
    b. bland diets.
    c. irregular defecation habits.
    d. exercise.

16. Which of the following feces consistency would be considered abnormal?
    a. Soft
    b. Moist
    c. Semisolid
    d. Dry

FOCUSED STUDY TIPS

1. Distinguish normal from abnormal characteristics and constituents of feces.

2. List the seven parts of the colon (large intestine).

3. Identify factors that influence fecal elimination and patterns of defecation.

4. Discuss the physiology of defecation.

5. Discuss regular exercise and how it helps clients develop a regular defecation pattern.

6. Discuss some of the ways to reduce or expel flatus.

7. Describe methods used to assess the intestinal tract.

8. Identify examples of nursing diagnoses, outcomes, and interventions for clients with elimination problems.

9. List and describe the three types of movements that occur in the large intestine.

10. Identify measures that maintain normal fecal elimination patterns.

11. Describe the purpose and action of commonly used enema solutions.

12. List four common problems that are related to fecal elimination.

13. Describe essentials of fecal stoma care for clients with an ostomy.

14. List and discuss the three primary sources of flatus.

15. Describe how to administer an enema.

CASE STUDY

A 37-year-old client has been experiencing diarrhea for the past 12 hours.

1. *Identify ways for the client to manage diarrhea.*
2. *Provide the client with information about healthy defecation.*
3. *Identify three major causes of diarrhea.*

NCLEX® REVIEW QUESTIONS

1. A gastrostomy is an opening:
   1. through the abdominal wall into the stomach.
   2. through the abdominal wall into the jejunum.
   3. into the colon (large bowel).
   4. into the ileum (small bowel).

2. Which type of enema is given primarily to expel flatus?
   1. Retention
   2. Carminative
   3. Return-flow
   4. Cleansing

3. Which of the following actions is NOT appropriate for the nurse removing a fecal impaction?
   1. Place a bedpad under the client's buttocks and a bedpan nearby to receive stool.
   2. Ask the client to assume a right side-lying position, with the knees flexed and the back toward the nurse.
   3. Drape the client for comfort and to avoid unnecessary exposure of the body.
   4. Gently insert the index finger into the rectum and move the finger along the length of the rectum.

4. A nurse is evaluating a client's understanding of healthy defecation. Which of the following statements indicates a need for further teaching?
   1. "I will include high-fiber foods, such as vegetables, fruits, and whole grains, in my diet."
   2. "I will maintain a fluid intake of 4,000 to 5,000 mL each day."
   3. "I will allow time to defecate, preferably at the same time each day."
   4. "I will avoid over-the-counter medications to treat constipation and diarrhea."

5. During discharge planning, the nurse is teaching the client how to manage diarrhea. Which of the following actions is NOT correct?
   1. Drink at least 8 glasses of water per day to prevent dehydration.
   2. Eat foods with sodium and potassium.
   3. Increase foods containing insoluble fiber, such as high-fiber whole-wheat and whole-grain breads and cereals, and raw fruits and vegetables.
   4. Limit fatty foods.

6. A nurse is evaluating a client's understanding of ostomy care. Which of the following statements indicates a need for further teaching?
   1. The pouch is emptied when it is 1/3 to 1/2 full.
   2. Ostomy appliances can be applied for up to 10 days.
   3. Most pouches contain odor barrier material.
   4. If the pouch overfills, it can cause separation of the skin barrier from the skin and stool can come in contact with the skin.

7. A nurse is evaluating a nursing student's understanding of colostomies. Which of the following statements demonstrates a need for further teaching?
   1. The single stoma is created when one end of bowel is brought out through an opening onto the anterior abdominal wall.
   2. In the loop colostomy, a loop of bowel is brought out onto the abdominal wall and supported by a plastic bridge, or a piece of rubber tubing.
   3. The divided colostomy consists of two edges of bowel brought out onto the abdomen but separated from each other.
   4. The loop colostomy is often used in situations where spillage of feces into the distal end of the bowel needs to be avoided.

8. The nurse is promoting regular defecation for a client whom she is taking care of. Which of the following actions by the nurse is NOT correct?
   1. A client should be encouraged to defecate when the urge is recognized.
   2. Regular exercise helps clients develop a regular defecation pattern.
   3. Although the squatting position best facilitates defecation, on a toilet seat the best position for most people seems to be leaning backward.
   4. For clients who have difficulty sitting down and getting up from the toilet, an elevated toilet seat can be attached to a regular toilet.

9. A primary care provider orders examination of stool for signs of intestinal infection. What color of stool would the nurse expect to see?
   1. Red
   2. Green
   3. Black
   4. White

10. A nurse is evaluating a nursing student's understanding of the actions of enema solutions. Which of the following statements demonstrates a need for further teaching?
    1. Hypertonic solutions draw water into the colon.
    2. Hypotonic solutions distend the colon, stimulate peristalsis, and soften feces.
    3. Isotonic solutions lubricate the feces and the colonic mucosa.
    4. Soapsud solutions irritate the mucosa and distend the colon.

CHAPTER 50

OXYGENATION

CHAPTER OUTLINE

MediaLink

www.prenhall.com/berman

DVD-ROM
- Audio Glossary
- NCLEX® Review
- Skills Checklists
- Video and Animations:
  - Carbon Dioxide Transport
  - Gas Exchange
  - Humidifier
  - Incentive Spirometry
  - Nasal Cannula
  - Nonrebreather Mask
  - Oxygen Transport
  - Pulmonary Diseases
  - Salmeterol
  - Slidenafil
  - Simple Mask

Companion Website
- Additional NCLEX® Review
- Case Study: Coping with Emphysema
- Care Plan Activity: Deep Breathing
  and Coughing
- Application Activities:
  - Learning About Lung Disease
  - Tracheostomy Nursing Care
- Links to Resources

234

KEY TOPIC REVIEW

1. Postural drainage is the drainage by gravity of secretions from various lung segments.
   a. True
   b. False
2. Suctioning is aspirating secretions through a catheter connected to a suction machine or wall suction outlet.
   a. True
   b. False
3. Hyperoxygenation involves giving the client breaths that are 1 to 1.5 times the tidal volume set on the ventilator through the ventilator circuit or via a manual resuscitation bag.
   a. True
   b. False
4. When air collects in the pleural space, it is known as a hemothorax.
   a. True
   b. False
5. Hyperinflation can be done with a manual resuscitation bag or through the ventilator and is performed by increasing the oxygen flow (usually to 100%) before suctioning and between suction attempts.
   a. True
   b. False
6. _____ is a clear odorless gas that constitutes approximately 21% of the air we breathe, and is necessary for proper functioning of all living cells.
7. _____ pressure (pressure within the lungs) always equalizes with atmospheric pressure.
8. _____ is a collapse of a portion of the lung.
9. _____ is the movement of gases or other particles from an area of greater pressure or concentration to an area of lower pressure or concentration.
10. _____ is the cessation of breathing.
11. Match the following terms with the correct definition.
    a. Surfactant
    b. Sputum
    c. Cyanosis
    d. Expectorate
    e. Hemoglobin
    f. Bradypnea
    g. Humidifiers
    h. Hypoxia
    i. Orthopnea
    j. Erythrocytes

    _____ a lipoprotein produced by specialized alveolar cells, acts like a detergent, reducing the surface tension of alveolar fluid.
    _____ oxygen-carrying red pigment.
    _____ red blood cells, or RBCs.
    _____ a condition of insufficient oxygen anywhere in the body, from the inspired gas to the tissues.
    _____ bluish discoloration of the skin, nailbeds, and mucous membranes, due to reduced hemoglobin-oxygen saturation.
    _____ an abnormally slow respiratory rate.
    _____ the inability to breathe except in an upright or standing position.
    _____ coughed-up material.
    _____ spit out.
    _____ devices that add water vapor to inspired air.

12. _____ is a series of vigorous quiverings produced by hands that are placed flat against the client's chest wall.
    a. Hemoglobin
    b. Hematocrit
    c. Oxyhemoglobin
    d. Vibration

13. _____ is the continual tendency of the lungs to collapse away from the chest wall.
    a. Atelectasis
    b. Lung recoil
    c. Diffusion
    d. Lung compliance

14. _____ is a condition of insufficient oxygen anywhere in the body, from the inspired gas to the tissues.
    a. Hypoxia
    b. Emphysema
    c. Hypercarbia
    d. Hypercapnia

15. _____ refers to reduced oxygen in the blood and is characterized by a low partial pressure of oxygen in arterial blood or a low hemoglobin saturation.
    a. Cyanosis
    b. Tachypnea
    c. Hypoxemia
    d. Bradypnea

16. Normal respiration (_____) is quiet.
    a. Orthopnea
    b. Apnea
    c. Dyspnea
    d. Eupnea

FOCUSED STUDY TIPS

1. Discuss what an obstructed airway is and how to assess and keep an airway open.

2. List and explain some of the types of medications that can be used for clients with oxygenation problems.

3. Explain how chest tubes are inserted.

4. Discuss the overall outcomes/goals for a client with oxygenation problems.

5. List and explain the nursing responsibilities regarding drainage systems.

6. Discuss some of the NANDA diagnostic labels for clients with oxygenation problems.

7. State outcome criteria for evaluating client responses to measures that promote adequate oxygenation.

8. Explain the use of therapeutic measures such as medications, inhalation therapy, oxygen therapy, artificial airways, airway suctioning, and chest tubes to promote respiratory function.

9. Describe nursing measures to promote respiratory function and oxygenation.

10. Identify common manifestations of impaired respiratory function.

11. Identify factors influencing respiratory function.

12. Explain the role and function of the respiratory system in transporting oxygen and carbon dioxide to and from body tissues.

13. Describe the processes of breathing (ventilation) and gas exchange (respiration).

14. Outline the structure and function of the respiratory system.

CASE STUDY

You are a nursing student's preceptor today. This is her first semester in nursing school. When she first arrives to the unit she asks you several questions:

1. *Which factors does adequate ventilation depend on?*
2. *Which factors affect the rate of oxygen transport from the lungs to the tissues?*
3. *Which factors influencing oxygenation affect the cardiovascular system as well as the respiratory system?*
4. *What are oxygen therapy safety precautions?*

NCLEX® REVIEW QUESTIONS

1. Which of the following does adequate ventilation not depend on?
   1. Clear airways
   2. Adequate pulmonary compliance and recoil
   3. An intact sympathetic nervous system and respiratory center
   4. An intact thoracic cavity capable of expanding and contracting

2. Eupnea means:
   1. a normal respiration that is quiet, rhythmic, and effortless.
   2. a rapid rate.
   3. an abnormally slow respiratory rate.
   4. the cessation of breathing.

3. Which of the following is marked rhythmic waxing and waning of respirations from very deep to very shallow breathing and temporary apnea?
   1. Biot's (cluster) respirations
   2. Orthopnea
   3. Cheyne-Stokes respirations
   4. Dyspnea

4. The nonrebreather mask delivers the highest oxygen concentration possible (95% to 100%) by means other than intubation or mechanical ventilation, at liter flows of _____ L per minute.
   1. 2 to 6
   2. 5 to 8
   3. 6 to 10
   4. 10 to 15

5. Which type of mask delivers oxygen concentrations varying from 24% to 40% or 50% at liter flows of 4 to 10 L per minute?
   1. Nonrebreather
   2. Venturi
   3. Simple face
   4. Partial rebreather

6. A nurse is evaluating a nursing student's understanding of endotracheal tubes. Which of the following statements indicates a need for further teaching?
   1. Endotracheal tubes are most commonly inserted for clients who have had general anesthetics or for those in emergency situations where mechanical ventilation is required.
   2. An endotracheal tube is inserted by the primary care provider, nurse, or respiratory therapist with specialized education.
   3. An endotracheal tube is inserted through the mouth or the nose and into the trachea with the guide of a laryngoscope.
   4. The client is able to speak while an endotracheal tube is in place.

7. Which of the following is the amount of air remaining in the lungs after maximal exhalation?
   1. TLC
   2. RV
   3. VC
   4. ERV

8. The spouse of a client is explaining to the nurse what she learned about a cough reflex. Which of the following indicates a need for further teaching? The spouse states:
   1. the epiglottis and glottis (vocal cords) close.
   2. a large inspiration of approximately 3.5 L occurs.
   3. nerve impulses are sent through the vagus nerve to the medulla.
   4. a strong contraction of abdominal and internal intercostal muscles dramatically raises the pressure in the lungs.

9. A nurse is evaluating a nursing student's understanding of oxygen therapy precautions. Which of the following statements indicates a need for further teaching?
   1. Place cautionary signs reading "No Smoking: Oxygen in Use" on the client's door, at the foot or head of the bed, and on the oxygen equipment.
   2. Be sure that electric monitoring equipment, suction machines, and portable diagnostic machines are all electrically grounded.
   3. Make known the location of fire extinguishers, and make sure personnel are trained in their use.
   4. The use of volatile, flammable materials, such as oils, greases, alcohol, ether, and acetone (e.g., nail polish remover), near clients receiving oxygen is acceptable with a physician order.

10. Which of the following actions is NOT appropriate for the nurse providing tracheostomy care?
    1. Clean the lumen and entire inner cannula thoroughly using a brush or pipe cleaners moistened with sterile normal saline.
    2. Rinse the inner cannula thoroughly in the sterile normal saline.
    3. After rinsing, gently tap the cannula against the inside edge of the sterile saline container.
    4. Put on sterile gloves. Keep your nondominant hand sterile during the procedure.

CHAPTER 51

CIRCULATION

CHAPTER OUTLINE

MediaLink

www.prenhall.com/berman

DVD-ROM
- Audio Glossary
- NCLEX® Review
- Skill Checklist
- Videos and Animations:
  - Atrial Contraction
  - Blood Flow Atria
  - Blood Pressure
  - Congenital Heart Defects
  - Coronary Artery Disease
  - Dysrhythmias
  - Heart Attack
  - Hemodynamics
  - Normal Sinus Rythym
  - Ventricular Contraction

Companion Website
- Additional NCLEX® Review
- Case Study: Client with Diabetes
- Care Plan Activity: Client Experiencing Pain from Walking
- Application Activity: Health Promotion for a Healthy Heart
- Links to Resources

V. Nursing Management
   A. Assessing
      1. Nursing History
      2. Physical Assessment
      3. Diagnostic Studies
         a. Cardiac Monitoring
         b. Blood Tests
         c. Hemodynamic Studies
   B. Diagnosing
   C. Planning
   D. Implementing
      1. Promoting Circulation
         a. Vascular
         b. Cardiac
      2. Medications
      3. Preventing Venous Stasis
         a. Sequential Compression Devices
            Skill 51-1 Sequential Compression Devices
      4. Cardiopulmonary Resuscitation
   E. Evaluating

KEY TOPIC REVIEW

1. Cardiac muscle contraction is a mechanical event that occurs in response to electrical stimulation.
   a. True
   b. False
2. Pulse rates are highest and most variable in adults.
   a. True
   b. False
3. Congenital heart disease affects less than 1% of all live births, but is the leading cause of early death from all congenital anomalies.
   a. True
   b. False
4. Among people in their 40s and 50s, women have a higher incidence of hypertension than men.
   a. True
   b. False
5. Recent studies suggest that moderate alcohol use (1 to 2 oz of alcohol per day) may actually reduce the risk of heart disease.
   a. True
   b. False
6. _____ is a lack of blood supply due to obstructed circulation.
7. The _____ is a hollow, cone-shaped organ about the size of a fist.
8. Cardiac output is calculated by _____ the stroke volume (SV), the amount of blood ejected with each contraction, times the heart rate (HR).
9. _____ is the degree to which muscle fibers in the ventricle are stretched at the end of the relaxation period (diastole) and largely depends on the amount of blood returning to the heart from the venous circulation.
10. _____ is the resistance against which the heart must pump to eject the blood into circulation. Blood flows from an area of higher pressure to an area of lower pressure.

11. Match the following terms with the correct definition.
    a. Blood pressure (BP)
    b. Hemoglobin
    c. Blood
    d. Atherosclerosis
    e. Systemic
    f. Cardiovascular
    g. Hemodynamics
    h. Hemoglobin
    i. Ischemia
    j. Respiratory

    _____ is a major component of red blood cells (erythrocytes), the predominant cell present in blood.

    _____, the buildup of fatty plaque within the arteries, is the major contributor to cardiovascular disease, the leading cause of death in North America.

    _____ serves as the transport medium within the cardiovascular system, bringing oxygen and nutrients from the environment (via the lungs and gastrointestinal system) to the cells.

    _____ A _____ arrest (pulmonary arrest) is the cessation of breathing.

    _____ is the study of the forces or pressures involved in blood circulation.

    _____ is a lack of blood supply due to obstructed circulation.

    _____ is the molecule that oxygen attaches to; it gives an indication of the oxygen-carrying capacity of the blood.

    _____ The heart and the blood vessels make up the _____ system that, together with blood, is the major system for transporting oxygen and nutrients to the tissues, and waste products away from the tissues for elimination.

    _____ is a type of blood vessel that carries blood to the tissues through a system of arteries, arterioles, and capillaries and returns it to the heart through the venules, veins, and the venae cavae.

    _____ the force exerted on arterial walls by the blood flowing within the vessel.

12. Electrocardiography most commonly uses _____ "leads" or different views of the heart.
    a. 6
    b. 8
    c. 10
    d. 12

13. Each health care facility has policies and procedures for announcing cardiac/respiratory arrest and initiating interventions. In many institutions this emergency is called a Code _____, and the announcement is referred to as "calling a code."
    a. Blue
    b. Red
    c. Green
    d. Yellow

14. Cardiac output (CO) is the amount of blood pumped by the ventricles in _____ minute.
    a. 1
    b. 2
    c. 3
    d. 4

15. With each contraction, a certain amount of blood, known as the stroke volume, is ejected from the ventricles into circulation. In adults, the average stroke volume is about _____ mL per beat.
    a. 40
    b. 50
    c. 60
    d. 70

16. Nearly _____% of the adult population of the United States is overweight or obese.
    a. 30
    b. 40
    c. 50
    d. 60

FOCUSED STUDY TIPS

1. Explain what a modifiable risk factor is and list several examples.

2. List the signs of anemia.

3. Explain arterial circulation.

4. Discuss cardiopulmonary resuscitation (CPR).

5. Describe the cardiac cycle.

6. Discuss the importance of homocysteine levels.

7. Summarize venous return.

8. What is cardiac monitoring and what is it used for?

9. List the signs of impaired peripheral arterial circulation.

10. Discuss physical assessment as it relates to the cardiovascular system.

11. Discuss life span considerations as they relate to the cardiovascular system.

12. Discuss serum lipid levels and coronary artery disease.

13. Explain what a nonmodifiable risk factor is and give some examples.

14. Define hypertension.

15. List the three cardinal signs of a cardiac arrest.

CASE STUDY

A 43-year-old female client has just been diagnosed with hypertension. She also has elevated serum lipid levels. The client asks you the following questions:

1. *Why is the physician concerned about my lipid levels being elevated?*
2. *What is hypertension?*
3. *What are the risk factors for coronary heart disease?*

NCLEX® REVIEW QUESTIONS

1. The spouse of a client is recalling the modifiable risk factors for coronary heart disease. Which of the following indicates a need for further teaching? Modifiable risk factors for coronary heart disease include all of the following EXCEPT:
   1. age.
   2. diabetes.
   3. obesity.
   4. sedentary lifestyle.

2. Which of the following conditions increases afterload?
   1. Hypertension
   2. Myocardial infarction
   3. Hypervolemia
   4. Mitral regurgitation

3. Normal changes of aging may contribute to problems of circulation in elders, even when there is no actual pathology. Which of the following is a correct statement?
   1. A decrease of muscle tone in the heart results in a decrease in cardiac output.
   2. Blood vessels become less elastic and have an increase in calcification.
   3. Impaired valve function in the heart is often the result of increased stiffness and calcification and results in a decrease in cardiac output.
   4. There is an increase in baroreceptor response to blood pressure changes, making the heart and blood vessels more responsive to exercise and stress.

4. A nurse is planning a seminar on promoting a healthy heart. Which of the following statements is incorrect?
   1. Reduce stress and manage anger.
   2. Exercise at least 20 minutes, three times a week.
   3. Do not smoke.
   4. Eat a diet low in total fat, saturated fats, and cholesterol.

5. A nurse is evaluating a nursing student's understanding of the heart. Which of the following statements demonstrates a need for further teaching?
   1. There are four hollow chambers within the heart; two upper atria and two lower ventricles are separated longitudinally by the interventricular septum, forming two parallel pumps.
   2. The heart is a hollow, cone-shaped organ about the size of a fist.
   3. The heart is located in the mediastinum, between the lungs and underlying the sternum.
   4. Deoxygenated blood from the veins enters the left side of the heart through the superior and inferior venae cavae.

6. Which of the following statements by the nurse is NOT correct?
   1. Systole is when the heart ejects (propels) the blood into the pulmonary and systemic circulations.
   2. At the end of the systolic phase the atria contract, adding an additional volume to the ventricles.
   3. The diastolic phase of the cardiac cycle is twice as long as the systolic phase.
   4. Diastole is largely a passive process.

7. The primary pacemaker of the heart is the:
   1. SA node.
   2. Bundle of His.
   3. AV node.
   4. Purkinje fibers.

8. PVR is determined by:
   1. blood vessel length.
   2. blood vessel diameter.
   3. the viscosity of the blood.
   4. the fineness of the blood.

9. During discharge planning, the nurse is teaching the client about homocysteine. Which of the following statements is correct?
   1. Homocysteine is an amino acid that has been shown to be decreased in many people with atherosclerosis.
   2. Clients with elevated homocysteine levels may have a decreased risk of myocardial infarction, coronary artery disease, cerebrovascular accidents (stroke), and peripheral vascular disease.
   3. Clients can reduce their homocysteine level by taking a multivitamin that provides folate, vitamin B_6, vitamin B_{12}, and riboflavin.
   4. Homocysteine circulates in the blood and is made up of cholesterol, triglycerides, and phospholipids.

10. Which of the following would be a sign of heart failure?
    1. Pulmonary congestion; adventitious lung sounds
    2. Decreased respiratory rate
    3. Warm, red extremities
    4. Decreased heart rate

CHAPTER 52

FLUID, ELECTROLYTE, AND ACID–BASE BALANCE

CHAPTER OUTLINE

MediaLink

www.prenhall.com/berman

DVD-ROM
- Audio Glossary
- NCLEX® Review
- Skills Checklists
- Animations:
  - Acid–Base Balance
  - Central Venous Line
  - Filtration Pressure
  - Fluid Balance
  - Furosemide
  - Membrane Transport

Companion Website
- Additional NCLEX® Review
- Case Study: Client with Suspected Electrolyte Imbalance
- Care Plan Activity: Client with Heart Failure
- Application Activities:
  - Determining Body Fluid Problems
  - Arterial Blood Gases and Acid–Base Balance
- Links to Resources

III. Factors Affecting Body Fluid, Electrolytes, and Acid–Base Balance
   A. Age
   B. Gender and Body Size
   C. Environmental Temperature
   D. Lifestyle
IV. Disturbances in Fluid Volume, Electrolyte, and Acid–Base Balance
   A. Fluid Imbalances
      1. Fluid Volume Deficit
         a. Third Space Syndrome
      2. Fluid Volume Excess
         a. Edema
      3. Dehydration
      4. Overhydration
   B. Electrolyte Imbalances
      1. Sodium
      2. Potassium
      3. Calcium
      4. Magnesium
      5. Chloride
      6. Phosphate
   C. Acid–Base Imbalances
      1. Respiratory Acidosis
      2. Respiratory Alkalosis
      3. Metabolic Acidosis
      4. Metabolic Alkalosis
V. Nursing Management
   A. Assessing
      1. Nursing History
      2. Physical Assessment
      3. Clinical Measurements
         a. Daily Weights
         b. Vital Signs
         c. Fluid Intake and Output
      4. Laboratory Tests
         a. Serum Electrolytes
         b. Complete Blood Count (CBC)
         c. Osmolality
         d. Urine pH
         e. Urine Specific Gravity
         f. Urine Sodium and Chloride Excretion
         g. Arterial Blood Gases
   B. Diagnosing
   C. Planning
      1. Planning for Home Care

D. Implementing
   1. Promoting Wellness
   2. Enteral Fluid and Electrolyte Replacement
      a. Fluid Intake Modifications
      b. Dietary Changes
      c. Oral Electrolyte Supplements
   3. Parenteral Fluid and Electrolyte Replacement
      a. Intravenous Solutions
      b. Venipuncture Sites
      c. Intravenous Equipment
      d. Starting an Intravenous Infusion
         Skill 52-1 Starting an Intravenous Infusion
      e. Regulating and Monitoring Intravenous Infusions
      f. Milliliters per Hour
      g. Drops per Minute
      h. Devices to Control Infusions
         Skill 52-2 Monitoring an Intravenous Infusion
      i. Changing Intravenous Containers, Tubing, and Dressings
         Skill 52-3 Changing an Intravenous Container, Tubing, and Dressing
         Skill 52-4 Discontinuing an Intravenous Infusion
         Skill 52-5 Changing an Intravenous Catheter to an Intermittent Infusion Lock
   4. Blood Transfusions
      a. Blood Groups
      b. Rhesus (Rh) Factor
      c. Blood Typing and Crossmatching
      d. Selection of Blood Donors
      e. Blood and Blood Products for Transfusion
      f. Transfusion Reactions
      g. Administering Blood
         Skill 52-6 Initiating, Maintaining, and Terminating a Blood Transfusion Using a Y-Set
E. Evaluating

KEY TOPIC REVIEW

1. The proportion of the human body composed of fluid is surprisingly large. Approximately 90% of the average healthy adult's weight is water, the primary body fluid.
   a. True
   b. False

2. The body fluid compartments are separated from one another by cell membranes and the capillary membrane.
   a. True
   b. False
3. Osmosis is the movement of water across cell membranes, from the less concentrated solution to the more concentrated solution.
   a. True
   b. False
4. Diffusion is the power of a solution to draw water across a semipermeable membrane.
   a. True
   b. False
5. The kidneys are the primary regulator of body fluids and electrolyte balance.
   a. True
   b. False
6. The most common electrolyte imbalances are deficits or excesses in sodium, potassium, and _____.
7. Fluid volume excess (FVE) is also referred to as _____ -volemia.
8. Human _____ is commonly classified into four main groups (A, B, AB, and O).
9. The number of drops delivered per milliliter of solution varies with different brands and types of infusion sets. This rate is called the _____ factor.
10. _____, or wing-tipped, needles with plastic flaps attached to the shaft are sometimes used for IV catheters.
11. Match the following terms with the correct definition.
    a. Extracellular fluid (ECF)
    b. Cations
    c. Milliequivalent
    d. Filtration
    e. Acid
    f. Buffers
    g. Hyponatremia
    h. Dehydration
    i. Bases or alkalis
    j. Diffusion

    _____ the chemical combining power of the ion, or the capacity of cations to combine with anions to form molecules.

    _____ the continual intermingling of molecules in liquids, gases, or solids brought about by the random movement of the molecules.

    _____ found outside the cells and accounts for about one-third of total body fluid.

    _____ have a low hydrogen ion concentration and can accept hydrogen ions in solution.

    _____ or hyperosmolar imbalance, occurs when water is lost from the body, leaving the client with excess sodium.

    _____ prevent excessive changes in pH by removing or releasing hydrogen ions.

    _____ a sodium deficit, or serum sodium level of less than 135 mEq/L, and is, in acute care settings, a common electrolyte imbalance.

    _____ a substance that releases hydrogen ions (H^+) in solution.

    _____ a process whereby fluid and solutes move together across a membrane from one compartment to another.

    _____ ions that carry a positive charge.

12. _____ is a potassium deficit or a serum potassium level of less than 3.5 mEq/L.
    a. Hypokalemia
    b. Hypocalcemia
    c. Hyperkalemia
    d. Hypercalcemia
13. Hypoventilation and carbon dioxide retention cause carbonic acid levels to increase and the pH to fall below 7.35, a condition known as _____.
    a. compensation
    b. respiratory acidosis
    c. hyperphosphatemia
    d. hypochloremia

14. _____ is an indicator of urine concentration that can be performed quickly and easily by nursing personnel.
   a. Arterial blood gases
   b. Hematocrit
   c. Specific gravity
   d. Volume expander

15. The _____ is inserted in the basilic or cephalic vein just above or below the antecubital space of the right arm. The tip of the catheter rests in the superior vena cava.
   a. central dripping catheter
   b. centrally elongated catheter
   c. central venous catheters
   d. peripherally inserted central venous catheter (PICC)

16. _____, or hyperosmolar imbalance, occurs when water is lost from the body, leaving the client with excess sodium.
   a. Edema
   b. Overhydration
   c. Pitting edema
   d. Dehydration

FOCUSED STUDY TIPS

1. Discuss the selection and screening of blood donors.

2. List several examples of cations.

3. Explain dehydration.

4. Discuss gender and body size and its effects on total body water.

5. List three simple clinical measurements that the nurse can initiate without a patient care provider's order.

6. Identify three factors that generally result in fluid volume deficit.

7. List three of the six measurements that are commonly used to interpret arterial blood gas tests.

8. What is a volume expander? Give one example.

9. List and discuss the three main mechanisms that can cause edema.

10. List several of the items usually included in infusion sets.

11. Discuss lifestyle and its affect on fluid, electrolyte, and acid–base balance.

12. Describe acid–base balance and its regulation.

13. List three of the four routes of fluid output.

14. List and explain the methods by which electrolytes and other solutes move.

15. List the four main groups that human blood is commonly classified into.

CASE STUDY

A 37-year-old male client has just been admitted to the unit. His fluid intake has been about 500 mL per day. He then tells you he is very thirsty but he believes someone is trying to contaminate his water and coffee.

1. *Why is water vital to health and normal cellular function?*
2. *Explain the thirst mechanism.*
3. *List the four routes of fluid output.*

NCLEX® REVIEW QUESTIONS

1. A nurse is evaluating a nursing student's understanding of body water. Which of the following statements indicates a need for further teaching?
   1. Approximately 60% of the average healthy adult's weight is water, the primary body fluid.
   2. Infants have the highest proportion of water, accounting for 70% to 80% of their body weight.
   3. Men have a lower percentage of body water than women.
   4. Water makes up a greater percentage of a lean person's body weight than an obese person's.

2. Which of the following information about osmosis is NOT correct?
   1. Osmosis is the continual intermingling of molecules in liquids, gases, or solids brought about by the random movement of the molecules.
   2. Osmosis is an important mechanism for maintaining homeostasis and fluid balance.
   3. Osmosis occurs when the concentration of solutes on one side of a selectively permeable membrane, such as the capillary membrane, is higher than on the other side.
   4. Osmolality is determined by the total solute concentration within a fluid compartment and is measured as parts of solute per kilogram of water.

3. Which of the following is a sodium deficit, or serum sodium level of less than 135 mEq/L, and is, in acute care settings, a common electrolyte imbalance?
   1. Hypernatremia
   2. Hypokalemia
   3. Hyponatremia
   4. Hyperkalemia

4. Which of the following events occurs when a person hyperventilates?
   1. Less carbon dioxide than normal is exhaled.
   2. Carbonic acid levels increase.
   3. pH rises to greater than 7.45.
   4. More oxygen than normal is exhaled.

5. The following are normal values of arterial blood gases EXCEPT:
   1. $PaO_2 = 50-70$ mm Hg.
   2. pH $= 7.35-7.45$.
   3. $PaCO_2 = 35-45$ mm Hg.
   4. $HCO_3^- = 22-26$ mEq/L.

6. Which of the following actions is NOT appropriate for the nurse who is starting an intravenous infusion? The nurse:
   1. adjusts the pole so that the container is suspended about 1 m (3 ft) above the client's head.
   2. completely fills the drip chamber with solution.
   3. uses the client's nondominant arm, unless contraindicated.
   4. cleans the skin at the site of entry with a topical antiseptic swab.

7. A nurse is planning a seminar on wellness care and promoting fluid and electrolyte balance. Which of the following statements is correct?
   1. Consume nine to ten glasses of water daily.
   2. Limit alcohol intake because it has a diuretic effect.
   3. Avoid excess amounts of foods or fluids high in salt, sugar, and caffeine.
   4. Increase fluid intake before, during, and after strenuous exercise.

8. The nurse who is starting an intravenous infusion should avoid using all of the following EXCEPT a vein that is:
   1. damaged by previous use, phlebitis, infiltration, or sclerosis.
   2. in an area of flexion.
   3. not as visible, because it will tend to roll away from the needle.
   4. continually distended with blood, or knotted or tortuous.

9. A nurse is evaluating a nursing student's understanding of blood transfusions. Which of the following statements demonstrates a need for further teaching?
   1. A blood transfusion is the introduction of whole blood or blood components into the venous circulation.
   2. To avoid transfusing incompatible red blood cells, both blood donor and recipient are typed and their blood is crossmatched.
   3. Stop the transfusion immediately if signs of a reaction develop.
   4. Human blood is commonly classified into four main groups: A, AB, O, and AO.

10. Which of the following actions is NOT appropriate for the nurse administering blood to a client?
    1. Blood is usually administered through a #18- to #20-gauge intravenous needle or catheter.
    2. Saline is used to prime the set and flush the needle before administering blood.
    3. A transfusion should be completed within 4 hours of initiation.
    4. An S-type blood transfusion set with an in-line or add-on filter is used when administering blood.

ANSWER KEY

Chapter 1
Key Topic Review Answers

1. Promote wellness, prevent illness, restore health, care of the dying
2. a, d 3. b 4. b
5. f, a, h, j, d, g, b, i, e, c
6. Consumer, patient, client
7. a, d
8. Professionalization
9. b 10. a
11. Diagnostic-related groups
12. c
13. The right to accept or refuse care; the ability to use advanced directives

Case Study Answers

1. *What role is the nurse acting in by representing the client's needs and wishes and when assisting the client in behavior modification plans?* The nurse is acting as a change agent in this role. Nurses are continually dealing with change in the health care system.

2. *The nurse is in the process of helping the client recognize and cope with both the asthma condition and the tobacco cessation program. The nurse is acting as a change agent, and what other role is the nurse representing?* The nurse is acting as a client advocate to protect the client. The nurse may represent the client's needs to other health care providers. The nurse may suggest some medications to assist the client in his smoking cessation program, such as Zyban.

3. *According to Benner's stages of nursing expertise, in what stage is the nurse functioning?* The nurse has been practicing for 4 years. The nurse is thus at Stage IV, Proficient. (Refer to Box 1–3 in the textbook.)

Review Question Answers

1. *Answer:* 1 (Objective: 2) *Rationale:* The traditional nursing role has always entailed humanistic caring, nurturing, comforting, and supporting. Religion has also played a significant role in the development of nursing. The Christian value of "love thy neighbor as thyself " and Christ's parable of the Good Samaritan both had a significant impact on the development of Western nursing. Wars accentuate the need for nurses. Greater financial support provided through public and private health insurance programs has increased the demand for nursing care. *Nursing Process:* Assessment *Client Need:* Safe, Effective Care Environment

2. *Answer:* 3 (Objective: 6) *Rationale:* A nurse who has an advanced education and is a graduate of a nurse practitioner program is considered a nurse practitioner. Nurse practitioners usually deal with non-emergency acute or chronic illness and provide primary ambulatory care. *Nursing Process:* Assessment *Client Need:* Safe, Effective Care Environment

3. *Answer:* 2 (Objective: 8) *Rationale:* Stage III, Competent, is able to coordinate multiple complex care demands and focuses on the important aspects of care. *Nursing Process:* Assessment *Client Need:* Safe, Effective Care Environment

4. *Answer:* 4 (Objective: 1) *Rationale:* Workplace issues include inadequate staffing, heavy workloads, increased use of overtime, and difficulty recruiting and retaining nurses. *Nursing Process:* Assessment *Client Need:* Safe, Effective Care Environment

5. *Answer:* 4 (Objective: 1) *Rationale:* The ANA is actively working to improve the image of nursing. The radio commercial will most likely include information to help shape the listener's image of contemporary nursing. *Nursing Process:* Assessment *Client Need:* Safe, Effective Care Environment

6. *Answer:* 2 (Objective: 2) *Rationale:* Preventing illness—The goal of illness prevention programs is to maintain optimal health by preventing disease. Nursing activities that prevent illness include immunizations, prenatal and infant care, and prevention of sexually transmitted disease. *Nursing Process:* Planning *Client Need:* Health Promotion and Maintenance

7. *Answer:* 1 (Objective: 4) *Rationale:* Protect the public—although nurse practice acts differ in various jurisdictions, they all have a common purpose: to protect the public. *Nursing Process:* Assessment *Client Need:* Safe, Effective Care Environment

8. *Answer:* 3 (Objective: 3) *Rationale:* The caregiver role has traditionally included those activities that assist the client physically and psychologically while preserving the client's dignity. *Nursing Process:* Assessment *Client Need:* Safe, Effective Care Environment

9. *Answer:* 2 (Objective: 9) *Rationale:* Professionalization is the process of becoming professional, that is, of acquiring characteristics considered to be professional. *Nursing Process:* Implementation *Client Need:* Safe, Effective Care Environment

10. *Answer:* 4 (Objective: 7) *Rationale:* Demography is the study of population, including statistics about distribution by age and place of residence, mortality (death), and morbidity (incidence of disease). From demographic data, population needs for nursing services can be assessed. *Nursing Processes:* Assessment *Client Need:* Safe, Effective Care Environment

Chapter 2
Key Topic Review Answers

1. Registered nurses
2. a. "Right not to be harmed" either physically, emotionally, legally, financially, or socially
   b. "Right to full disclosure" without deception about what participating in a study would involve
   c. "Right to self determination" without feeling pressured to participate in studies and without constraints, coercion, or any undue influence to participate in a study
   d. "Right to privacy and confidentiality," such as ensuring anonymity of the participant
3. Confidentiality
4. Research is the application of the scientific approach to generate empirical knowledge.
5. Research
6. a. 2; b. 2; c. 1; d. 2; e. 1
7. a, b, c, e
8. i, c, a, f, j, h, d, g, e, b
9. c, d, a, b, e
10. a. mean: a measure of central tendency, computed by summing all scores and dividing by the number of subjects

   b. median: measure of central tendency, representing the exact middle score or value in a distribution of scores; the median is the value above and below which 50% of the scores lie.
   c. mode: the score or value that occurs most frequently in a distribution of scores
   d. range: a measure of variability, consisting of the difference between the highest and lowest values or dispersion, equal to the square of the standard deviation
   e. variance: a measure of variance or dispersion, equal to the square of the standard deviation
   f. standard deviation: the most frequently used measure of variability, indicating the average from which scores deviate from the mean

11. b   **12.** a   **13.** b
14. Feasibility
15. Pilot study

Case Study Answers

1. *Which theorist and theory is used as a framework to explore the concept of spirituality? Why do you think that the author used that theorist?* The framework used was Watson's theory of caring. The caring theory encompasses a humanitarian, human science orientation to human caring processes, phenomena, and experiences. Caring science includes arts and humanities as well as science.

2. *What was the purpose of this pilot study? Why did the authors use a pilot study instead of doing a more in-depth research study?* The purpose of the pilot study was to determine the perception and current practice of nursing students regarding spirituality in an attempt to identify areas of improvement within the framework of a caring nursing curriculum. The pilot study was used to test the validity of the tools and review the preliminary findings of the pilot study to see if the research questions were valid and the findings were significant to warrant a larger, in-depth study. In addition, the study tested the student population to see if spirituality was being addressed in the classroom.

3. *What were the indications for further study?* Educators need to work with the students to increase knowledge of how to identify the clients' spiritual needs, increase knowledge of different religions among the student populations, identify multidisciplinary resources, facilitate time management, and identify resources within a clinical facility for the client's spiritual needs.

4. *What tools were used in this pilot study? What was the reliability of this study?* The *Spiritual Care Inventory* (SCI) developed by Garner, Gray, Snow, and Wright (1994) was used in the pilot study after seeking permission to use the tool from the authors. This tool used qualitative and quantitative methods to assess the students' perceptions of spiritual care and the current practice of supporting spiritual care in nursing. Reliability in this study was measured by Cronbach's alpha (r = 0.8351).

Review Question Answers

1. *Answer:* 3 (Objective: 1) ***Rationale:*** Licensed practical nurses practice under the supervision of a registered nurse in a hospital, nursing home, rehabilitation center, or home health agency. LPNs (LVNs) usually provide basic direct technical care to clients. The registered nurse, who has the knowledge and skill to make more sophisticated nursing judgments, is responsible for assessing the client's condition, planning care, and evaluating the effect of care provided. ***Nursing Process:*** Implementation ***Client Need:*** Safe, Effective Care Environment

2. *Answer:* 3 (Objective: 5) ***Rationale:*** Qualitative study is not linear like quantitative research. The intent of qualitative research is to describe and then explain a phenomenon. The technique most often used to collect data for this type of research is interviews. Quantitative research progresses through systematic, logical steps according to a specific plan to collect numerical information, often under conditions of considerable control that is analyzed using statistical procedures. Ethnographic inquiry is related to selective topics specific to a group with the same beliefs or lifestyles. Pilot studies are often a tentative probe to see if further research study is needed on a topic. ***Nursing Process:*** Assessment ***Client Need:*** Safe, Effective Care Environment

3. *Answer:* 1, 2, 4 (Objective: 4) ***Rationale:*** All of the choices listed are examples of the professional nurse's activities in nursing research. One of the nurse's responsibilities with research is in safeguarding the rights of the client, which include informed consent. ***Nursing Process:*** Implementation ***Client Need:*** Safe, Effective Care Environment

4. *Answer:* 4 (Objective: 1) ***Rationale:*** The nursing student should not document any identifiers on paperwork that would be made public or could cause potential embarrassment to the client. The use of identifiers would violate the right of privacy and confidentiality for the client. ***Nursing Process:*** Implementation ***Client Need:*** Safe, Effective Care Environment

5. *Answer:* 3 (Objective: 2) ***Rationale:*** Fire safety is a mandatory in-service program for most facilities to meet insurance and safety standards. In-service education programs are administered by employers to increase the knowledge and/or skills of the employees. The term *continuing education* (CE) refers to formalized experiences designed to enlarge the knowledge or skills of practitioners that keep nurses informed of new techniques and knowledge, assist nurses in attaining expertise in a specialized area of practice, and provide nurses with information essential to nursing practice. ***Nursing Process:*** Implementation ***Client Need:*** Safe, Effective Care Environment

6. *Answer:* 1, 3 (Objective: 3) ***Rationale:*** The most appropriate assignment for the RN would be the newly diabetic patient and the patient receiving TPN due to the complexity of the care. The administration of an IV medication such as TPN needs to be done by an RN since the RN does client assessment, while the LPN can collect the data for the lab test and assist with personal care such as toileting and ambulation. ***Nursing Processes:*** Assessment, Implementation ***Client Needs:*** Safe, Effective Care Environment; Physiological Integrity; Health Promotion and Maintenance

7. *Answer:* 1, 2 (Objective: 3) ***Rationale:*** New scientific knowledge acquired with new discoveries regarding health and cultural changes that are continuously changing as time progresses are two reasons for continually revising nursing education curricula. Disease and treatments evolve as time passes so nurses must keep up to date on all medical breakthroughs. ***Nursing Process:*** Assessment ***Client Need:*** Health Promotion and Maintenance

8. *Answer:* 1 (Objective: 6) ***Rationale:*** Scientific and technological advances are key factors in keeping abreast of the changing healthcare environment. ***Nursing Process:*** Assessment ***Client Need:*** Health Promotion and Maintenance

9. *Answer:* 1, 3, 4, 5 (Objective: 7) ***Rationale:*** The research process involves identifying the problem or question, collecting the data, and analyzing the data. ***Nursing Process:*** Assessment ***Client Need:*** Health Promotion and Maintenance

10. *Answer:* 2 (Objective: 6) ***Rationale:*** All nurses involved in research have a role in safeguarding the client's rights. ***Nursing Process:*** Implementation ***Client Need:*** Safe, Effective Care Environment

Chapter 3
Key Topic Review Answers

1. *Theory* has been defined as a supposition or system of ideas that is proposed to explain a given phenomenon.

    a. It is an articulated idea about something important.

    b. Theories are also used to describe, predict, and control phenomena.

    c. Theories offer ways of looking at or conceptualizing the central interests of a discipline.

2. In the practice disciplines, the main function of theory (and research) is to provide new possibilities for understanding the discipline's practice (music, art, management, and nursing).

3. b

4. Soft; hard

5. Concepts

6. Conceptual framework; grand; conceptual model

7. Paradigm

8. a. Person or client, the recipient of nursing care (includes individuals, families, groups, and communities).

    b. Environment, the internal and external surroundings that affect the client. This includes people in the physical environment, such as families, friends, and significant others.

    c. Health, the degree of wellness or well-being experienced by the client.

    d. Nursing, the attributes, characteristics, and actions of the nurse providing care on behalf of or in conjunction with the client.

9. Nightingale's theories, interactive theories, systems theories, and developmental theories

10. b, a, c, c, a, b, c, b, c, a, b

11. Florence Nightingale

12. Philosophy

13. a

14. a. Client (person): recipient of nursing care (individuals, families, groups)

    b. Environment: internal/external surroundings that affect the client (includes people in the physical environment—families, friends, significant others)

    c. Health: degree of wellness and well-being experienced by the client

    d. Nursing: attributes, characteristics, and actions of the nurse providing care on behalf of or in conjunction with the client

15. Nursing is considered to be a practice discipline because the central focus is performance of a professional role (nursing, teaching, management, music).

Case Study Answers

1. *Choose the best nursing theory on which to base the philosophy of nursing for this particular facility.* Imogene King's theory of goal attainment would work well in a long-term facility and the assisted living facility. King developed a transactional model of interaction between the nurse and client. Her theory is based on systems theory and the behavioral sciences. However, there may be several different theories that would work in this situation.

2. *Explain the rationale for using the theory that you have choosen.* The rationale for the theory should be based on the main ideals supported by the concepts. The answer will depend on which theory the student chooses.

Review Question Answers

1. *Answer:* 2 (Objective: 1) *Rationale: Theory* is defined as a supposition or system of ideas that is proposed to explain a given phenomenon. Concepts are called the "building blocks" of theories and are difficult to explain or define. *Paradigm* refers to a pattern of shared understandings and assumptions about reality and the world. *Conceptual models* or *frameworks* are defined as a group of related ideas, statements, or concepts. They articulate a broad range of the significant relationships among the concepts of a discipline. *Nursing Process:* Assessment *Client Need:* Safe, Effective Care Environment

2. *Answer:* 2 (Objective: 3) *Rationale:* Concepts are labels given to ideas, objects, and/or events—a summary of thoughts or a way to categorize thoughts or ideas. Intelligence, motivation, learned helplessness, and/or obesity are examples of construct, which is a group of concepts. A theory is the organization of concepts or constructs that shows the relationship of the ideas with the intent of describing, explaining, or predicting. An example of a theory includes: self-care, adaptation, caring, behavioral system, unitary man, hierarchy of needs, interpersonal relationships, humanistic, and/or nurse-client transactions. *Nursing Process:* Assessment *Client Need:* Safe, Effective Care Environment

3. *Answer:* 4 (Objective: 2) *Rationale:* Jean Watson's theory is based on a humanistic and caring

concept of nursing. The holistic outlook addresses the impact and importance of altruism, sensitivity, trust, and interpersonal skills. Imogene King's theory is based on systems theory and the behavioral sciences. A transactional model of interaction between the nurse and client was developed. Creation spirituality, the client, and the environment are the basis of Roy's model of nursing. Orem's theory of nursing is based on self-care and restoring the client to the highest level of functioning. *Nursing Process*: Planning *Client Need:* Psychosocial Integrity

4. *Answer:* 4 (Objective: 3) *Rationale:* Peplau's psychodynamic nursing model is an example of a middle-range theory. Watson's, Orem's, and King's theories are considered grand theories. *Nursing Process:* Assessment *Client Need:* Safe, Effective Care Environment

5. *Answer:* 4 (Objective: 3) *Rationale:* Virginia Henderson's theory explains the 14 essential functions toward independence that a client must meet to achieve the highest level of health. Myra Estrin Levine's theory was based on four conservation principles of inpatient client resources. Dorthea Orem uses nursing interventions to meet clients' self-care needs. Madeline Leininger's theory uses transcultural nursing and caring nursing, in which the concepts are aimed toward caring and the components of a culture care theory. *Nursing Process:* Assessment *Client Need:* Safe, Effective Care Environment

6. *Answer:* 1 (Objective: 4) *Rationale:* Maintenance of system equilibrium is one of the goals of Betty Neuman's nursing theory. Orem's model is based on assisting the client to achieve the highest level of self-care. Internal and external stimuli are based on Roy's adaptation model. The last choice in this grouping of answers is not a factor in any of the nursing theories. *Nursing Process:* Planning *Client Need:* Psychosocial Integrity

7. *Answer:* 2 (Objective: 4) *Rationale:* It was an early effort to define nursing phenomena that serves as the basis for later theoretical formulations. *Nursing Process:* Assessment *Client Need:* Safe, Effective Care Environment

8. *Answer:* 3 (Objective: 5) *Rationale:* Disciplines without a strong theory and research base historically were referred to as "soft," a negative comparison with the "hard" natural sciences. Many of the soft disciplines attempted to emulate the sciences, so theory and scientific research became a more important part of academic life, both in the practice disciplines and in the humanities. *Nursing Process:* Assessment *Client Need:* Safe, Effective Care Environment

9. *Answer:* 1 (Objective: 1) *Rationale:* A conceptual framework is a group of related ideas, statements, or concepts. A philosophy is a belief system, often an early effort to define nursing phenomena, and serves as the basis for later theoretical formulations. A paradigm refers to a pattern of shared understandings and assumptions about reality and the world. *Nursing Process:* Assessment *Client Need:* Safe, Effective Care Environment

10. *Answer:* 1, 2, 3, and 5 (Objective: 4) *Rationale:* The four major concepts are considered to be: person or client, the recipient of nursing care (includes individuals, families, groups, and communities); the environment, the internal and external surroundings that affect the client—the enviroment includes people in the physical environment, such as families, friends, and significant others; health, the degree of wellness or well-being that the client experiences; and nursing, the attributes, characteristics, and actions of the nurse providing care on behalf of or in conjunction with the client. *Nursing Process:* Planning *Client Need:* Psychosocial Integrity

Chapter 4
Key Topic Review Answers

1. It is important because nurses are accountable for their professional judgments and actions.

2. Accountability is an essential concept of professional nursing practice and the law. Knowledge of laws that regulate and affect nursing practice is needed for two reasons:

a. To ensure that the nurse's decisions and actions are consistent with current legal principles.

b. To protect the nurse from liability.

3. Two functions of laws in nursing are:

a. They provide a framework for establishing the nursing actions while caring for clients.

b. They differentiate the nurse's responsibility from those of other members of the health care team.

4. b   **5.** a

6. a. Public law refers to the body of law that deals with relationships between individuals and the government and/or governmental agencies.

b. Criminal law deals with actions against the safety and welfare of the public.

7. b, d, e

8. Litigation

9. a; e; d; b; c

10. a, b, c, and d

11. b

12. Mutual recognition; interstate

13. Certification

14. Standards of care are the skills and learning commonly possessed by members of a profession. The purpose is to protect the consumer.

    a. Internal standards

    b. External standards

15. Four examples of external standards of care are:

    a. Nurse practice acts

    b. Professional organizations

    c. Nursing specialty-practice organizations

    d. Federal organizations and federal guidelines

16. a

17. A contract is considered to be expressed when the two parties discuss and agree, either orally or in writing, to terms and conditions during the creation of the contract. One example of a contract is when a travel nurse works at a hospital for a stated length of time and under stated conditions. An implied contract is one that has not been explicitly agreed to by the parties but that the law nevertheless considers as existing. An example of an implied contract is when a nurse is expected to be competent and to follow hospital policies and procedures even though the expectations were not written or discussed.

18. A right is a privilege or fundamental power to which an individual is entitled unless it is revoked by law or given up voluntarily. A responsibility is the obligation associated with a right. See Table 4–2 in Chapter 4 of the textbook for examples of the responsibilities and rights associated with each role.

19. Strike

20. a. Informed consent is an agreement by a client to accept a course of treatment or a procedure after being provided complete information, including the benefits and the risks of treatment, alternatives to the treatment, and prognosis if left untreated. Usually the client or the client's representative signs a form provided by the institution that is considered a record of informed consent.

    b. Implied consent is when the client's behavior indicates agreement or when a medical emergency occurs and the client cannot express consent.

21. b

22. The nurse's signature confirms three things:

    a. The client gives consent voluntarily after receiving enough information to give consent.

    b. The signature is authentic.

    c. The client appears competent to give consent.

23. The actions of the nurse include verification that the client is aware of the pros and cons of refusal and is making an informed decision. Documentation is essential and must include notification of the health care provider, the concerns of the client, the understanding of refusal of the client, and any witnesses to the refusal.

24. The nurse needs to know the State Practice Act because it will assist her in delegation of duties among the various personnel and also in the recognition of what is involved in the scope of nursing practice.

25. a

26. The Americans with Disabilities Act prohibits discrimination on the basis of disability in employment, public services, and public accommodations. The nurse assists individuals with disabilities to comprehend the opportunities provided by law. Also, the nurse needs to be familiar with this law because disabled nurses may be refused employment opportunities inappropriately, and the nurse manager must know the laws in order to avoid discrimination of others.

27. b

28. Stress

29. The definitions of the following terms and certain responsibilities of nurses are:

    a. Advance directives: allows persons to specify aspects of care that they wish to receive should they become unable to make or communicate their preferences. Nurses need to assess whether clients and families have an accurate understanding of advance directives and give instructions as necessary. Also, nurses must know the laws in their practicing states regarding patient self-determination.

    b. Autopsies: also called postmortem examinations. An autopsy is an examination of the body after death and is only performed in certain cases. It examines the organs and tissues to establish the exact cause of death. The nurse needs to ensure that the consent forms are signed.

    c. Certification of death: is the formal determination of death or pronouncement that must be performed by a physician, a coroner, or a nurse. The granting of the authority to nurses to pronounce death is regulated by the state or province. It is necessary by law to complete this form.

    d. Do-Not-Resuscitate orders (DNRs): are generally written by the provider when the client or proxy has expressed the wish for no resuscitation in the event of respiratory or cardiac arrest. It is written to indicate that the goal of treatment is a comfortable, dignified death and that further life-sustaining measures are not indicated. The nurse can request for a change in assignment if a DNR is contrary to the nurse's personal beliefs. The responsibility of the nurse is to make sure that the health care team is aware of any DNR orders.

e. Euthanasia: is the act of painlessly putting to death persons suffering from incurable or distressing disease. It is illegal in both Canada and the United States to perform any type of euthanasia. Some states have right-to-die statutes and honor living wills. These states legally recognize the right-to-die statutes as the client's right to refuse treatment. Nurses must know their state's policies and the Nurse Practice Acts in order to make any decisions regarding this matter.

f. Inquests: are legal inquiries into the cause or manner of a death. An inquest is usually performed when the death is a result of an accident to determine any blame. Agency policy dictates who is responsible for reporting deaths to the coroner or medical examiner.

g. Organ donation: is the donation of organs that a person 18 years or older and of sound mind can endorse. They can make a gift of any organs or their body for the following purposes: medical or dental education and research, the advancement of medical or dental science, therapy, and/or transplantation. Nurses may serve as witnesses for people consenting to donate organs.

30. Tort

31. c, d

32. HIPAA is the first nationwide legislation to protect the privacy of health information. The four specific areas of HIPAA include:

a. The electronic transfer of information among organizations

b. Standardized numbers for identifying providers, employers, and health plans

c. Security rules providing for a uniform level of protection of all health care information

d. Privacy rules that set standards defining appropriate disclosure to protect health information

33. Nurses should question any order a client questions, any order if the client's condition has changed, any verbal orders to avoid miscommunications, and any orders that are illegible, unclear, or incomplete.

Case Study Answers

1. *Did the surgeon adhere to the signed consent form that the client signed before the surgery?* No, the surgeon did not adhere to the signed consent form because the appendix was not listed in the original signed consent.

2. *Under the circumstances, what type of tort is the surgeon liable for?* Battery is the type of tort because the surgeon has intentionally and wrongfully performed an act without the client's permission.

3. *What was the operating nurse's role in this incident?* The operating nurse should have questioned the removal of the appendix since it is assumed that she reviewed the informed consent and is considered the patient's advocate.

Review Question Answers

1. *Answer:* 4 (Objective: 2) *Rationale:* The nurse with a master's degree and a certificate in maternal-infant nursing is deemed an expert in that field because of the advanced preparation. The other choices do not address the needed expertise. *Nursing Process:* Assessment *Client Needs:* Safety; Management of Care

2. *Answer:* 2, 5 (Objective: 4) *Rationale:* Of these options, the parents of the 14-year-old child and the competent older client would be the best persons to make health care decisions. The other responses are incorrect due to the altered mental state and age of consent limitations. If the child with the laceration was hemorrhaging, implied consent would be adequate enough in order to save the child's life. *Nursing Process:* Assessment *Client Need:* Safe, Effective Care Environment

3. *Answer:* 1 (Objective: 1) *Rationale:* Failing to provide discharge instructions is a form of malpractice. The nurse should document in the client's chart that discharge instructions were given verbally, the client expressed understanding of the discharge instructions, and/or a copy of the discharge instructions were given to the client or caregiver. *Nursing Process:* Implementation *Client Need:* Safe, Effective Care Environment

4. *Answer:* 3 (Objective: 4) *Rationale:* The client can give a verbal explanation for the surgical procedure and has verbalized understanding of the procedure and the physician's explanation of the surgery. Express consent is an oral or written agreement. *Nursing Process:* Assessment *Client Needs:* Safety; Safe, Effective Care Environment

5. *Answer:* 1 (Objective: 7) *Rationale:* A living will provides specific instructions about what medical treatment the client chooses to omit or refuse in the event that the client is unable to make those decisions. A durable power of attorney for health care is a notarized or witnessed statement that appoints someone to make health care decisions when the client is unable to do so. *Nursing Process:* Assessment *Client Need:* Safe, Effective Care Environment

6. *Answer:* 4 (Objective: 11) *Rationale:* Assault is the attempt or threat to touch another person unjustifiably. It often precedes battery. Battery is the willful touching of a person that may or may not cause harm. *Nursing Process:* Assessment *Client Needs:* Planning; Management of Care; Safety

7. *Answer:* 2, 5 (Objective: 1) *Rationale:* Libel is defamation by means of print, writing, or pictures. Slander is defamation by the spoken word, stating unprivileged or false works by which a reputation is damaged. Unprofessional conduct includes incompetence or gross negligence, conviction for practicing without a license, falsification of client records, illegally obtaining, using, or possessing controlled substances. According to the *Code of Ethics for Nurses,* nurses are responsible for retaining their professional boundaries. *Nursing Process:* Implementation *Client Need:* Management of Care

8. *Answer:* 3 (Objective: 1) *Rationale:* Unprofessional conduct is defined by the *Code of Ethics for Nurses.* Unethical conduct may also be addressed in nurse practice acts. It includes violation of professional ethical codes, breach of confidentiality, fraud, or refusing to care for clients of specific socioeconomic or cultural origins. *Nursing Process:* Assessment *Client Needs:* Safety; Safe, Effective Care Environment

9. *Answer:* 2 (Objective: 15) *Rationale:* The conscience clauses give hospitals the right to deny admission to abortion clients and give health care personnel, including nurses, the right to refuse to participate in abortions. When these rights are exercised, the statutes also protect the agency and employee from discrimination or retaliation. *Nursing Process:* Implementation *Client Need:* Management of Care

10. *Answer:* 4 (Objective: 2) *Rationale:* Hospital policies are not included in the laws of nursing. The other three items are functions of nursing laws. *Nursing Process:* Assessment *Client Need:* Management of Care

Chapter 5
Key Topic Review Answers

1. Values are enduring beliefs or attitudes about the worth of a person, object, idea, or action. Values are important because they influence decisions and actions, including nurses' ethical decision making.

2. Beliefs (or opinions) are interpretations that people accept as true. Beliefs do not always involve values. Values give direction to life and form the basis of behavior.

3. Attitudes

4. a. altruism b. autonomy c. human dignity d. integrity e. social justice.

5. Whenever clients hold detrimental or conflicting values regarding their health, the nurse could use values clarification as a nursing intervention.

6. Bioethics or nursing ethics

7. Morality

8. b

9. a. B; b. A; c. C; d. B; e. A; f. A; g. C; h. B

10. A statement on compassion has been added and the duty to protect patients has been broadened to include all patient rights.

11. To reach a mutual peaceful agreement that is in the best interests of the client

12. Inform, support, and mediate

13. Beneficence

14. Justice

15. Veracity

16. Accountability; responsibility

Case Study Answers

1A. *What considerations should you take into account in assisting the client to make those decisions?* You should consider the client and family's outlook and past experiences, the client's fears about and abilities to cope with this disorder, and the client's religious beliefs. As the nurse, you could use the seven questions to facilitate values clarification for the client. The process is listed in the textbook.

1B. *In what way could you assist the client in reaching decisions about further health care?* You need to let the client and family make their own choices, help guide the client and family in working through their emotions, maintain professional relationships with both the client and the family, and be aware of your own thoughts and feelings regarding this issue. You should be sure not to impose your own feelings on the client or family members.

1C. *Would an ethics committee be involved in this matter?* The ethics committee would be helpful in the decision-making process and would give recommendations. The committee is a multidisciplinary team and assists with ethical issues, client values, and professional obligations.

1D. *What principles of autonomy are applied to this situation?* Autonomy is defined as having independence or freedom from control by external forces. The final decision regarding the extent of life-promoting activities is in the hands of the client. The nurse could inform the client about advance directives and other methods that may be helpful in this matter.

2A. *What are his rights as a client?* According to the patient's Bill of Rights and HIPAA regulations, he should have a right to privacy and anonymity as a client in the hospital.

2B. *Could he take legal actions?* He would have the right to sue the hospital for privacy invasion. It would have to be proven in a court of law.

Review Question Answers

1. *Answer:* 1 (Objective: 1) *Rationale:* Laws reflect the moral values of a society, and can be offered as guidance in determining what is moral. An action can be legal but not moral. *Nursing Process:* Assessment *Client Need:* Psychosocial and Emotional Equilibrium

2. *Answer:* 4 (Objective: 3) *Rationale:* Altruism is a concern for the welfare and well-being of others. In professional practice, altruism is reflected by the nurse's concern for the welfare of patients, other nurses, and other health care providers. *Nursing Process:* Assessment *Client Need:* Psychosocial and Emotional Equilibrium

3. *Answer:* 3 (Objective: 2) *Rationale:* When clients hold unclear or conflicting values that are detrimental to their health, the nurse should use values clarification as an intervention. The behaviors listed ignore a health professional's advice, demonstrate inconsistent communication or behavior, or have confusion or uncertainty about which course of action to take in given situations. *Nursing Process:* Planning *Client Needs:* Safe, Effective Care Environment; Education and Health Promotion

4. *Answer:* 1 (Objective: 4) *Rationale:* Ethics committees include nurses and can be asked to provide guidance to a competent client, an incompetent client's family, or health care providers. They ensure that relevant facts of a case are brought out, provide a forum in which diverse views can be

expressed, provide support for caregivers, and can reduce the institution's legal risks. *Nursing Process:* Assessment *Client Need:* Safe, Effective Care Environment

5. *Answer:* 1 (Objective: 7) *Rationale:* The relationships-based (caring) theories stress courage, generosity, commitment, and the need to nurture and maintain relationships. *Nursing Process:* Implementation *Client Need:* Safe, Effective Care Environment

6. *Answer:* 2 (Objective: 6) *Rationale:* Unintentional harm occurs when the risk could not have been anticipated. The other examples are examples of intentional harm. Harm can be intentionally causing harm, placing someone at risk of harm, and unintentionally causing harm. A client may be at risk of harm as a known consequence of a nursing intervention that is intended to be helpful. *Nursing Process:* Implementation *Client Need:* Safe, Effective Care Environment

7. *Answer:* 1, 3, 4 (Objective: 5) *Rationale:* Invasion of privacy is an intentional tort and nurses and nursing staff can be held liable if convicted. HIPAA, the American Health Insurance Portability and Accountability Act of 1996, requires that health information about clients be secured in such a way that only those with the right and need to acquire the information are able to do so. The clinical faculty would already know the client they had assigned to the student. The nurse should not randomly discard any items of a client's without express permission. If the cousin is not listed on a signed release from the client and hospital, then the cousin nor other family members should not be allowed to review the client's record. *Nursing Process:* Implementation *Client Need:* Safe, Effective Care Environment

8. *Answer:* 3 (Objective: 6) *Rationale:* The nurse should inform the physician about the lack of education and/or experience and refuse to do the procedure or task. All of the other answers would make the nurse and physician negligent. However, if the nurse does not inform the physician, only the nurse would be liable. *Nursing Process:* Implementation *Client Need:* Safe, Effective Care Environment

9. *Answer:* 1 (Objective: 2) *Rationale:* All facts and information regarding a person's condition, treatment, care, progress, refusal or consent of treatment, and response to illness and treatment should be documented in the chart. *Nursing Process:* Assessment *Client Need:* Safe, Effective Care Environment

10. *Answer:* 2, 3 (Objective: 2) *Rationale:* The National Organ Transplant Act prohibits the selling of organs and/or marketing of body parts.

The other examples are acceptable. *Nursing Process:* Assessment *Client Need:* Safe, Effective Care Environment

Chapter 6
Key Topic Review Answers

1. The correct responses are:
   a. Primary prevention
   b. Secondary prevention
   c. Tertiary prevention
2. a   **3.** b   **4.** b
5. a. increase quality and years
   b. eliminate health disparities
6. a
7. Public Health Service (PHS) of the U.S. Department of Health and Human Services
8. Occupational health clinics are an important setting for employee health care. They are responsible for worker safety, health education, annual employee health screening for tuberculosis, and maintenance of immunization information. Other screenings for health concerns can be conducted at the discretion of the nurse or companies.
9. Factors affecting health care delivery include the following:
   a. Increasing number of elderly
   b. Advances in technology
   c. Economics
   d. Women's health
   e. Uneven distribution of services
   f. Access to health insurance
10. Fastest; 76.5 million; 90 million by 2030
11. One of the major alterations in how health care is practiced in this country may be attributed to the Health Insurance Portability and Accountability Act of 1996 (HIPAA). The new regulations were instituted to protect the privacy of individuals by safeguarding individually identifiable health care records, including electronic media. Violations of HIPAA regulations by health care providers or agencies can result in heavy fines for this breach of trust.
12. Case management may be used as a cost-containment strategy in managed care. Both of the systems often use critical pathways to track the client's progress. A critical pathway is an interdisciplinary plan or tool that specifies interdisciplinary assessments, interventions, treatments, and outcomes for health-related conditions across a time line.

Case Study Answers

1A. *What type of health care coverage could she have at this point?* The client could have private pay, Medicare, Medicaid, or Supplemental Security Income.

1B. *If the client's income is below the poverty level, what type of coverage could also be included in the health care coverage plan?* Supplemental Security Income is available for persons with disabilities or those who are blind or not eligible for Social Security.

2A. *What roles do the two providers fulfill?* The physical therapy could be performed by the physical therapist. Physical therapists treat movement dysfunctions by means of heat, water, exercise, massage, and electric current. They also assess client mobility and strength, provide therapeutic measures, and teach new skills. A dietitian has special knowledge about the diets required to maintain health and treat disease.

2B. *Where could the client receive the services, and what type of coverage could possibly pay for these services?* The patient could receive the services at a long-term care facility that has rehabilitative services or home health care that offers those services. Medicare Part B and the SSI could supplement it as needed.

3A. *How was the quality of care measured?* The quality of care was measured through the patient outcomes: rates of medication errors, falls, and certain infections.

3B. *What types of models were used? Define each of those types of models.* These models included total care (case method), which is defined as a client-centered model. One nurse is assigned to and is responsible for the comprehensive care of a group of clients during an 8- to 12-hour shift. Team nursing is the delivery of individualized nursing care to clients by a team led by a professional nurse. The nursing team consists of registered nurses, licensed practical nurses, and unlicensed assistive personnel. Primary nursing is a system in which one nurse is responsible for overseeing the total care of a number of clients 24 hours a day, 7 days a week, even if he or she does not personally deliver all care.

3C. *How was quality, coordination, and communication in the units affected?* The results were higher on those units that had all registered-nurse staffing as opposed to staffing that included unlicensed assistive personnel and practical nurses. The total care delivery model had the lowest quality.

3D. *Why is this type of research important in today's health care delivery systems?* It shows a relationship between the composition of the nursing staff and the quality of patient care. It is important to continue to examine delivery models and their effectiveness in order to allow optimal deployment of registered nurses in a time of nursing shortage.

Review Question Answers

1. *Answer:* 1, 4 (Objective: 5) *Rationale:* Managed care and team nursing are used as frameworks for care in today's health care system. *Nursing Process:* Assessment *Client Need:* Safe, Effective Care Environment

2. *Answer:* 3 (Objective: 5) *Rationale:* The Medicare plan is divided into two parts, Part A and Part B. Part A is available to people with disabilities and people 65 years and over. It provides insurance toward hospitalization, home care, and hospice care. Part B is voluntary and provides partial coverage of outpatient and physician services to people eligible for Part A. Part D is the voluntary prescription drug plan begun in January 2006. Medicaid is a federal public assistance program paid out of general taxes to people who require financial assistance, such as people with low incomes. *Nursing Process:* Assessment *Client Need:* Psychosocial Integrity

3. *Answer:* 2 (Objective: 5) *Rationale:* The Medicare plan is divided into two parts, Part A and Part B. Part A is available to people with disabilities and people 65 years and over. It provides insurance toward hospitalization, home care, and hospice care. Part B is voluntary and provides partial coverage of outpatient and physician services to people eligible for Part A. Part D is the voluntary prescription drug plan begun in January 2006. Medicaid is a federal public assistance program paid out of general taxes to people who require financial assistance, such as people with low incomes. *Nursing Process:* Assessment *Client Need:* Psychosocial Integrity

4. *Answer:* 1 (Objective: 5) *Rationale:* The Medicare plan is divided into two parts, Part A and Part B. Part A is available to people with disabilities and people 65 years and over. It provides insurance toward hospitalization, home care, and hospice care. Part B is voluntary and provides partial coverage of outpatient and physician services to people eligible for Part A. Part D is the voluntary prescription drug plan begun in January 2006. Medicaid is a federal public assistance program paid out of general taxes to people who require financial assistance, such as people with low incomes. *Nursing Process:* Assessment *Client Need:* Psychosocial Integrity

5. *Answer:* 4 (Objective: 5) *Rationale:* The Medicare plan is divided into two parts, Part A and Part B. Part A is available to people with disabilities and people 65 years and over. It provides insurance toward hospitalization, home care, and hospice care. Part B is voluntary and provides partial coverage of outpatient and physician services to people eligible for Part A. Part D is the voluntary prescription drug plan begun in January 2006. Medicaid is a federal public assistance program paid out of general taxes to people who require financial assistance, such as people with low incomes. *Nursing Process:* Assessment *Client Need:* Psychosocial Integrity

6. *Answer:* 1, 2, 3, 5 (Objective: 5) *Rationale:* Supplemental Security Income (SSI) is for persons with disabilities, individuals who are blind, or those who may not be eligible for Social Security. The benefits are not restricted to health care costs. Clients often use this money to purchase medicines or to cover costs of extended health care. *Nursing Process:* Assessment *Client Need:* Psychosocial

7. *Answer:* 4 (Objective: 5) *Rationale:* Diagnosis-related groups (DRGs) are a prospective payment system limiting the amount paid to hospitals that are reimbursed by Medicare. The system has categories that establish pretreatment diagnosis billing categories. *Nursing Process:* Assessment *Client Need:* Psychosocial Integrity

8. *Answer:* 1 (Objective: 4) *Rationale:* Private health insurance pays either the entire bill or 80% of the costs of health care services. *Nursing Process:* Assessment *Client Need:* Psychosocial

9. *Answer:* 3 (Objective: 2) *Rationale:* Prepaid group plans include HMOs, PPOs, PPAs, IPAs, and PHOs. Medicare and Medicaid are government programs and Blue Cross and Blue Shield are private pay insurance plans. *Nursing Process:* Assessment *Client Need:* Psychosocial Integrity

10. *Answer:* 1 (Objective: 1) *Rationale:* Immunization is not a secondary prevention, rehabilitation is a tertiary prevention, and palliative care provides comfort for the dying. *Nursing Process:* Assessment *Client Need:* Health Promotion and Maintenance

Chapter 7

Key Topic Review Answers

1. a, c, d
2. Primary care consists of:
   a. Community participation is provider directed.
   b. Professional's role is expert, provider, authority, and team leader.

c. Collaboration occurs among members of the health care team.

d. The individual of the family is the focus.

e. Access is limited.

f. Health care is available within given health care institutions.

g. Empowerment is a provider-assisted process.

3. Primary health care consists of:

a. Community participation is client directed.

b. The professional's role is facilitator, consultant, and resource.

c. Collaboration goes beyond the health care sector.

d. The community or some aggregate is the focus.

e. Access is universal.

f. Health care is available where people live and 'work.

g. Empowerment is a collaborative, enabling process.

4. CBHC is a primary health care system that provides health-related services within the context of people's daily lives—that is, in places where people spend their time, for example, in the home, in shelters, in long-term care residences, at work, in schools, in senior citizens centers, in ambulatory settings, and in hospitals. The care is directed toward a specific group within the geographical neighborhood. A physical boundary, an employer, a school district, a managed care insurance provider, or a specific medical need or category may establish the group. Community-based care is holistic and involves a broad range of services designed not only to restore health but also to promote health, prevent illness, and protect the public.

5. Community

6. Population

7. a. integrated health care system: makes all levels of care available in an integrated form—primary care, secondary care, and tertiary care. The goals are to facilitate care across settings, recovery, positive health outcomes, and the long-term benefits of modifying harmful lifestyles through health promotion and disease prevention.

b. community initiatives: are being sponsored by some hospitals or local community agencies. These initiatives, called healthy cities and healthier communities, involve members of the community to establish health priorities, set measurable goals, and determine actions to reach these goals. If a community agency is initiating this project, the associated hospital generally contributes human resources to assist in the endeavor.

c. community coalitions: bring together individuals and groups for the shared purpose of improving the community's health. Nurses are major participants and contributors in these coalitions and often assume leadership positions.

d. managed care: a common model in health care restructuring. Health care providers (hospitals, physicians, nurse practitioners, insurance carriers, and so on) join to meet health needs across the care continuum. The managed care organization serves as a "go-between" or "gatekeeper" with the client, provider, and payer. Providers are organized into groups and the client must select one from the group to which they belong. Managed care aims in this way to enhance the quality and cost-effectiveness of health care.

e. case management: is an integrative health care model that tracks client needs and services through a variety of care settings to ensure continuity. The case manager is familiar with clients' health needs and resources available through their insurance coverage so they can receive cost effective care. Another important aspect of case management is assisting the client and family to understand and navigate their way through the health care system.

f. outreach programs: using lay health workers, a method of linking underserved or high-risk populations with the formal health care system. They can minimize or reduce barriers to health care, increase access to services, and thus improve the health status of the community. They involve partnerships between nurses and members of the community.

8. a.   9. a, c, d   10. a.

Case Study Answers

1. *What are some types of community nursing that could be considered?* Occupational health nursing, school nursing, parish nursing, telehealth, public health nursing, correctional nursing, camp nurse, home health, or community nursing centers are all possible options.

2. *What skills would be needed for community nursing that might not be used in the pediatric unit?* The nurse would need to utilize roles of the nurse such as collaborator, educator, advocate, manager, and clinician. With the experience from the pediatric

ward, the nurse should consider the school nurse position role.

Review Question Answers

1. *Answer:* 2 (Objective: 7) *Rationale:* This means a collegial working relationship with another health care provider in the provision of client care. It requires the discussion of client diagnosis and cooperation in the management and delivery of care. *Nursing Process:* Planning *Client Needs:* Safety Management of Care

2. *Answer:* 1 (Objective: 6) *Rationale:* The nurse collaborator shares personal expertise with other nurses and elicits the expertise of others to ensure quality client care. The nurse also develops a sense of trust and mutual respect with peers and recognizes their unique contributions. The other responses are the interactions with other health care professionals, nursing organizations, and legislators. *Nursing Process:* Planning *Client Need:* Management of Care

3. *Answer:* 1 (Objective: 5) *Rationale:* The nurse role is diverse and comprehensive in various practice settings. The nurse providing care to individuals, families, groups, and the general community must be flexible in order to accommodate the various locations. The community may include schools, rural areas, public health, home health, camp nursing, parish nursing, and occupational health sites. *Nursing Process:* Planning *Client Need:* Management of Care

4. *Answer:* 2 (Objective: 9) *Rationale:* Discharge planning needs to begin when a client is admitted to an agency, especially in hospitals where stays are considerably shortened. Effective discharge planning involves ongoing assessment to obtain comprehensive information about the client's ongoing needs and nursing care plans to ensure those needs are met. *Nursing Process:* Assessment *Client Need:* Safe, Effective Care Environment

5. *Answer:* 2, 4, 5 (Objective: 4) *Rationale:* A home health hazard appraisal includes all areas listed, including self-care barriers, lack of wheelchair access to bathroom or home, lack of space for required equipment, or other hazards identified by the nurse. *Nursing Processes:* Planning *Client Need:* Safe, Effective Care Environment

6. *Answer:* 1 (Objective: 8) *Rationale:* The elderly client without caregivers would need a referral to meet his or her health care needs. The nurse would assess the client's personal and health data; ability to perform the activities of daily living; any physical,

cognitive, or other functional limitations; adequacy of financial resources; and any other factors. *Nursing Process:* Planning *Client Need:* Safe, Effective Care Environment

7. *Answer:* 2 (Objective: 5) *Rationale:* Community health nursing involves continuous primary health care, provides autonomy to nurses in their practice, utilizes interdisciplinary approaches, and involves other factors. *Nursing Process:* Planning *Client Need:* Safe, Effective Care Environment

8. *Answer:* 1, 3 (Objective: 3) *Rationale:* Communication needs to flow among all the citizens of a healthy community. In addition, health promotion must be promoted among all the members of the community. *Nursing Process:* Assessment *Client Need:* Safe, Effective Care Environment

9. *Answer:* 4 (Objective: 2) *Rationale:* The parish nurse serves as a personal health counselor to that community within the congregation. *Nursing Process:* Planning *Client Need:* Safe, Effective Care Environment

10. *Answer:* 3 (Objective: 2) *Rationale:* The homeless population has benefited from advanced practice nurses being in the community. Such nurses provide easier access to health care. *Nursing Process:* Implementation *Client Need:* Health Promotion and Maintenance

Chapter 8
Key Topic Review Answers

1. A number of factors have contributed to this trend, among them are rising health care costs, an aging population, and a growing emphasis on managing chronic illness and stress, preventing illness, and enhancing the quality of life. Four factors that have influenced home health growth are an increase in the elderly population, third-party payers that favor home health to control costs, the ability of agencies and institutions to successfully deliver high-technology services in the home, and consumers who prefer to receive care in the home rather than an institution.

2. Home care today involves a wide range of health care professionals providing services in the home setting to people recovering from an acute illness/injury, those who are disabled, or those with a chronic condition.

3. Hospice

4. Some of the advantages of home health nursing include the intimacy and familiarity of the home setting. There is a sharing between the client, nurse, and family members. The nurse functions independently.

5. The disadvantages of home health nursing are lack of available resources in the event of a crisis. Also, the burden of caregiving and family dynamic roles are often more apparent to the home health nurse. Nurses enter homes where the living conditions are less than desirable. (for example, no running water or electricity)

6. The home health nurse performs a variety of duties or functions:

    a. Perform physical assessments

    b. Change wound dressings

    c. Insert and maintain intravenous access for various therapies

    d. Establish and monitor indwelling urinary catheters

    e. Monitor exercise or nutritional therapies

7. a

8. Home health is reimbursed by private pay, third-party reimbursement, or a combination of sources.

9. c, b, d, a

Case Study Answers

1. *What were the community concerns with the nurse's safety?* Eighty-three rehabilitation nurses were surveyed regarding safety. They identified poor communication systems, delayed notification of dangerous situations, dangerous neighborhoods, and driving in hazardous conditions as primary concerns.

2. *What are some additional measures that could be carried out in order to promote the safety of the home health personnel?* As a preventive measure, the personnel should be trained in self-defense measures, safety issues in driving, and emergency preparedness. Communication devices such as radio or telephones, global positioning systems (GPS), reporting of any unsafe home situations, and providing an escort to dangerous neighborhoods are just a few of the examples that might be used in order to promote the safety of the staff.

Review Question Answers

1. *Answer:* 3 (Objective: 3) *Rationale:* A durable medical equipment (DME) company supplies health care equipment for the client at home. *Nursing Process:* Assessment *Client Need:* Safe, Effective Care Environment

2. *Answer:* 3 (Objective: 5) *Rationale:* The major roles of the home health nurse are those of advocate, caregiver, educator, and case manager. The nurse that is instructing the client on the diabetic diet in the role of an educator. Caregiver is an example of changing the foley, documenting the care is an example of case

management, and advocate is referring the client for a social work consultation. *Nursing Process:* Assessment *Client Need:* Safe, Effective Care Environment

3. *Answer:* 2 (Objective: 4) *Rationale:* The major roles of the home health nurse are those of advocate, caregiver, educator, and case manager. The nurse that is instructing the client on the diabetic diet in the role of an educator. Caregiver is an example of changing the Foley, documenting the care is an example of case management, and advocate is referring the client for a social work consultation. *Nursing Process:* Assessment *Client Need:* Safe, Effective Care Environment

4. *Answer:* 1 (Objective: 4) *Rationale:* The major roles of the home health nurse are those of advocate, caregiver, educator, and case manager. *Nursing Process:* Assessment *Client Need:* Safe, Effective Care Environment

5. *Answer:* 4 (Objective: 5) *Rationale:* Education is ongoing and can be considered the crux of home care practice; its goal is to help clients learn to manage as independently as possible. *Nursing Process:* Assessment *Client Need:* Health Promotion and Maintenance

6. *Answer:* 2 (Objective: 2) *Rationale:* The person receiving the care is considered the primary recipient of care, while the family members are considered to be secondary clients. *Nursing Process:* Assessment *Client Need:* Safe, Effective Care Environment

7. *Answer:* 1, 2, 4 (Objective: 7) *Rationale:* Signs of caregiver overload include all listed, except the caregiver may have feelings of anger and depression, rather than feelings of joy and happiness. There might be a dramatic change in the home environment's appearance. *Nursing Process:* Assessment *Client Need:* Safe, Effective Care Environment

8. *Answer:* 3 (Objective: 1) *Rationale:* Daily wound care is a skilled nursing task. The other tasks are not dependent on nursing care. *Nursing Process:* Assessment *Client Need:* Safe, Effective Care Environment

9. *Answer:* 3 (Objective: 3) *Rationale:* Hospice nursing is the support and care of the dying person and family. Hospice services are frequently delivered to terminally ill clients in their residence. *Nursing Process:* Assessment *Client Need:* Psychosocial Integrity

10. *Answer:* 3 (Objective: 8) *Rationale:* Discharge teaching should begin on hospital admission. However, the clients should have a choice for the home health care provided by the hospital personnel. *Nursing Process:* Assessment *Client Need:* Psychosocial Integrity

Chapter 9
Key Topic Review Answers

1. a. Central processing unit
   b. Memory and storage
   c. Keyboard and other input devices
   d. Monitor
   e. Output devices
2. Privacy, confidentiality
3. Word processors, databases, spreadsheets, communication and graphic presentation programs
4. a. Hardware: the physical part of the computer that allows the user to enter data into the computer, performs the actions of the computer's processing, and produces the computer output.
   b. Central processing unit (CPU): is in the box that contains the computer hardware necessary to process and store data.
   c. Peripherals: are located with the CPU and consist of the power supply, disk drives, chips, and connections for all the other computer hardware.
   d. Random-access memory (RAM): data and instructions for the computer are located in the RAM.
5. Portable laptop; notebook, tablet, handheld computers
6. Online; network
7. a. Word processing: ability to save and manipulate words; probably the most used computer application. It can be used in any facility in the health care setting.
   b. Databases: used to manage detailed information. One example of a database is that of a pharmacy that lists the mediation it has in stock and the strength, quantity, locations, price, and manufacturer for each of the medications.
   c. Spreadsheets: programs that manipulate words and numbers. The data is arranged into columns and rows. It can be used to manage budgets for a health care facility.
   d. Communications: these devices require software to guide the computer in connecting to a remote device and knowing what data to send or receive. An important type of communications software is electronic mail (e-mail). E-mail has become a standard method of communication worldwide.
   e. Presentation graphics programs: software programs to create charts, graphs, tables, pictures, videos, audio, and other nontext files have become increasingly popular. Users can create so-called "slide shows" for use in teaching or research presentations.
8. a. Admissions
   b. Medial records
   c. Clinical laboratory
   d. Pharmacy
   e. Finance
9. Health Insurance Portability and Accountability Act of 1996 (HIPAA)
10. a. Access to literature
    b. Computer-assisted instruction (CPI)
    c. Classroom technologies
    d. Strategies for learning at a distance

Case Study Answers

1. *If the client's results are entered into computer-based patient records (CPRs), who would be able to legally access her medical information?* Any member of the health care team can access the CPRs with the necessary passwords.

2. *The chest x-ray is abnormal and the physician wishes to consult a respiratory specialist. If he sends the x-ray film electronically to the consulting physician, that is an example of what type of medicine?* Telemedicine.

3. *What are the advantages of this type of consultation?* By using telemedicine, the client does not physically have to be seen by the specialist unless it is deemed necessary. It could possibly save time and resources, and enable quicker health care.

4. *Does the client have to sign any consent forms in regard to her electronic medical record?* The client has a right to confidentiality and privacy. The hospital should have a consent form that should be signed prior to the entering of any data into the system.

Review Question Answers

1. *Answer:* 1 (Objective: 4) *Rationale:* Paper records have already been tested by the legal community and are already understood. There are years of cost analysis from using the paper medical records to analyse and provide data regarding cost of care. Computer documentation systems are relatively new and there is not much background data found in the legal histories. *Nursing Process:* Assessment *Client Need:* Safe, Effective Care Environment

2. *Answer:* 2 (Objective: 1) *Rationale:* The World Wide Web (www) refers to the complex links among Web pages or websites, accessed through "addresses" called universal resource locators (URLs). URLs

begin with the designation http://, often followed by www. URLs end with a designation that denotes the type of site. *Nursing Process:* Assessment *Client Need:* Psychosocial Integrity

3. *Answer:* 3 (Objective: 1) *Rationale:* "Addresses" are called universal resource locators (URLs). URLs begin with the designation http://, often followed by www. URLs end with a designation that denotes the type of site. *Nursing Process:* Assessment *Client Need:* Psychosocial Integrity

4. *Answer:* 3 (Objective: 5) *Rationale:* Telemedicine uses technology to transmit electronic data about clients to persons at distant locations. However, there are legal and ethical concerns over the use of telemedicine, despite the advantages to remote locations. *Nursing Process:* Assessment *Client Need:* Safe, Effective Care Environment

5. *Answer:* 2 (Objective: 4) *Rationale:* The World Wide Web (www) refers to the complex links among Web pages or websites, accessed through "addresses" called universal resource locators (URLs). URLs begin with the designation http://, often followed by www. URLs end with a designation that denotes the type of site. For example, .com is used for commercial sites, .org for organizations, .edu for educational institutions, and .gov for government facilities. *Nursing Process:* Assessment *Client Need:* Psychosocial Integrity

6. *Answer:* 2 (Objective: 3) *Rationale:* Synchronous distance learning is used as one method of distance learning. *Nursing Process:* Assessment *Client Need:* Safe, Effective Care Environment

7. *Answer:* 2 (Objective: 6) *Rationale:* A nurse administrator may use a computer system to manage personnel, budgets, human resources, staffing, and other measures. The other tasks may be performed by a nurse administrator but they do not fit within that role for the nurse. *Nursing Process:* Assessment *Client Need:* Safe, Effective Care Environment

8. *Answer:* 1 (Objective: 3) *Rationale:* Software programs enhance the education of nurses and assist them in meeting educational needs for credentialing. *Nursing Process:* Assessment *Client Need:* Safe, Effective Care Environment

9. *Answer:* 4 (Objective: 4) *Rationale:* Confidentiality and privacy are major concerns in any health-care-related field. Nurses should participate in the ongoing debate about and development of federal laws designed to ensure patient privacy and confidentiality. HIPAA plays a major role in establishing privacy for health care

clients. *Nursing Process:* Planning *Client Need:* Safe, Effective Care Environment

10. *Answer:* 2 (Objective: 7) *Rationale:* Maintaining privacy and security of health care data is a significant issue. Additional policies and procedures are needed for protecting the confidentiality of electronic medical records. There are no national standards at this time. *Nursing Process:* Implementation *Client Need:* Safe, Effective Care Environment

Chapter 10
Key Topic Review Answers

1. Problem solving and decision making
2. a. Trial and error: a number of approaches are tried until a solution is found. Trial and error can be dangerous because the client might suffer harm if an approach is inappropriate.
   b. Intuition: the understanding or learning of things without the conscious use of reasoning also known as the sixth sense. Its use is not recommended for novices or students.
   c. Nursing Process: a systemic, rational method of planning and providing individualized nursing care. The phases of the nursing process are assessing, diagnosing, planning, implementing, and evaluating.
   d. Scientific method: most useful when the researcher is working in a controlled situation. Refer to Table 10–4 of the textbook for further information.
   e. Modified scientific method: a formalized, logical, systematic approach to solving problems that is often used by health care professionals. Refer to Table 10–4 in the textbook for further information.
3. Critical thinking
4. Inductive reasoning moves from specific examples (premises) to a generalized conclusion. Deductive reasoning is reasoning from the general premise to the specific conclusion.
5. Socratic questioning
6. Independence, fair-mindedness, insight, intellectual humility, intellectual courage to challenge the status quo and rituals, integrity, perseverance, confidence, and curiosity
7. Reflection
8. a. Identify the purpose
   b. Set the criteria
   c. Weigh the criteria
   d. Seek alternatives
   e. Examine alternatives

f. Project

g. Implement

h. Evaluate the outcome

9. Decision making is a critical-thinking process for choosing the best actions to meet a desired goal. For example, the individual who wishes to become a nurse in the United States has several possible courses of action: a diploma program, an associate degree program, or a baccalaureate program. Prospective students must choose between the options. Therefore, they must evaluate the different types of programs, as well as personal circumstances, to make a decision appropriate to their situations.

10. b.

Case Study Answers

1. *A close friend states that she is habitually overdrawing her bank checking account. She has asked you for advice with this problem. Using the Socratic questions listed in Box 10–2 of the textbook, analyze this problem*

a. Questions about the question or problem: This problem about lack of financial planning is correctly identified, important, and clear.

b. Questions about assumptions: Your friend seems to be assuming that she is always overdrawn at the bank. Is that so?

c. Questions about point of view: Can this be seen in any other way? There are two possible ways that this could be viewed. One, your friend is spending more money than she puts into her checking account. Two, your friend may not be listing all the checks and/or service fees correctly in her checkbook.

d. Questions about evidence and reasons: The evidence is the bank statement and your friend's stating the fact that she has trouble managing her checking account. What do the past 12 months' banking statements reflect in this matter?

e. Questions about implications and consequences: The implications are that her credit could be ruined and she will pay more money in overdraft fees.

Review Question Answers

1. *Answer:* 3 (Objective: 1) *Rationale:* Assumptions are not used in the nursing process. *Nursing Process:* Assessment *Client Need:* Safe, Effective Care Environment

2. *Answer:* 4 (Objective: 3) *Rationale:* Trial-and-error methods of problem solving involve trying a number of approaches until a successful one is found. This technique lacks precision and may be time consuming while trying the various approaches, the situation is not always evaluated, and the potential consequences of each option are not always considered. *Nursing Process:* Assessment *Client Need:* Safe, Effective Care Environment

3. *Answer:* 1 (Objective: 3) *Rationale:* The scientific method is logical, organized, and systematic. It is used most often to discover relationships between what is observed and the explanation for what has been observed. It is most effective in controlled situations. *Nursing Process:* Assessment *Client Need:* Safe, Effective Care Environment

4. *Answer:* 2, 3, 4 (Objective: 2) *Rationale:* The modified scientific method as used in nursing involves the interaction between client and nurse as they work together. It is used to identify potential or actual health care needs, set goals, devise a plan to meet the client's needs, and evaluate that plan's effectiveness. The process is not always linear and steps may overlap somewhat. *Nursing Process:* Assessment *Client Need:* Safe, Effective Care Environment

5. *Answer:* 4 (Objective: 4) *Rationale:* Critical thinking enables the nurse to respond quickly even when unexpected situations arise. It enables the nurse to adapt interventions to meet specific client needs. *Nursing Process:* Assessment *Client Need:* Safe, Effective Care Environment

6. *Answer:* 3 (Objective: 4) *Rationale:* Implementation of client interventions requires critical thinking and creativity. *Nursing Process:* Planning *Client Need:* Health Promotion and Maintenance

7. *Answer:* 1 (Objective: 1) *Rationale:* Intuition is the understanding or learning of things without the conscious use of reasoning, whereas research process is a formalized, logical, systematic approach to problem solving. Intuition is also known as the "sixth sense." *Nursing Process:* Assessment *Client Need:* Safe, Effective Care Environment

8. *Answer:* 3 (Objective: 3) *Rationale:* Inductive reasoning generalizations are formed from a set of facts or observations. *Nursing Process:* Assessment *Client Need:* Safe, Effective Care Environment

9. *Answer:* 1 (Objective: 4) *Rationale:* Discussing any problems in a collegial way creates the environment to support critical thinking. A nurse cannot develop or maintain critical-thinking attitudes in a vacuum. Nurses should encourage colleagues to examine evidence carefully before they come to conclusions and to avoid group thinking. *Nursing Process:* Planning *Client Need:* Safe, Effective Care Environment

10. *Answer:* 4 (Objective: 3) *Rationale:* The nursing process is defined as a systematic, rational method of planning and providing individualized nursing care. *Nursing Process:* Assessment *Client Need:* Safe, Effective Care Environment

Chapter 11
Key Topic Review Answers

1. The purpose of the nursing process is to identify a client's health status and actual or potential health care problems or needs, to establish plans to meet the identified needs, and to deliver specific nursing interventions to meet these identified needs.

2. a.

3. a.

4. The four different types of assessment are:

   a. Initial assessment

   b. Problem-focused assessment

   c. Emergency assessment

   d. Time-lapped reassessment

5. The assessment should be completed within 24 hours according to JACHO standards.

6. The four activities involved in the nursing process are:

   a. Collecting data

   b. Organizing data

   c. Validating data

   d. Documenting data

7. S, O, S, O, O, O

8. s, p, s, p

9. c

10. interview

Case Study Answers

1. *What is the objective data?* The objective data is what the medical surgical nurse observes on her initial assessment.

2. *What is the subjective data?* The recovery room nurse's report is considered subjective. The client's reporting of pain is also considered subjective data.

3. *Who is considered the primary source?* The client.

4. *Who is considered the secondary source?* The recovery room nurse.

Review Question Answers

1. *Answer:* 1, 2 (Objective: 6) *Rationale:* Vision and smell would be used. The color of the sputum and any smell associated with it may be important cues to the disease process. *Nursing Process:* Assessment *Client Need:* Safe, Effective Care Environment

2. *Answer:* 1 (Objective: 7) *Rationale:* When a person is hospitalized, he or she loses control over even the most basic decisions of daily life. Some coping mechanisms to deal with this sense of loss may be anger, or micromanaging the few things over which the person does have control. *Nursing Process:* Planning *Client Need:* Safe, Effective Care Environment

3. *Answer:* 3 (Objective: 10) *Rationale:* The distance between the interviewer and interviewee should be neither too small nor too great because people feel uncomfortable when talking to someone who is too close or too far away. The Japanese culture has an accepted difference of 36 inches, while clients from Arab countries maintain a distance of 8 to 12 inches. (Refer to Box 11–3 in the textbook.) *Nursing Process:* Assessment *Client Need:* Psychosocial Integrity

4. *Answer:* 4 (Objective: 8) *Rationale:* Open-ended questions are those questions that allow the interviewee to do the talking. They are easy to answer and are nonthreatening. (Refer to Box 11–2 in the textbook.) *Nursing Process:* Planning *Client Need:* Health Promotion and Maintenance

5. *Answer:* 3 (Objective: 3) *Rationale:* The cephalocaudal or head-to-the-toe approach begins the examination at the head; progresses to the neck, thorax, abdomen, and extremities; and ends at the toes. *Nursing Process:* Assessment *Client Need:* Health Promotion and Maintenance

6. *Answer:* 2 (Objective: 10) *Rationale:* Gordon's functional health pattern framework collects data about functional and dysfunctional behaviors. Orem delineates eight universal self-care requisites of humans. Roy uses the adaptation model and classifies observable behaviors into four categories: physiologic, self-concept, role functions, and interdependence. *Nursing Process:* Planning *Client Need:* Health Promotion and Maintenance

7. *Answer:* 2 (Objective: 2) *Rationale:* Diagnosing is analyzing data; identifying health problems, risks, and strengths; and formulating diagnostic statements. *Nursing Process:* Assessment *Client Need:* Safe, Effective Care Environment

8. *Answer:* 1 (Objective: 1) *Rationale:* The first step in the nursing process is assessment, the process of collecting data. The other processes rely on

accurate and complete data. *Nursing Process:*
Assessment *Client Need:* Safe, Effective Care
Environment

9. *Answer:* 1 (Objective: 3) *Rationale:* The
ongoing evaluation is done while or immediately
after implementing the nursing intervention.
Intermittent evaluation is performed at specified
intervals, while terminal evaluation indicates the
client's condition at the time of discharge. *Nursing
Process:* Evaluation *Client Need:* Safe, Effective
Care Environment

10. *Answer:* 2 (Objective: 5) *Rationale:* Data that
is measurable is objective data. The client's
statements and complaints of symptoms are
documented as subjective data. *Nursing Process:*
Assessment *Client Need:* Safe, Effective Care
Environment

Chapter 12
Key Topic Review Answers

1. Assessment
2. Diagnosis
3. Taxonomy
4. a. Diagnostic—statement or conclusion
   regarding the nature of a phenomenon
   b. Diagnostic labels—standardized NANDA
   names for the diagnoses
   c. Client problem statement—consists of
   diagnostic label plus the etiology (causal
   relationship between a problem and its related or
   risk factors); is called a nursing diagnosis
5. b   6. a
7. a. actual; b. risk; c. wellness; d. possible;
   e. syndrome
8. Specific
9. a. deficient; b. impaired; c. decreased;
   d. ineffective; e. compromised
10. Etiology identifies one or more probable causes
of the health problem. It gives direction to the
required nursing therapy and enables the nurse to
individualize the client's care.
11. a   12. a

Case Study Answers

1. *What is an actual nursing diagnosis for this
client?* Ineffective Therapeutic Regimen
Management

2. *What is a potential nursing diagnosis for this
client?* Risk for Peripheral Neurovascular
Dysfunction

3. *Identify one subjective and one objective
assessment to substantiate the nursing diagnosis.*
Subjective data: "I use the bathroom about 8 times
per day."
Objective data: Fingerstick blood sugar = 213 mg/dl

4. *What is the outcome goal for the patient?*
Effective Therapeutic Regimen Management for
Type II diabetes

Review Question Answers

1. *Answer:* 3 (Objectives: 2 and 4) *Rationale:* The
identification of the actual or potential health
problems of the client is the end result of the data
assessment. *Nursing Process:* Assessment *Client
Need:* Safe, Effective Care Environment

2. *Answer:* 3 (Objective: 1) *Rationale:* The
potential for sleep-pattern disturbances is a nursing
diagnosis while the other three are considered
medical diagnoses. *Nursing Process:* Planning
Client Need: Safe, Effective Care Environment

3. *Answer:* 3 (Objectives: 4 and 6) *Rationale:* The
client's problem statement consists of the diagnostic
label plus etiology, which is the causal relationship
between a problem and its related or risk factors.
Nursing Process: Diagnosis *Client Need:* Safe,
Effective Care Environment

4. *Answer:* 1, 3, 5 (Objectives: 6 and 2) *Rationale:*
All of the listed activities are part of the diagnosing
component in the nursing diagnosis except obtaining a
nursing health history and reviewing the client records
and nursing literature. *Nursing Process:* Assessment
Client Need: Safe, Effective Care Environment

5. *Answer:* 1 (Objective: 8) *Rationale:* Clarifying
the gaps and inconsistencies in the data is one of the
three continuous and sequential activities involved in
the diagnostic process. *Nursing Process:* Assessment
Client Need: Safe, Effective Care Environment

6. *Answer:* 1 (Objective: 3) *Rationale:* Some
diagnostic statements, such as wellness diagnoses
and syndrome nursing diagnoses, consist of a
NANDA label only. *Nursing Process:* Assessment
Client Need: Safe, Effective Care Environment

7. *Answer:* 2 (Objective: 7) *Rationale:* This
statement is considered a two-part statement and lists
the diagnosis with the related factors and
characteristics. *Nursing Process:* Diagnosis *Client
Need:* Safe, Effective Care Environment

8. *Answer:* 3 (Objective: 5) *Rationale:* A
collaborative problem is a type of potential problem
that nurses manage using both independent and
physician-prescribed interventions. *Nursing Process:*
Diagnosis *Client Need:* Safe, Effective Care
Environment

9. *Answer:* 1 (Objective: 5) ***Rationale:*** The basic three-part nursing diagnosis statement is called the PES format and includes the problem, etiology, and signs and symptoms. The signs and symptoms have been identified, and the PES system is ideal for beginning nursing students. ***Nursing Process:*** Diagnosis ***Client Need:*** Safe, Effective Care Environment

10. *Answer:* 3 (Objective: 6) ***Rationale:*** Qualifiers are words that have been added to some NANDA labels to give additional meaning to the diagnostic statement. ***Nursing Process:*** Diagnosis ***Client Need:*** Safe, Effective Care Environment

11. *Answer:* 1, 3, 4 (Objective: 9) ***Rationale:*** A taxonomy is a classification system or set of categories arranged based on a single principle or set of principles. The members of NANDA include staff nurses, clinical specialists, faculty, directors of nursing, deans, theorists, and researchers. The group has currently approved more than 170 nursing diagnoses labels for clinical use and testing. Physicians do not use nursing diagnoses in their practice. ***Nursing Process:*** Planning ***Client Need:*** Safe, Effective Care Environment

12. *Answer:* 1, 2, 3, 4, 5 (Objective: 2) ***Rationale:*** A nursing diagnoses has three components and consists of all of the above except the medical conditions. A medical diagnosis is made by a physician and refers to a condition that only a physician can treat. ***Nursing Process:*** Planning ***Client Need:*** Safe, Effective Care Environment

Chapter 13
Key Topic Review Answers

1. Nursing intervention

2. Planning is a deliberative, systematic phase of the nursing process that involves decision making and problem solving. Planning begins with the first client contact and continues until the nurse–client relationship ends, usually when the client is discharged from the health care agency.

3. The nurse who performs the admission assessment usually develops the initial comprehensive plan of care. Planning should be initiated as soon as possible after the initial assessment, especially because of the trend toward shorter hospital stays.

4. All nurses who work with the client do ongoing planning. As nurses obtain new information and evaluate the client's responses to care, they can individualize the initial care plan further. Ongoing planning also occurs at the beginning

of a shift as the nurse plans the care to be given that day. Using ongoing assessment data, the nurse carries out daily planning for the following purposes:

    a. To determine whether the client's health status has changed

    b. To set priorities for the client's care during the shift

    c. To decide which problems to focus on during the shift

    d. To coordinate the nurse's activities so that more than one problem can be addressed at each client contact

5. a. Prioritize problems/diagnosis.

    b. Formulate goals/desired outcomes.

    c. Select nursing interventions.

    d. Write nursing orders.

6. b, a, d, c

7. a. complete list of client problems

    b. Kardex cards for client profile, basic needs, and collaborative plans

    c. preprinted plans to address client problems

    d. critical pathways

    e. addendum to discharge plan

    f. addendum to teaching plan

    g. individualized nursing care plans for nursing diagnoses

8. Standards of care are developed and accepted by the nursing staff in order to ensure that minimally acceptable standards are met and promote efficient use of nurses' time by removing the need to author common activities that are done over and over for many of the clients in a nursing unit. The advantages of standards of care are that they promote efficient use of nurses' time, they describe achievable rather than ideal nursing care, they do not contain medical interventions, and they define the interventions for which nurses are held accountable. The disadvantages are that standards of care are not individualized and communicate the minimal acceptable standards.

9. Students are often asked to complete pathophysiology flow sheets or concept maps as a method of learning and demonstrating the linkages among disease processes, laboratory data, medications, signs and symptoms, risk factors, and other relevant data (see Figure 13–5). A rationale is the scientific principle given as the reason for selecting a particular nursing intervention. Students may also be required to cite supporting literature for

their stated rationale. Another method of organizing and representing care plan information is the use of a concept map. A concept map is a visual tool in which ideas or data are enclosed in circles or boxes and relationships between these are indicated by connecting lines or arrows. Concept maps are creative endeavors. They can take many different forms and encompass various categories of data, according to the creator's interpretation of the client or health condition.

10. On a care plan, the goals/desired outcomes describe, in terms of observable client responses, what the nurse hopes to achieve by implementing the nursing interventions. The terms *goal* and *desired outcome* are used interchangeably in this text, except when discussing and using standardized language. Some references also use the terms *expected outcome, predicted outcome, outcome criterion,* and *objective.* They are sometimes combined into one statement linked by the words "as evidenced by." The Nursing Outcomes Classification (NOC) is designed for describing client outcomes that respond to nursing interventions.

Case Study Answers

1a. *What is the first action to take at this point?* Designate a person to call 911.

1b. *If the client does not respond, what should the next action be?* Position client on the back, open airway and look for foreign obstruction; if seen perform a finger sweep; if not then face the victim and kneel astride the victim's hips. With one of your hands on top of the other, place the heel of your bottom hand on the upper abdomen below the rib cage and above the navel. Use your body weight to press into the victim's upper abdomen with a quick upward thrust. Repeat until object is expelled. If the victim has not recovered, then proceed with CPR. Continue these directions until the ambulance arrives.

1c. *What has the nurse done to assess the situation?* The nurse has identified the signs of choking in an adult victim and applied critical-thinking skills.

1d. *What parts of the nursing process are being carried out?* Assessment of the situation, making a diagnoses (actual airway obstruction), planning, implementation, reassess the situation, and evaluation.

2a. *What is the subjective and objective data?*

(O) stage 4 pressure ulcers on the coccyx, left and right malleolus, and both heels

(O) unable to turn himself in the bed

(S) "This happened so suddenly; he did not have these sores until he had the stroke and quit eating."

(O) elderly

(O) emaciated

(O) bedfast client

2b. *What nursing diagnosis will fit this situation?* Impaired skin integrity related to pressure and inadequate circulation as manifested by evidence of pressure ulcer.

2c. *What are the realistic short-term and long-term goals for this client?* Some examples of short-term goals for this client are: No further deterioration of the ulcer stage, reduce or eliminate the factors leading to the pressure ulcers, not develop an infection in the pressure ulcer. Some examples of long-term goals for this client is to have healing of pressure ulcers and/or no recurrence of pressure ulcers.

2d. *What are four nursing orders or interventions that can be used for this client?*

1. assess causative factors such as limited activity, limited mobility, any presence or absence of sensory deficits, altered nutrition and hydration status, oxygenation, any circulatory concerns, incontinence issues, etc.

2. use of pressure related devices such as foam overlays for the mattress, float the heels, etc.

3. Turn q 2 hours and have client sit up for short intervals

4. Assess stages of wounds, measure length, width, depth and locations, assess for signs of infection, amount of granulation tissue, or other abnormal findings

Review Question Answers

1. *Answer:* 2 (Objective: 8) *Rationale:* Short-term goals are useful for clients who require health care for a short time and for those who are frustrated by long-term goals that seem difficult to attain and who need the satisfaction of achieving a short-term goal. *Nursing Process:* Planning *Client Need:* Psychosocial Integrity

2. *Answer:* 1 (Objectives: 6 and 7) *Rationale:* Long-term goals are often used for clients who live at home and have chronic health problems and for clients in nursing homes, extended care facilities, and rehabilitation centers. *Nursing Process:* Planning *Client Need:* Psychosocial Integrity

3. *Answer:* 1 (Objectives: 1 and 2) *Rationale:* This intervention is known as an independent intervention. These are activities that nurses are licensed to initiate on the basis of their knowledge and skills. ***Nursing Process:*** Planning ***Client Need:*** Safe, Effective Care Environment

4. *Answer:* 3 (Objectives: 4, 5, and 6) ***Rationale:*** Prevention interventions prescribe the care needed to avoid complications or reduce risk factors. ***Nursing Process:*** Planning ***Client Need:*** Safe, Effective Care Environment

5. *Answer:* 2 (Objective: 5) ***Rationale:*** A licensed practical/vocational nurse has the necessary skills and training to insert Foley catheters. ***Nursing Process:*** Planning ***Client Need:*** Psychological Integrity

6. *Answer:* 3 (Objective: 7) ***Rationale:*** Selecting nursing interventions based on the assessment findings and nursing diagnosis is the next step in the nursing process. ***Nursing Process:*** Planning ***Client Need:*** Safe, Effective Care Environment

7. *Answer:* 1 (Objectives: 1 and 2) ***Rationale:*** This is a short-term nursing goal. It is useful for clients who require health care for a short period of time and clients who are frustrated by long-term goals that seem difficult for them to attain and who need the satisfaction of completing a short-term goal. ***Nursing Process:*** Implementation ***Client Need:*** Safe, Effective Care Environment

8. *Answer:* 4 (Objective: 2) ***Rationale:*** On the initial contact with the client, the nursing assessment begins and continues throughout the hospital stay, with reassessment during the stay and after the nursing interventions. ***Nursing Process:*** Assessment ***Client Need:*** Safe, Effective Care Environment

9. *Answer:* 2 (Objective: 10) ***Rationale:*** The client care plan is a permanent part of the record. The protocols and procedures are not part of the permanent record. The nurse's notes are sometimes called the nurse's "brain." The nurse may write down short notes about any events that happen during the shift to help the nurse to correctly document events in the client's chart. ***Nursing Process:*** Implementation ***Client Need:*** Safe, Effective Care Environment

10. *Answer:* 3 (Objective: 2) ***Rationale:*** Implementation of the nursing care plan is part of the nursing process to achieve the goals and/or outcomes. Reassessment continues at this time to see if the interventions are working effectively. The plan of care may be altered at any time during the client's stay at the facility as needed. ***Nursing Process:*** Assessment ***Client Need:*** Safe, Effective Care Environment

11. *Answer:* 1, 2, 3, 4, 5 (Objective: 11) ***Rationale:*** All of the selections are correct. Refer to Box 13–4 in the textbook. The benefits of specific nursing interventions enable nursing professionals to

provide anticipated changes in the clients. ***Nursing Process:*** Assessment ***Client Need:*** Safe, Effective Care Environment

12. *Answer:* 2 (Objective: 9) ***Rationale:*** A taxonomy of nursing outcome statements, the Nursing Outcomes Classification (NOC) has been developed to describe measurable states, behaviors, or perceptions that respond to nursing interventions. Each has a definition, a measuring scale, and indicators. ***Nursing Process:*** Assessment ***Client Need:*** Safe, Effective Care Environment

Chapter 14
Key Topic Review Answers

1. Action; client centered; outcome
2. Implementing
3. Cognitive, interpersonal, technical
4. It terminates with the documentation of the nursing activities and client responses.
5. Assessing, diagnosing, and planning

6. b	**7.** a	**8.** a	**9.** b
10. c	**11.** b	**12.** b	**13.** c

14. a. Reassessing the client
    b. Determining the nurse's need for assistance
    c. Implementing the nursing interventions
    d. Supervising the delegated care
    e. Documenting nursing activities

15. a

Case Study Answers

1. *List different potential nursing diagnoses for Mr. Sanchez, give an example of subjective and objective data, and list one nursing intervention for each diagnosis.*

    a. Grieving RT terminal illness, impending death, and overwhelming grief

    b. Subjective data: "I do not want to see my family."

    c. Objective data: client refuses to talk with family members or staff.

    d. Intervention: Provide opportunities for the client and family members to vent feelings; discuss the loss openly. Employ empathetic sharing and acknowledge the grief by sitting with client silently or talking with client during care.

2. *List other comfort measures that the nurse may implement for Mr. Sanchez.* The nurse can provide accurate information whenever the client asks questions, provide privacy during periods

of acute pain, assess response to medication administration 30 minutes after the dose was given, reposition the client, splint the area of pain, employ distraction techniques, and utilize massage and music therapy.

Review Question Answers

1. *Answer:* 3 (Objective: 10) *Rationale:* An audit means the examination or review of records. A concurrent audit is the evaluation of a client's health care while the client is still receiving care from the agency. A retrospective audit is the evaluation of a client's record after discharge from an agency. Another type of evaluation is the peer review that involves other nurses reviewing the care based on preestablished standards or criteria. *Nursing Process:* Assessment *Client Need:* Safe, Effective Care Environment

2. *Answer:* 1 (Objective: 1) *Rationale:* Nursing interventions are based on scientific knowledge, nursing research, and evidenced-based practice. The nurse implements the interventions and evaluates the desired outcomes. Based on this evaluation, the plan of care is modified, continued, or modified. Refer to Chapter 13 of the textbook. *Nursing Process:* Implementation *Client Need:* Physiological Integrity

3. *Answer:* 1 (Objective: 5) *Rationale:* Evaluating is a planned, ongoing, purposeful activity in which clients and health care professionals determine the client's progress toward achievement of goals/outcomes and the effectiveness of the nursing care plan. *Nursing Process:* Assessment *Client Need:* Safe, Effective Care Environment

4. *Answer:* 4 (Objective: 8) *Rationale:* Conclusions are drawn when the nurse uses judgments about the goal achievement status. The nurses determine whether the care plan needs to be modified. *Nursing Process:* Evaluation *Client Need:* Safe, Effective Care Environment

5. *Answer:* 1, 5 (Objective: 2) *Rationale:* One of the steps during the implementation of the plan of care is to supervise delegated care of unlicensed personnel such as nursing assistants or patient care technicians. The nurse does not supervise and direct care of the physician. *Nursing Process:* Planning *Client Need:* Safe, Effective Care Environment

6. *Answer:* 2 (Objective: 3) *Rationale:* Interpersonal skills are the combination of verbal and nonverbal activities persons use when interacting with one another. *Nursing Process:* Implementation *Client Need:* Safe, Effective Care Environment

7. *Answer:* 4 (Objective: 2) *Rationale:* The nurse would need assistance during transfer of a bilateral amputee in order to provide safe care. The nurse needs to be holistic, implement safe care, adapt activities to the individual clients, and clearly understand the needed nursing interventions. *Nursing Process:* Implementation *Client Need:* Safe, Effective Care Environment

8. *Answer:* 4 (Objective: 6) *Rationale:* Evaluating and assessing are two nursing phases of the nursing process that often overlap because the nurse is evaluating the plan of care and assessing the client's responses to it. *Nursing Process:* Assessment *Client Need:* Safe, Effective Care Environment

9. *Answer:* 2 (Objective: 8) *Rationale:* The evaluation statement consists of two parts, conclusion and supporting data. The conclusion is a statement that the goal or desired outcome was met, partially met, or not met. Supporting data are the list of client responses that support the conclusion. Reexamining the client care plan is a process of making decisions about problem status and critiquing each phase of the nursing process. *Nursing Process:* Implementation *Client Need:* Safe, Effective Care Environment

10. *Answer:* 1, 2, 3 (Objective: 9) *Rationale:* A quality assurance program is an evaluation which includes the consideration of the structures, processes, and outcomes of nursing care. Quality improvement is a philosophy and process internal to the institution, and does not rely on inspections by an external agency. *Nursing Process:* Implementation *Client Need:* Safe, Effective Care Environment

Chapter 15

Key Topic Review Answers

1. d
2. Legal; ethical duty
3. a. communication
   b. planning client care
   c. auditing health agencies
   d. research
   e. education
   f. reimbursement
   g. legal documentation
   h. health care analysis
4. a. timely
   b. complete
   c. accurate
   d. confidential
   e. client specific

5. The fax cover sheet should contain instructions that the faxed material is to be given only to the named recipient. Consent is needed from the client to fax information. All personally identifiable information (name, Social Security number, etc.) should be removed. Be sure to check that the fax number is correct, check the number twice, and get a confirmation sheet to place in the chart.

6. b

7. The traditional client record is called a source-oriented record. Each department makes notations in separate areas of the chart. Narrative charting is a traditional part of source-oriented records.

8. Advantages: It is convenient because of the forms used and it is easy to locate each department's notes regarding the client.

   Disadvantages: The information about a particular problem is scattered throughout the chart and often is not in chronological order. It can lead to decreased communication with the health care team.

9. a. The data in the chart are arranged according to the client's problems. The health care members contribute to the problem list, plan of care, and progress notes.

   b. The four basic components are the database, problem list, plan of care, and progress notes.

10. Advantages: It encourages collaboration, and the problem lists in the front of the chart alert health care members to the client's needs and make it easier to track the status of the problem.

    Disadvantages: The caregivers differ in their ability to use the required charting format, it takes vigilance to maintain the problem lists, and it is somewhat inefficient because assessments and interventions that apply to more than one problem have to be repeated.

11. a. SOAP is an acronym for subjective data (S), objective data (O), assessment (A), and plan (P) of care designed to resolve the stated problem.

    b. The SOAP format has been changed over the years to include (I) interventions, (E) evaluations of client's responses to the interventions, and (R) revision of the plan of care.

12. Charting by exception (CBE) is a documentation system in which only abnormal or significant findings or exceptions to norms are recorded. There are three key elements to CBE:

    1. use of flow sheets
    2. standards of nursing care
    3. bedside access to chart forms

Many nurses believe the saying "not charted, not done," and they may be uncomfortable with the CBE system.

13. Advantages: The case management model emphasizes quality, cost-effective care delivered within an established length of stay. It promotes collaboration and teamwork among caregivers, helps to decrease the length of stay, and makes efficient use of time.

    Disadvantages: Clients with multiple diagnoses or those with an unpredictable course of symptoms are difficult to document on a critical path.

Case Study Answers

1. *Demonstrate the correct way to correct the following note:*

   > 12/04/06 09:10am Pt stated "I am coughing so bad I am coughing junk up."—respirations 28 breaths/minute; temp 101 degrees orally; 140/76 Lt arm, sitting; pulse 96 per min—no use of accessory muscles noted. D. Smith, RN BSN
   >
   > 12/04/06 09:15am. Correction to above note-Temp 98 degrees orally-D. Smith, RN BSN

The way to correct an error made in notes is dependant on the facility policy. There are several ways to correct errors within written nurses' note. Draw a line through the mistaken entry, initial, and time corrected. Another way to correct a mistaken entry is to make an addendum or correction to the above note with date and time corrected, corrected information and nurse's signature. Refer to textbook for further information regarding documentation.

2. *What should be included in the shift report for the next shift?* Room number _____ is Michael Johnson, a 47-year-old male admitted for treatment of delirium tremens secondary to alcohol abuse. He is awake, alert, and oriented to person, place, and situation but has begun hallucinations this shift. He did become apprehensive during his care. He has a saline lock in his right forearm that is patent. He has an ulcer on the sole of his right foot (give orders for dressings, dimensions, etc.). His B/P is running around 190/104, pulse 104, respirations 22, and oral temperature is 99.3°F. He has an order for 2 mg. of Ativan prn [state order details and if he had any medications, his response to the medications].

Review Box 15–3 in the textbook for key elements of a change-of-shift report.

Review Question Answers

1. *Answer:* 4 (Objective: 4) *Rationale:* The Kardex is used to provide quick access to client information. It should be kept updated at all times. *Nursing Process:* Assessment *Client Need:* Safe, Effective Care Environment

2. *Answer:* 2, 4 (Objective: 6) *Rationale:* Skilled care clients require more extensive nursing with specialized nursing skills. The intermediate care focus is on clients with chronic illnesses. *Nursing Process:* Assessment *Client Need:* Physiological Integrity

3. *Answer:* 4 (Objective: 6) *Rationale:* The 55-year-old male with an MI would require more frequent charting due to the unstable changes occurring after a major MI. *Nursing Process:* Implementation *Client Need:* Physiological Integrity

4. *Answer:* 2 (Objective: 7) *Rationale:* Draw a line through it and write the words "mistaken entry" above or next to the original entry with your name or initials. Do not erase, blot out, or use correction fluid. Avoid writing the word "error" when recording that a mistake has been made. *Nursing Process:* Implementation *Client Need:* Physiological Integrity

5. *Answer:* 1 (Objective: 7) *Rationale:* The documentation is complete and states that education was given informing the client of consequences of refusal. *Nursing Process:* Assessment *Client Need:* Physiological Integrity

6. *Answer:* 2, 3, 5 (Objective: 2) *Rationale:* The main purposes of charting are to communicate care, help identify patterns of responses and changes in status, provide a basis for evaluation, provide a legal document, and supply validation for insurance purposes. *Nursing Process:* Assessment *Client Need:* Safe, Effective Care Environment

7. *Answer:* 4 (Objective: 3) *Rationale:* The student nurse needs to read the charts and ask questions such as "What are the diagnoses?" "What are they doing to treat the client?" "How is the client responding?" *Nursing Process:* Assessment *Client Need:* Safe, Effective Care Environment

8. *Answer:* 1 (Objective: 7) *Rationale:* The charting is specific, concise, descriptive, and nonjudgmental. The other three examples are vague. *Nursing Process:* Assessment *Client Need:* Physiological Integrity

9. *Answer:* 2 (Objective: 8) *Rationale:* When giving the change-of-shift report, the nurse should use a guide, begin by giving background information of the client, be specific, describe abnormal findings and provide supporting evidence, and stress any abnormal findings. *Nursing Process:* Implementation *Client Need:* Safe, Effective Care Environment

10. *Answer:* 4 (Objective: 1) *Rationale:* Flow-sheet charting allows nurses to record nursing data quickly and concisely. It provides an easy-to-read record of the client's condition over time. *Nursing Process:* Implementation *Client Need:* Physiological Integrity

11. *Answer:* 1, 2, 3, 5 (Objective: 1) *Rationale:* The nurse has a legal and ethical duty to maintain confidentiality of the client's record. The client's record should never be discarded into a trash can, it should be shredded or disposed of per the facility policies. The Social Security numbers are not used because the clients' are given a hospital number. *Nursing Process:* Assessment *Client Need:* Safe, Effective Care Environment

12. *Answer:* 1, 3, 4, 5 (Objective: 5) *Rationale:* The client's status or care should never be discussed in situations where other persons may overhear the privileged information. Nurses have a legal and ethical duty to maintain confidentiality of the client's record, personal information, and any other information that relates to that individual's health care. *Nursing Process:* Assessment *Client Need:* Safe, Effective Care Environment

Chapter 16
Key Topic Review Answers

1. a. They are self-regulating.
   b. They are compensatory.
   c. They tend to be regulated by negative feedback systems.
   d. They may require several feedback mechanisms to correct only one physiologic imbalance.

2. Health promotion, health maintenance, health education, illness prevention, and restorative-rehabilitation care

3. a. Physiological needs—air, food, H_2O, shelter, rest, sleep, activity, and temperature maintenance are crucial for survival.
   b. Safety and security needs—client needs to feel safe in both physical environments and in relationships.
   c. Love and belonging needs—giving and receiving affection, attaining a place in a group, and maintaining the feeling of belonging.
   d. Self-esteem needs—feelings of independence, competence, and self-respect and esteem from others such as recognition, respect, and appreciation.

e. Self-actualization—when self-esteem is satisfied, the individual strives for the innate need to develop one's maximum potential and realize one's abilities and qualities.

4. He added an additional category between the physiologic needs and the safety and security needs. This level includes sex, activity, exploration, manipulation, and novelty.

5. b

6. a. "Increase quality and years of healthy life" indicates the aging of the population

b. "Eliminate health disparities" reflects the diversity of the population. The two goals reflect the nation's changing demographics.

7. a

8. The health promotion plans need to fit the desires and priorities of the client.

9. The nurse acts as a resource person in a nonjudgmental manner.

10. All of the selections except the marital status would be relevant to the lifestyle assessment.

Case Study Answers

Answers will vary depending on each individual. Refer to the textbook and the MediaLinks for suggestions for the various health promotion activities that you have identified as concerns.

NCLEX® Review Question Answers

1. *Answer:* 5 (Objective: 10) *Rationale:* In the precontemplation stage, the person does not change his/her behavior in the next 6 months. In this stage, the client tends to avoid reading, talking, or thinking about his or her high-risk behaviors. *Nursing Process:* Assessment *Client Need:* Psychosocial Integrity

2. *Answer:* 1, 5 (Objective: 11) *Rationale:* Information dissemination is the most basic type of health promotion program. Examples are billboards, posters, brochures, newspapers, books, and health fairs. It raises the level of knowledge and awareness of individuals and groups about healthy behaviors. *Nursing Process:* Implementation *Client Need:* Health Promotion and Maintenance

3. *Answer:* 3 (Objective: 8) *Rationale:* Tertiary care begins after an illness, when a disability is fixed, stabilized, or determined to be irreversible. The focus is to assist rehabilitation and restore clients to the highest level of functioning. *Nursing Process:* Implementation *Client Need:* Health Promotion and Maintenance

4. *Answer:* 1 (Objective: 11) *Rationale:* Primary prevention is generalized health promotion and

specific protection against diseases or specific accidents targeted to a specific group. This intervention precedes disease or dysfunction and is applied to generally healthy individuals or groups. Secondary prevention emphasizes early detection of disease, prompt intervention, and health maintenance for individuals experiencing health problems. Tertiary prevention begins after an illness, when a defect or disability is fixed, stabilized, or determined to be irreversible. Its focus is to help the client rehabilitate and be restored to an optimum level of functioning within the constraints of disability. There is not limited prevention. *Nursing Process:* Implementation *Client Need:* Health Promotion and Maintenance

5. *Answer:* 3 (Objective: 13) *Rationale:* Primary prevention is generalized health promotion and specific protection against diseases or specific accidents targeted to a specific group. This intervention precedes disease or dysfunction and is applied to generally healthy individuals or groups. Secondary prevention emphasizes early detection of disease, prompt intervention, and health maintenance for individuals experiencing health problems. Tertiary prevention begins after an illness, when a defect or disability is fixed, stabilized, or determined to be irreversible. Its focus is to help the client rehabilitate and be restored to an optimum level of functioning within the constraints of disability. There is not limited prevention. *Nursing Process:* Implementation *Client Need:* Health Promotion and Maintenance

6. *Answer:* 1 (Objective: 11) *Rationale:* Primary prevention is generalized health promotion and specific protection against diseases or specific accidents targeted to a specific group. This intervention precedes disease or dysfunction and is applied to generally healthy individuals or groups. Secondary prevention emphasizes early detection of disease, prompt intervention, and health maintenance for individuals experiencing health problems. Tertiary prevention begins after an illness, when a defect or disability is fixed, stabilized, or determined to be irreversible. Its focus is to help the client rehabilitate and be restored to an optimum level of functioning within the constraints of disability. There is not limited prevention. *Nursing Process:* Implementation *Client Need:* Health Promotion and Maintenance

7. *Answer:* 1, 2, 3 (Objective: 6) *Rationale:* All of the individuals listed are engaging in health promotion activities. However, the overweight 29-year-old who engages in risky behaviors is not engaged in health promotion activity. *Nursing Process:* Assessment *Client Need:* Health Promotion and Maintenance

8. *Answer:* 4 (Objective: 10) *Rationale:* The termination stage is when the individual has complete confidence that the problem is no longer a temptation or threat. The preparation stage occurs when the person intends to take action in the immediate future. The action stage occurs when the person actively implements the changes needed to interrupt the previous risky behaviors. The maintenance stage is when the person is striving to prevent relapse by integrating newly adopted behaviors into his or her lifestyle. *Nursing Process:* Evaluation *Client Need:* Health Promotion and Maintenance

9. *Answer:* 1 (Objective: 10) *Rationale:* The maintenance stage is when the person is striving to prevent relapse by integrating newly adopted behaviors into his or her lifestyle. The termination stage is when the individual has complete confidence that the problem is no longer a temptation or threat. The preparation stage occurs when the person intends to take action in the immediate future. The action stage occurs when the person actively implements the changes needed to interrupt the previous risky behaviors. *Nursing Process:* Implementation *Client Need:* Health Promotion and Maintenance

10. *Answer:* 3 (Objective: 11) *Rationale:* The client develops his or her own plan with some assistance from the other team members as needed. *Nursing Process:* Assessment *Client Need:* Health Promotion and Maintenance

Chapter 17
Key Topic Review Answers

1. Illness is usually associated with disease but may occur independently of it. Illness is a highly personal state in which the person feels unhealthy or ill. Disease alters body functions and results in a reduction of capacities or a shortened life span.

2. b, a

3. An individual's usual pattern of behavior changes with illness and hospitalization, which disrupt a person's privacy, autonomy, lifestyle, roles, and finances. Nurses need to be aware that the illness of one member of a family affects all other members.

4. Internal variables include biologic, psychologic, and cognitive dimensions. The biologic dimension includes genetic makeup, sex, age, and developmental level. The psychologic dimension includes mind–body interactions and self-concept. The cognitive dimension includes lifestyle choices and spiritual and religious beliefs.

5. a, c—A person's decision to implement health behaviors or to take action to improve health depends on such factors as the importance of health to the

person, perceived threat of a particular disease or severity of the health care problems, perceived benefits of preventive or therapeutic actions, inconvenience and unpleasantness involved, degree of lifestyle change necessary, cultural ramifications, and cost.

6. External variables influencing health are physical environment, standards of living, family and cultural beliefs, and social support networks.

7. The seven dimensions of wellness are the physical, social, emotional, intellectual, spiritual, occupational, and environmental dimensions.

8. Etiology

9. a. Clients are not held responsible for their condition.

b. Clients are excused from certain social roles and tasks.

c. Clients are obliged to try to get well as quickly as possible.

d. Clients or their families are obliged to seek competent help.

10. a. Locus of control (LOC): a concept from social learning theory that nurses can use to determine whether clients are likely to take action regarding health—that is, whether clients believe that their health status is under their own or others' control.

b. Exacerbation: an increase in the severity of a disease or any of its signs or symptoms.

c. Health behaviors: the actions people take to understand their health state, maintain an optimal state of health, prevent illness and injury, and reach their maximum physical and mental potential.

d. Health beliefs: concepts about health that an individual believes are true.

e. Health status: level of health of an individual person, a group, or a population as assessed by that individual or by objective measures.

f. Acute illness: typically characterized by severe symptoms of relatively short duration, for example, appendicitis.

g. Remission: abatement or lessening in severity of the symptoms of a disease.

h. Risk factors: practices that have potentially negative effects on health, for example, overeating.

Case Study Answers

1. *With the goals of* Healthy People 2010, *how can the nurse assist the client?* The goals are to increase the length and quality of life and to eliminate health disparities within populations.

When the client decides to quit smoking, she will reduce her risks of many of the diseases associated with smoking. The nurse could supply the client with smoking cessation information, refer her to social support groups, and notify the physician of the client's desires.

NCLEX® Review Question Answers

1. *Answer:* 3 (Objective: 3) *Rationale:* The role performance model identifies health as the ability of an individual to fulfill societal roles, such as performing his or her own work. People are viewed as physiologic systems with related functions, and health is identified by the absence of signs and symptoms of disease or injury, in the clinical model. In the adaptive model, health is a creative process; disease is a failure in adaptation, or maladaption. The eudemonistic model incorporates a comprehensive view of health. Health is seen as a condition of actualization or realization of a person's potential. In this model the highest aspiration of people is fulfillment and complete development, which is actualization. Illness, in this model, is a condition that prevents self-actualization. *Nursing Process:* Assessment *Client Need:* Health Promotion and Maintenance

2. *Answer:* 4 (Objective: 3) *Rationale:* The role performance model identifies health as the ability of an individual to fulfill societal roles, such as performing his or her own work. People are viewed as physiologic systems with related functions, and health is identified by the absence of signs and symptoms of disease or injury, in the clinical model. In the adaptive model, health is a creative process; disease is a failure in adaptation, or maladaption. The eudemonistic model incorporates a comprehensive view of health. Health is seen as a condition of actualization or realization of a person's potential. Actualization is the apex of the fully developed personality, described by Abraham Maslow. In this model the highest aspiration of people is fulfillment and complete development, which is actualization. Illness, in this model, is a condition that prevents self-actualization. *Nursing Process:* Evaluation *Client Need:* Health Promotion and Maintenance

3. *Answer:* 2 (Objective: 4) *Rationale:* Gender influences the distribution of disease. Certain acquired and genetic diseases are more common in one sex than in the other. Genetic makeup influences biologic characteristics, innate temperament, activity level, and intellectual potential. Age is also a significant factor. The distribution of disease varies with age. Developmental level has a major impact on health status. *Nursing Process:* Assessment *Client Need:* Health Promotion and Maintenance

4. *Answer:* 4 (Objective: 5) *Rationale:* Gender influences the distribution of disease. Certain acquired and genetic diseases are more common in one sex than in the other. Genetic makeup influences biologic characteristics, innate temperament, activity level, and intellectual potential. Age is also a significant factor. The distribution of disease varies with age. Developmental level has a major impact on health status. *Nursing Process:* Assessment *Client Need:* Health Promotion and Maintenance

5. *Answer:* 2 (Objective: 9) *Rationale:* Emotional responses to stress affect body function. For example, a student who is extremely anxious before a test may experience urinary frequency and diarrhea. A person worried about the outcome of surgery or about the behavior of a teenager may chain-smoke. Prolonged emotional distress may increase susceptibility to organic disease or precipitate it. Emotional distress may influence the immune system through central nervous system and endocrine alterations. *Nursing Process:* Assessment *Client Need:* Health Promotion and Maintenance

6. *Answer:* 2, 3, 4 (Objective: 6) *Rationale:* Lifestyle choices refer to a person's general way of living that are influenced by sociocultural factors and personal characteristics. Lifestyle choices have either a positive or negative effect on health. Practices that have potentially negative effects on health are often referred to as risk factors. *Nursing Process:* Assessment *Client Need:* Health Promotion and Maintenance

7. *Answer:* 1 (Objective: 3) *Rationale:* Rosenstock's health belief model is intended to predict which individuals would or would not use preventive measures. Becker added positive health motivation to that belief model. *Nursing Process:* Assessment *Client Need:* Health Promotion and Maintenance

8. *Answer:* 2 (Objective: 4) *Rationale:* Physical wellness is the ability to carry out daily tasks and practice positive lifestyle habits. Social wellness is the ability to interact successfully with people and within the environment. Emotional wellness is the ability to manage stress and express emotions appropriately. Intellectual wellness is the ability to learn and use that information positively. *Nursing Process:* Assessment *Client Need:* Health Promotion and Maintenance

9. *Answer:* 2 (Objective: 5) *Rationale:* Many factors influence adherence to healthy practices. Role modeling by the nurse is a very important aspect when teaching clients about healthier choices. ***Nursing Process:*** Implementation ***Client Need:*** Health Promotion and Maintenance

10. ***Answer:*** 3 (Objective: 6) ***Rationale:*** Illness is a highly personal state in which the person's physical, emotional, intellectual, social, developmental, or spiritual functioning is diminished. Acute illness is typically characterized by severe symptoms of relatively short duration. Disease can be described as an alteration in body functions resulting in a reduction of capacities or a shortening of the normal life span. The causation of a disease is called its etiology. A chronic illness is one that lasts for an extended period, usually 6 months or longer, and often for the person's life. ***Nursing Process:*** Assessment ***Client Need:*** Health Promotion and Maintenance

Chapter 18
Key Topic Review Answers

1. a. Culture can be defined as the nonphysical traits, such as values, beliefs, attitudes, and customs that are shared by a group of people and passed from one generation to the next. It is also considered the "thoughts, communications, actions, customs, beliefs, values, and institutions of racial, ethnic, religious, or social groups.

    b. It defines how health is perceived, how health care information is received, how rights and protections are exercised, how a health problem is defined, how concerns are expressed, who should provide treatment, and how and what kind of treatment should be given.

2. Heritage

3. The U.S. Department of Health and Human Services (DHHS) houses the Office of Minority Health "to improve and protect the health of racial and ethnic minority populations through the development of health policies and programs that will eliminate health disparities. In collaboration with other organizations, it developed the *National Standards for Culturally and Linguistically Appropriate Services in Health Class* (CLAS). Culture and language have a considerable impact on how clients access and respond to health care services.

4. The Centers for Disease Control (CDC) has an Office of Minority Health to "promote health and quality of life by preventing and controlling the disproportionate burden of disease, injury and disability among racial and ethnic minority populations."

5. The purpose of the National Center on Minority Health and Health Disparities (NCMHD) in the National Institutes of Health is to promote minority health and to lead, coordinate, support and assess the NIH effort to reduce and ultimately eliminate health disparities.

6. The nursing profession plays a major role in REACH by striving to eliminate racial and ethnic disparities in infant mortality; in screening and management of breast and cervical cancer, cardiovascular diseases, diabetes, and HIV infections/AIDS; and in child and adult immunizations.

7. One of the major goals of *Healthy People 2010* is to eliminate health disparities by gender, race or ethnicity, education, income, disability, geographic location, and sexual orientation.

8. It influences nursing in ways because it includes a comprehensive overview of disparities in health care among racial, ethnic, and socioeconomic groups in the general U.S. population and among priority populations.

9. Culturally sensitive nursing implies basic knowledge of and constructive attitudes toward the health traditions observed among the diverse cultural group found in the setting in which the nurse is practicing.

Culturally appropriate nursing implies that nurses apply the underlying background knowledge that must be possessed to provide the client with the best possible health care.

Culturally competent nursing implies that the nurse understands and attends to the total content of the client's situation and uses a complex combination of knowledge, attitudes, and skills. Providing nursing care within these three parameters is critical.

10. Madeline Leininger

Case Study Answers

1a. *If the nurse is culturally competent, what would be an appropriate comment?* "Are these areas from using traditional treatments to aid in healing your illness?"

1b. *If the nurse has xenophobia, what comment might the nurse make regarding the coining or cupping that occurred?* "You appear to be too smart to believe cupping will actually cure you!"

1c. *Give an example of an ethnocentric statement from the nurse.* "An antibiotic would treat you quicker than these bruises. We have a better success rate with antibiotics, and it's less painful!"

1d. *What nurse action would be considered discrimination?* Denying the client basic care or any medical treatment that one might offer other clients.

2a. *If the client does not return direct eye contact, is this indicative of a cultural difference or a result of a "shifty," evasive client?* Hispanic culture does not always use direct eye contact. The nurse must meet all clients with a nonjudgmental attitude.

2b. *The client's family desires to spend as much time with him as possible, including staying after hours. How does the nurse handle this situation?* The nurse should use her own judgment and see if the family members are hindering the client's recovery process. It may be necessary to obtain a physician's order or the supervisor's permission for the family to remain after hours. If the family members are disturbing other clients, they may need to leave, or have only one or two family members remain with the client.

2c. *The client does not want to take his preventative medication (Reglan) to prevent stress ulcers. He stated that his life and recovery status were in God's hands, and that he had "no need of pharmaceutical medications." What action should the nurse take at this time?* Notify the physician of the client's wishes to decline the medication and explain the consequences of the medication refusal to the client.

NCLEX® Review Question Answers

1. *Answer:* 1, 3 (Objective: 1) *Rationale:* The demographic changes in the overall population of the United States and the influence of immigration on health services are two major reasons for the immense need for culturally focused nursing care. *Nursing Process:* Assessment *Client Need:* Psychosocial Integrity

2. *Answer:* 1 (Objective: 9) *Rationale:* Bicultural is used to describe a person with dual patterns of identification who crosses two cultures, lifestyles, and sets of values. *Nursing Process:* Assessment *Client Need:* Psychosocial Integrity

3. *Answer:* 3 (Objective: 8) *Rationale:* Diversity refers to the fact or state of being different. Many factors account for diversity: race, gender, sexual orientation, culture, ethnicity, socioeconomic status, educational attainment, religious affiliation, and so on. *Nursing Process:* Assessment *Client Need:* Psychosocial Integrity

4. *Answer:* 2 (Objective: 8) *Rationale:* Acculturation is the involuntary process that occurs when people adapt to or borrow traits from another culture. *Nursing Process:* Assessment *Client Need:* Psychosocial Integrity

5. *Answer:* 3 (Objective: 9) *Rationale:* Assimilation is the process by which an individual develops a new cultural identity. It means the person becomes similar to the members of the dominant culture. *Nursing Process:* Assessment *Client Need:* Psychosocial Integrity

6. *Answer:* 3 (Objective: 5) *Rationale:* Stereotyping is assuming that all members of a culture or ethnic group are alike, instead of unique individuals. *Nursing Process:* Assessment *Client Need:* Psychosocial Integrity

7. *Answer:* 4 (Objective: 2) *Rationale:* Exorcism is considered both a mental and spiritual method of maintaining health, protecting health, and restoring health. *Nursing Process:* Assessment *Client Need:* Psychosocial Integrity

8. *Answer:* 1 (Objective: 3) *Rationale:* Massage is an example of complementary and alternative medicine (CAM) that is being used as an alternative to Western medical treatment. *Nursing Process:* Assessment *Client Need:* Psychosocial Integrity

9. *Answer:* 4 (Objective: 3) *Rationale:* An interpreter is "an individual who mediates spoken or signed communication between people speaking different languages, without adding, omitting, or distorting material from one language to another. *Nursing Process:* Planning *Client Need:* Psychosocial Integrity

10. *Answer:* 1 (Objective: 6) *Rationale:* Stereotyping is assuming that all members of a culture or ethnic group are alike. Stereotyping that is unrelated to reality may be based on racism or discrimination. *Nursing Process:* Assessment *Client Need:* Safe, Effective Care Environment

11. *Answer:* 2, 3, 5 (Objective: 9) *Rationale:* Health beliefs and practices, family patterns, communication style, space and time orientation, and nutritional patterns may influence the relationship between the nurse and the client who have different cultural backgrounds. Avoid slang words and do not use a member of the client's family to act as an interpreter because the client may not want the family to know about his condition. *Nursing Process:* Assessment *Client Need:* Safe, Effective Care Environment

12. *Answer:* 1, 3, 4 (Objective: 7) *Rationale:* Nurses are encouraged to integrate cultural skills, encounters, desires, awareness, and knowledge. Methods to obtain the integration include in-services, community events that entertain other cultures, and by reviewing professional nursing journals that include cultural awareness topics. *Nursing Process:* Assessment *Client Need:* Safe, Effective Care Environment.

Chapter 19

Key Topic Review Answers

1. Holism
2. The focus of the AHNA is to enhance the healing of the whole person from birth to death.
3. When the nurse takes time to be with clients in deeply caring ways and balance technology and compassion, that nurse creates a healing environment.
4. a. Identify behaviors that indicate over involvement (example = saying yes instead of no, feeling selfish when you do say no).
   b. Perform relaxation exercises on a regular basis.
   c. Maintain and enhance your physical health.
   d. Develop support networks with other nurses or health care workers.
5. a, d, e
6. Energy
7. Chiropractic
8. b, d, e, a, c, f
9. Pregnancy, pacemakers, implanted defibrillators, aneurysm clips in the brain, cochlear implants, or other implanted electric devices are contraindications for magnetic therapy, the emerging science that studies how living organisms interact with electromagnetic fields.
10. Chelatin therapy is the introduction of chemicals into the bloodstream that bind with heavy minerals in the body.

Case Study Answers

1. *During the initial assessment interview with an elderly client, what type of questions should the nurse ask to investigate the use of complementary and alternative therapies?* What alternative therapies have you used, such as acupuncture, touch therapies, herbs, or dietary supplements? Tell me about any teas, herbs, vitamins, or other natural products you use to improve your health.

2. *What popular herbal preparation could affect bruising and cause a decrease in antihypertensive medication effectiveness?* Garlic increases the anticoagulant effects of aspirin and may also decrease the effects of the antihypertensive medication.

NCLEX® Review Question Answers

1. *Answer:* 1, 2, 3 (Objective: 1) *Rationale:* Holism is a combination of mental, emotional, spiritual, relationship, and environmental components. Humanism perspective includes propositions such as the mind and body are indivisible and well-being is a combination of personal satisfaction and contributions to the larger community. Balance is a concept that consists of mental, physical, emotional, spiritual, and environmental components. *Nursing Process:* Assessment *Client Need:* Psychosocial Integrity

2. *Answer:* 1 (Objective: 4) *Rationale:* Naturopathic medicines are a system of medicine and a way of life. Naturopathic medicine may be the model health system of the future. It is the restoration of health and normal body function, rather than the application of a particular therapy. Homeopathy is a self-healing system, assisted by small doses of remedies or medicines, which is useful in a variety of acute and chronic disorders. Nutritional therapy consists of the consumption of several kinds of diets. Chiropractic practitioners believe that health is a state of balance, especially of the nervous and musculoskeletal systems. *Nursing Process:* Assessment *Client Need:* Health Promotion and Maintenance

3. *Answer:* 3 (Objective: 7) *Rationale:* Hydrotherapy and colonic are not recommended for those populations. Nurses should not "prescribe" any types of alternative treatments without discussing with the client and health care members. Clients may not always recognize that certain herbs or teas may interfere with other prescriptions being taken. *Nursing Process:* Assessment *Client Need:* Safe, Effective Care Environment

4. *Answer:* 3 (Objective: 3) *Rationale:* Pilates is a method of physical movement and exercise designed to stretch, strengthen, and balance the body. Increased lung capacity, improved flexibility and joint health, improved muscular coordination, increased bone density, and better posture and balance are possible benefits. *Nursing Process:* Planning *Client Need:* Health Promotion and Maintenance

5. *Answer:* 3 (Objective: 8) *Rationale:* Infrared photoenergy therapies improve sensory impairment associated with peripheral neuropathy. The treatment is believed to work by increasing energy inside the cells. *Nursing Process:* Planning *Client Need:* Physiological Integrity

6. *Answer:* 4 (Objective: 10) *Rationale:* Humor and laughter in nursing is defined as helping the client "to perceive, appreciate, and express what is funny, amusing, or ludicrous in order to establish relationships, relieve tension, release anger, facilitate learning or cope with painful feelings" (Docihterman & Bulecheck, 2004, p. 422). *Nursing Process:* Planning *Client Need:* Psychosocial Integrity

7. Answer: 3 (Objective: 10) **Rationale:** The program consists of 110 hours of in-depth, hands-on training to provide nurses with training in relaxation and therapeutic imagery skills. **Nursing Process:** Assessment **Client Need:** Physiological Integrity.

8. Answer: 1 (Objective: 7) **Rationale:** Physical resting and rhythmic breathing are used in all three modalities of CAM. Meditation is a general term for a wide range of practices that involve relaxing the body and easing the mind. Guided imagery is a two-way communication between the conscious and unconscious mind and involves the whole body and all of its senses. It is a state of focused attention that encourages changes in attitudes, behaviors, and physiologic reactions. Biofeedback is a method for learned control of physiologic responses of the body. **Nursing Process:** Planning **Client Need:** Physiological Integrity

9. Answer: 3 (Objectives: 2 and 3) **Rationale:** Music without words is often used to relax and distract clients in a variety of settings, such as operating rooms and birthing rooms. **Nursing Process:** Implementation **Client Need:** Physiological Integrity

10. Answer: 3, 5, 6 (Objective: 2) **Rationale:** Massage aids in the relief of muscle tension, reduces muscle spasms, and increases relaxation. Music without words is often used to relax and distract clients in a variety of settings. Guided imagery is a two-way communication between the conscious and unconscious mind and involves the whole body and all of its senses. It is a state of focused attention that encourages changes in attitudes, behaviors, and physiologic reactions. **Nursing Process:** Implementation **Client Need:** Physiological Integrity

Chapter 20
Key Topic Review Answers

1. Growth is defined as physical change and increase in size. Some indicators of growth include height, weight, bone size, and dentition.

2. Development is an increase in the complexity of function and skill progression. It is the capacity and skill of a person to adapt to the environment and is the behavior aspect of growth.

3. Genetics, temperament, family influence, adequate nutrition, environmental conditions, the state of the individual's health, and cultural influences all affect development.

4. Psychosocial development refers to the development of personality.

5. Defense mechanisms, or adaptive mechanisms, as they are more commonly called today, are the result of

conflicts between the id's impulses and the anxiety created by the conflicts due to social and environmental restrictions. The third aspect of the personality, according to Freud, is the superego. The superego contains the conscience and the ego ideal. The conscience consists of society's "do not's," usually as a result of parental and cultural expectations. The ego ideal comprises the standards of perfection toward which the individual strives. Freud proposed that the underlying motivation to human development is a dynamic, psychic energy, which he called libido.

6. Social learning theory states that learning can occur by observation. Role modeling and learning from watching role models are a part of social learning theory. Attention and cognitive function, in which the individual thinks about the behavior of self and others, as well as the expected rewards and punishments for certain behaviors, are important to social learning.

7. Moral development—a complex process not fully understood—involves learning what ought not to be done. Kohlberg's theory focuses on the reason an individual makes a decision.

8. Behaviorist learning theory emphasizes stimulus-response and either positive or negative reinforcement as the basis for learning and behavior change.

9. Fowler and Westerhoff are two theorists who describe stages of spiritual development or faith. The spiritual component of growth and development refers to individuals' understanding of their relationship with the universe and their perceptions about the direction and meaning of life.

10. a. Accommodation is a process of change whereby cognitive processes mature sufficiently to allow the person to solve problems that were unsolvable before.

   b. Adaptation, or coping behavior, is the ability to handle the demands made by the environment.

   c. Assimilation is the process through which humans encounter and react to the new situations by using the mechanisms they already possess.

   d. Developmental task is a task which arises at or about a certain period in the life of an individual, successful achievement of which leads to his happiness and to success with later tasks, while failure leads to unhappiness in the individual, disapproval by society, and difficulty with later tasks.

Case Study Answers

1. *What topics are listed on this website?*
The NICHD maintains and is involved in a number

of health communication campaigns and programs. For more information on the projects, visit the website.

2. *What other information could be obtained from the site?* Information about different developmental tasks that should occur during childhood is noted on this site, and information about clinical trials is also given. It provides regularly updated information about federally and privately supported clinical research in human volunteers. This would be a great site to use for later reference.

NCLEX® Review Question Answers

1. *Answer:* 4 (Objective: 2) *Rationale:* The cephaolocaudal direction of growth starts at the head and moves to the trunk, legs, and the feet. This pattern is very obvious at birth, when the head of the infant is larger than the body. Proximodistal describes growth from the center of the body outward. *Nursing Process:* Assessment *Client Need:* Physiological Integrity

2. *Answer:* 3 (Objective: 10) *Rationale:* The preconceptual phase is from age 2–4 years. The significant behavior at this phase is when toddlers associate words with objects and everything relates to "me." The toddler associates the nurse with the needle and pain. Primary circular reaction is stage 2 from ages 1–4 months where the significant behavior is perception of events are centered on the body and objects are extension of self. Intuitive through phase is ages 2–4 years and the significant behavior uses an egocentric approach to accommodate the demands of an environment. Concrete operations phase is ages 7–11 years and the significant behaviors includes solving concrete problems, etc. Refer to Table 20–6 in the textbook. *Nursing Process:* Implementation *Client Need:* Physiological Integrity

3. *Answer:* 2 (Objective: 9) *Rationale:* According to Peck, preoccupation with declining body functions reduces happiness and satisfaction with life. The individual is adjusting to decreasing physical capacities and maintaining feelings of well-being. Ego differentiation versus work-role perception is when an adult's identity and feelings of worth are highly dependent on that person's work role. Body transcendence versus body preoccupation and this task calls for the individual to adjust to decreasing physical capacities and at the same time maintain feelings of well-being. Preoccupation with declining body functions reduces happiness and satisfaction with life. Integrity versus despair is Erikson's stage of development that deals with maturity. *Nursing Process:* Assessment *Client Need:* Physiological Needs

4. *Answer:* 1 (Objective: 8) *Rationale:* Adolescents are achieving new and mature relations. The other answers apply to other stages of development that take place after adolescents. Havighurst believed learning is basic to life and that people continue to learn throughout life. His developmental tasks provide a framework that the nurse can use to evaluate a person's general accomplishments. *Nursing Process:* Assessment, Evaluation *Client Need:* Health Promotion and Maintenance

5. *Answer:* 1 (Objective: 11) *Rationale:* Morals means relating to "both right and wrong" and morality refers to the requirements that are necessary for people to live together in society. Moral behaviors are how the client perceives morality and responds to it, while moral development is the pattern of changes while aging in moral behavior. *Nursing Process:* Assessment *Client Need:* Health Promotion and Maintenance

6. *Answer:* 4 (Objective: 9) *Rationale:* Peck's theory believes mental and social capacities tend to increase in the later part of life. In Freud's theory of psychosexual development, the personality develops in five overlapping stages from birth to adulthood. Piaget's theory deals with the child's cognitive ability. Kohlberg's theory deals with males and is not applicable. *Nursing Process:* Assessment *Client Need:* Safe, Effective Care Environment

7. *Answer:* 3 (Objective: 9) *Rationale:* Stage 4 is when marriages and careers are established. The other answers apply to other stages. *Nursing Process:* Assessment *Client Need:* Health Promotion and Maintenance

8. *Answer:* 2 (Objective: 11) *Rationale:* In this stage, women feel the need for a caring relationship. Stage 1 is when women feel more isolated and selfish. Stage 3 is when women identify the need for balance between caring for self and others. There is an increased awareness of responsibility. *Nursing Process:* Assessment *Client Need:* Psychosocial Integrity

Chapter 21
Key Topic Review Answers

1. Prenatal or intrauterine development lasts approximately 9 calendar months (10 lunar months) or 38 to 40 weeks, depending on the method of calculation.

2. Trimesters; 3

3. a. Embryonic phase is first semester—the fertilized ovum develops into an organism.

   b. Fetal phase is second trimester—rapid growth of fetus occurs and it resembles a small baby.

c. Third trimester—the baby is approximately 20 inches in length and approximately 7 pounds in weight

4. 1. Underweight before pregnancy

    2. Less than 21 pounds gained during pregnancy

    3. Low socioeconomic level

    4. High stress levels, including physical or emotional abuse

    5. History of abortion

5. Doubles; 5th; triples; 12

6. Interactions between individual and environment

7. Voluntary control increases and they learn to walk and speak, learn to control their bladder and bowels, and learn about their environment.

8. Initiative versus guilt and shame

9. a

10. a, c, e

Case Study Answers

1a. *What reflex disappears after 8 months?* The plantar reflex disappears after 8 months.

1b. *If this reflex persists after 1 year and remains positive, what does that indicate?* If the Babinski reflex persists after 1 year, it could indicate possible upper motor neuron damage.

2a. *Each year, how many children under the age of 5 die due to environment-related diseases?* Each year, 3 million children under the age of 5 die to environment-related diseases.

2b. *What are the three leading causes of death for children under the age of 5?* The three leading causes of death are acute respiratory infections, diarrheal diseases related to contaminated water and poor sanitation, and malaria.

NCLEX® Review Question Answers

1. *Answer:* 1 (Objectives: 8 and 10) *Rationale:* Significant changes in maternal temperature can alter the amniotic fluid and fetus which may result in birth defects. Temperature maintenance is one of the areas of health promotion. Oxygen, nutrition and fluids, rest, safe activities, and safety are also areas of instruction for pregnant mothers in order to promote a safe pregnancy and delivery of a healthy child. *Nursing Process:* Assessment and Implementation *Client Needs:* Safe, Effective Care Environment, Health Promotion and Maintenance

2. *Answer:* 4 (Objective: 4) *Rationale:* According to Piaget, school-age children begin the phase of concrete operations. Children learn about cause and effect during this time and learn to distinguish fantasy from fact. *Nursing Process:* Assessment *Client Need:* Psychosocial Integrity

3. *Answer:* 2 (Objective: 8) *Rationale:* The increasing number of overweight children contributes to an increasing incidence of hypertension and type 2 diabetes. Falls occur more often in the late adult stage, while colic is seen in infants. Unprotected sex occurs more often in the adolescence period. *Nursing Process:* Assessment *Client Need:* Health Promotion and Maintenance

4. *Answer:* 2 (Objective: 1) *Rationale:* The fetus starts to move around 5 months and the mother may feel the movements. All the other responses are incorrect based on normal prenatal development. The fetal heartbeat may also be heard around this time. *Nursing Process:* Assessment *Client Need:* Physiological Integrity

5. *Answer:* 2, 3, 4, 5 (Objective: 7) *Rationale:* The Denver Developmental Screening Test (DDST-II) is used to screen children from birth to 6 years of age. The test compares the abilities of the child with an average group of children of the same age. Four main areas of development screened are personal-social, fine-motor adaptive, language, and gross motor. *Nursing Process:* Assessment *Client Need:* Physiological Integrity

6. *Answer:* 3 (Objective: 2) *Rationale:* The heads of many newborn babies are misshapen because of head molding that occurs during vaginal deliveries. Fontanels are unossified membranous gaps in the bone structure of the skull. Sutures are junction lines of the skull bones that override to provide flexibility for molding of the head. The head usually regains its symmetry in approximately one week. All other responses are incorrect responses to the new mother. *Nursing Process:* Assessment *Client Need:* Health Promotion and Maintenance

7. *Answer:* 3 (Objective: 7) *Rationale:* Stroking the side of the foot elicits the Babinski reflex. Touching or stroking the baby's cheek causes the rooting reflex, the head turns to the touched side. It will disappear after 4 months. The stepping reflex can be elicited by holding the baby upright so that the feet touch a flat surface. The legs move up and down as if walking. This reflex disappears around 2 months. The plantar reflex occurs when an object is placed just beneath the toes and causes the toes to curl around it. This reflex disappears after 8–10 months. *Nursing Process:* Assessment *Client Need:* Physiological Integrity

8. *Answer:* 1 (Objectives: 2 and 7) *Rationale:* The toddler can walk, stand, dress self, and recognize and delay elimination. By 3 years of age, most children are toilet trained, although they may still have the occasional "accident." At 2 years of age, the toddlers can run, ride tricycles, and balance on one foot. According to Freud, the ages of 2 and 3 years represent the anal phase of development. Separation anxiety, regression, and self-concept are concerns at this age group. *Nursing Process:* Planning *Client Need:* Physiological Integrity

9. *Answer:* 4 (Objectives: 1 and 3) *Rationale:* Teenagers respond more readily if they know they are alone and other teens have the same issues. Adolescents do not routinely want their parents present. Any instructional material should be age appropriate. *Nursing Process:* Implementation *Client Need:* Psychosocial Integrity

10. *Answer:* 2 (Objectives: 6 and 8) *Rationale:* The parents have the right to request that the child be circumcised on that date. The nurse needs to inform the physician and obtain orders to carry out the request. *Nursing Process:* Implementation *Client Need:* Psychosocial Integrity

Chapter 22
Key Topic Review Answers

1. Adulthood is categorized into emerging adulthood (18–25), young adulthood (25–40), and middle (40–65).

2. Three distinct generations are included in adulthood: Baby Boomers, Generation X's, and Generation Y's.

3. Lifestyle, behaviors

4. Maturity

5. Generativity

6. Adjusting to aging parents, valuing work as a central theme, achieving social and civic responsibility, and establishing and maintaining an economic standard of living

7. Cancer and heart disease

8. b

9. Generativity versus stagnation—they look back for a sense of successfully having met goals they developed earlier in life.

10. a. marriage/building a family

b. complete education—advanced degrees

c. career choices—occupation

Case Study Answers

1. *What health problem could Lou be at risk for, especially since Mary reported to you that he has been staying out late and arrives home with alcohol on his breath?* Lou could be at risk for alcoholism.

2. *How can the nurse help clients and their families in dealing with this concern?* The nurse can provide information about the dangers of excessive alcohol use, help the client clarify values about health, and refer the client and/or family to special groups such as Alcoholics Anonymous.

3. *What other resources might help the couple resolve their other issues?* Marriage counseling, pastor counseling, or a support group could be beneficial, among other options.

NCLEX® Review Question Answers

1. *Answer:* 1 (Objective: 7) *Rationale: Healthy People 2010* reports that this is the leading cause of death in the age group of 1 to 44 years of age. *Nursing Process:* Assessment *Client Need:* Psychosocial Integrity

2. *Answer:* 1 (Objective: 1) *Rationale:* There are several contributing factors such as high housing costs, maladaptive behaviors, and substance abuse issues. *Nursing Process:* Evaluation *Client Need:* Psychosocial Integrity

3. *Answer:* 3 (Objective: 7) *Rationale:* Many of the causes of hypertension are unknown. Contributing factors include smoking, obesity, high-sodium diet, and high stress levels. *Nursing Process:* Assessment *Client Need:* Physiological Integrity

4. *Answer:* 1 (Objective: 9) *Rationale:* Young men should be instructed in how to perform testicular self-examination. The other types of cancer listed are not the most common. *Nursing Process:* Assessment *Client Need:* Health Promotion and Maintenance

5. *Answer:* 2 (Objective: 2) *Rationale:* The average age for menopause is 47 years. Menopause refers to the so-called change-of-life in women. The other responses would not be relevant to the symptoms the client reported. *Nursing Process:* Assessment *Client Need:* Physiological Integrity

6. *Answer:* 1 (Objective: 2) *Rationale:* Decreased metabolic and physical activity means a decrease in caloric need. The nurse should counsel clients about reducing caloric intake and exercising regularly. *Nursing Process:* Implementation *Client Need:* Health Promotion and Maintenance

7. *Answer:* 1 (Objective: 8) *Rationale:* According to Havighurst, achieving adult civic and social responsibility is a developmental milestone for middle-aged adults. *Nursing Process:* Assessment *Client Need:* Psychosocial Integrity

8. *Answer:* 2 (Objective: 8) *Rationale:* The young adult group has several psychosocial development tasks to meet, such as feeling independent from parents yet interacting well with the family. Young adults should like their lives and demonstrate emotional, social, and economic responsibility for their own lives. *Nursing Process:* Assessment *Client Need:* Psychosocial Integrity

9. *Answer:* 3 (Objective: 1) *Rationale:* Baby Boomers were born in years 1945–1964; Generation X's were born in 1965–1978; Generation Y's were born in 1979–2000; and Boomerang Kids are young adults who have returned home to live. *Nursing Process:* Assessment *Client Need:* Psychosocial Integrity

10. *Answer:* 1 (Objective: 3) *Rationale:* Some of the factors contributing to the "boomerang" trend are high housing costs, high divorce rates, high unemployment rates, problems from substance abuse, and maladaptive behaviors. *Nursing Process:* Assessment *Client Need:* Psychosocial Integrity

11. *Answer:* 1, 4, 5 (Objectives: 5 and 6) *Rationale:* The middle-aged adult has work as a central theme instead of leisure time activities. Kohlberg is a moral developmental theorist and that answer does not address the psychosocial development. *Nursing Process:* Assessment *Client Needs:* Psychosocial Integrity, Health Promotion and Maintenance

Chapter 23
Key Topic Review Answers

1. With advancements in disease control, living conditions, and health technology, people are living longer.

2. The elderly and young people

3. People 85 years and older are the fastest growing of all age groups in the country, numbering 4.6 million in 2002 and projected to reach 9.6 million by the year 2030.

4. a. 65 to 75 years
   b. Old
   c. old, 85, 100
   d. old, 100

5. a. food safety
   b. diabetes
   c. oral health
   d. tobacco use
   e. vision and hearing

6. b   7. b   8. b

9. Gerontology, geriatrics

10. Gerontological nursing involves advocating for the health of older persons at all levels of prevention (Mauk, 2006, p. 9). Practicing gerontological nurses can obtain gerontological nursing certification through the American Nurses Association. Advanced practice in gerontological nursing requires a master's degree in nursing, of which there are two options: the gerontological clinical nurse specialist and the gerontological nurse practitioner.

11. Strategies to enhance an increased sense of control and autonomy for the elder include providing adequate information in a timely manner, allowing participation in the scheduling of activities, explaining any changes in the plan of care, and viewing hospitalized elders as individuals who wish to regain their autonomy and dignity.

12. The objective of long-term care is to provide a place of safety and care to attain optimal wellness and independence for each individual. Long-term care includes many different levels of care. These may include assisted living, intermediate care, skilled care, and Alzheimer's units.

13. Many long-term care facilities offer specialized units for clients with Alzheimer's disease (AD), which involves progressive dementia, memory loss, and inability to care for oneself. The gerontological nurses working in Alzheimer's units have specialized knowledge and help family members understand and cope with the disease process affecting their loved ones.

14. This theory proposes that humans, like automobiles, have vital parts that run down with time, leading to aging and death. The theory proposes that the faster an organism lives, the quicker it dies. It proposes that cells wear out through exposure to internal and external stressors, including trauma, chemicals, and buildup of natural wastes.

Case Study Answers

1. *What age category of the aging population is this widow currently in?* The client belongs in the old-old age population.

2. *What is the myth of aging that her children are subscribing to? What is the reality?* The myth is that older people are depressed and should be allowed to withdraw from society. The reality of that myth is that only about one-third of older people exhibit depressive symptoms. However, depression is very treatable at any age.

3. *According to Erikson, what developmental task occurs at this phase?* The developmental task at this time is ego integrity versus despair.

NCLEX® Review Question Answers

1. *Answer:* 2 (Objective: 8) *Rationale:* By age 80, nearly all elders have some lens opacity or

cataracts that reduce visual acuity. Presbyopia is the inability to focus or accommodate due to loss of flexibility in the lens, causing a decrease in near vision. Presbycusis is having vision loss, while glaucoma is a different visual concern. *Nursing Process:* Planning *Client Need:* Physiological Integrity

2. *Answer:* 1, 3, 4, 5 (Objective: 15) *Rationale:* The working capacity of the heart diminishes with age. The heart rate at normal rest may decrease with age and is slower to respond to stress or after physical activity. There is reduced arterial elasticity in the arteries. Orthostatic hypotension may place the elderly client at risk for falls due to sudden changes in position. *Nursing Process:* Assessment *Client Need:* Physiological Integrity

3. *Answer:* 2 (Objective: 9) *Rationale:* The activity theory suggests that the best way to age healthily is to stay active and socially stimulated. The disengagement theory allows that the aged withdraw from others. The continuity theory states that people continue their values, behaviors, and habitats in older age. *Nursing Process:* Implementation *Client Need:* Psychosocial Integrity

4. *Answer:* 1 (Objective: 6) *Rationale:* Many nursing homes offer respite care for caregivers. Assisted living, adult day care, and leaving the client alone would not provide around-the-clock supervision and the type of assistance an Alzheimer's client would need. *Nursing Process:* Planning *Client Need:* Psychosocial Integrity

5. *Answer:* 3 (Objective: 15) *Rationale:* *Healthy People 2010* reports that falls account for more injuries in the older population. All other choices apply to other age groups. *Nursing Process:* Planning *Client Need:* Health Promotion and Maintenance

6. *Answer:* 4 (Objective: 2) *Rationale:* The older adults are the fastest growing population group in the United States today. All other responses are incorrect. *Nursing Process:* Assessment *Client Need:* Health Promotion and Maintenance

7. *Answer:* 2, 3 (Objective: 15) *Rationale:* Elder mistreatment may affect either sex; however, the victims most often are women over 75 years of age, the physically or mentally impaired, and those dependent for care on the abuser. The abuse may involve physical, psychological, or emotional abuse; sexual abuse; financial abuse; violation of human or civil rights; and active or passive neglect. Others are beaten and even raped by family members. Most victims experience two or more forms of abuse. Elder abuse or neglect may occur in private homes, senior citizen's homes, nursing homes, hospitals, and long-term care facilities. *Nursing Process:* Assessment *Client Need:* Safe, Effective Care Environment

8. *Answer:* 1 (Objective: 15) *Rationale:* By increasing roughage and fluids in the diet, constipation may be prevented. The other answers are not correct for this particular diagnosis. *Nursing Process:* Planning *Client Need:* Physiological Integrity

9. *Answer:* 2 (Objective: 7) *Rationale:* The endocrine theory is concerned with hormone production and response. The idea that the faster an organism lives, the faster it dies is a proposal of the wear-and-tear theory. The genetic theory proposes that organisms are programmed for a predetermined number of cell divisions, after which the cells die. The immunological theory suggests that the immune system declines with age. *Nursing Process:* Assessment *Client Need:* Physiological Integrity

10. *Answer:* 1, 2, 3, 5 (Objective: 16) *Rationale:* All of the measures listed except for removing the carpet and waxing the floors are measures to prevent falls. With aging comes the gradual reduction in the speed and power of skeletal or voluntary muscle contractions and sustained muscular effort. The client's reaction time slows with aging. *Nursing Process:* Assessment *Client Need:* Psychological Integrity

Chapter 24
Key Topic Review Answers

1. Family
2. System
3. Systems theory
4. The purpose of family assessment is to determine the level of family functioning, to clarify family interaction patterns, to identify family strengths and weaknesses, and to describe the health status of the family and its individual members.
5. Finding affordable, quality child care
6. Interrupted Family Processes; Readiness for Enhanced Family Coping; Disabled Family Coping; Impaired Parenting; Impaired Home Maintenance; and Caregiver Role Strain
7. 9% (12 million), 9% (12 million), 10 million, 2 million
8. Child care concerns, financial concerns, role overload and fatigue in managing daily tasks, and social isolation
9. Feedback
10. Structural–functional theory

Case Study Answers

1. *What would be the best interventions by the nurse in this situation?* The nurse could attempt to talk with the client alone by sending her husband on an errand or insisting that he step out of the room while she is being examined, and then perform a thorough physical examination, attempting to ascertain the extent of the current injuries and also looking for any previous injuries (scarring, old bruising, prior injuries). The nurse needs to verbalize concerns to the physician so he also can evaluate for signs of abuse. The nurse could also place a small brochure about battered women's shelters within reach of the client so she might place the item in her purse or pocket.

2. *What should the nurse be observing during the interactions between herself, the client, and the spouse?* Communications between all three individuals should be observed, including nonverbal communications.

NCLEX® Review Question Answers

1. *Answer:* 3 (Objective: 6) *Rationale:* The mother is demonstrating the inability to create, maintain, or regain an environment that promotes the optimum growth and development of children. The other diagnoses are not appropriate based on the information given. *Nursing Process:* Assessment *Client Need:* Health Promotion and Maintenance

2. *Answer:* 2 (Objective: 5) *Rationale:* Persons born into families with a history of certain diseases, such as diabetes or cardiovascular disease, are at greater risk of developing these conditions. Some family units or family members may be at risk of developing a disease by reason of gender or race. Many diseases are preventable, the effects of some diseases can be minimized, or the onset of disease can be delayed through lifestyle modifications. Families with members at both ends of the age continuum are at risk of developing health problems. *Nursing Process:* Assessment *Client Need:* Health Promotion and Maintenance

3. *Answer:* 4 (Objective: 6) *Rationale:* Many diseases are preventable, the effects of some diseases can be minimized, or the onset of disease can be delayed through lifestyle modifications. Persons born into families with a history of certain diseases, such as diabetes or cardiovascular disease, are at greater risk of developing these conditions. Some family units or family members may be at risk of developing a disease by reason of gender or race. Families with members at both ends of the age continuum are at risk of developing health problems. *Nursing*

Process: Assessment *Client Need:* Health Promotion and Maintenance

4. *Answer:* 3 (Objective: 2) *Rationale:* In this case, the grandparents live with and care for their grandchild but the child's parents are not a part of this family. Foster families contain children who can no longer live with their birth parents and require placement with a family that has agreed to include them temporarily. Traditional families are viewed as an autonomous unit in which both parents reside in the home with their children, the mother often assuming the nurturing role and the father providing the necessary economic resources. Cohabiting (or communal) families consist of unrelated individuals or families who live under one roof. *Nursing Process:* Assessment *Client Need:* Health Promotion and Maintenance

5. *Answer:* 3 (Objective: 4) *Rationale:* Family assessment gives an overview of the family process and helps the nurse identify areas that need further investigation. Nurses carry out a detailed assessment in specific target areas as they become more acquainted with the family and begin to understand family needs and strengths more fully. In planning interventions, nurses need to focus not only on problems but also on family strengths and resources as part of the nursing care plan. Family assessment includes: family structure, roles and functions, physical health status, interaction patterns, family values, and coping resources. *Nursing Process:* Assessment *Client Need:* Psychosocial Integrity

6. *Answer:* 1 (Objective: 4) *Rationale:* Family assessment gives an overview of the family process and helps the nurse identify areas that need further investigation. Nurses carry out a detailed assessment in specific target areas as they become more acquainted with the family and begin to understand family needs and strengths more fully. In planning interventions, nurses need to focus not only on problems but also on family strengths and resources as part of the nursing care plan. Family assessment includes: family structure, roles and functions, physical health status, interaction patterns, family values, and coping resources. *Nursing Process:* Assessment *Client Need:* Psychosocial Integrity

7. *Answer:* 1 (Objective: 7) *Rationale:* The incidence of family violence has increased in recent years. Statistics are not accurate because many cases remain unreported. Family violence includes abuse between intimate partners, child abuse, and elder abuse, and may include physical, mental, and verbal abuse, as well as neglect. Early symptoms are evident in burns, cuts, fractures, and even death. Other manifestations often seen are depression, alcohol and substance abuse, and suicide attempts. Nurses should be alert to the symptoms of family violence and take appropriate measures to report it and obtain resources for the family. *Nursing Process:* Assessment *Client Need:* Health Promotion and Maintenance

8. *Answer:* 2 (Objective: 6) *Rationale:* Nurses committed to family-centered care involve both the ailing individual and the family in the nursing process. Through their interaction with families, nurses can give support and information. Nurses make sure that not only the individual but also each family member understands the disease, its management, and the effect of these two factors on family functioning. *Nursing Process:* Assessment *Client Need:* Health Promotion and Maintenance

9. *Answer:* 4 (Objective: 4) *Rationale:* Nurses assess and plan health care for three types of clients: the individual, the family, and the community. The beliefs and values of each person and the support he or she receives come in large part from the family and are reinforced by the community. Thus an understanding of family dynamics and the context of the community assists the nurse in planning care. When a family is the client, the nurse determines the health status of the family and its individual members, the level of family functioning, family interaction patterns, and family strengths and weaknesses. *Nursing Process:* Assessment *Client Need:* Health Promotion and Maintenance

10. *Answer:* 3 (Objective: 6) *Rationale:* One of the main rationales for health promotions in schools is to increase students' knowledge about personal hygiene. *Nursing Process:* Assessment *Client Need:* Health Promotion and Maintenance

Chapter 25
Key Topic Review Answers

1. Caring, central
2. Connection between individuals, mutual recognition and involvement of both client and nurse
3. a. moral imperative
   b. affect
   c. human trait
   d. interpersonal relationships
   e. therapeutic intervention
4. a 5. g 6. e 7. a
8. b 9. d 10. f 11. c
12. Aesthetic knowing
13. A balanced diet, regular exercise, adequate sleep and rest, recreational activities, meditation and prayer

14. Reflection
15. b

Case Study Answers

1a. *What are two additional interventions to provide comfort measures?* Any of the following are appropriate responses: (1) Turn every 2 hours while in bed if client is immobile; (2) offer fluids/refreshments every 2–4 hours unless contraindicated; (3) provide privacy to the client during care.

2a. *As a student nurse assigned to this client, which of the six C's of caring in nursing do you want to incorporate in your interventions?* You would want to incorporate compassion, competence, confidence, conscience, commitment, and comportment (all six of the six C's).

2b. *If you were using the caring processes from Swanson's theory of caring, on what five processes would you base your nursing interventions for this client?* The processes are knowing, being with, doing for, enabling, and maintaining belief.

2c. *What type of knowing would you demonstrate if you are observing and documenting phenomena as it is occurring in this case?* This would demonstrate empirical knowing—the science of nursing.

NCLEX® Review Question Answers

1. *Answer:* 4 (Objective: 2) *Rationale:* Leininger believes the health care personnel should work toward an understanding of care and values from different cultures. Miller believes that caring validates the humanness of both client and caregiver. Watson views caring as the moral ideal of nursing. Swanson focuses on caring processes as nursing interventions. *Nursing Process:* Assessment *Client Need:* Psychosocial Integrity

2. *Answer:* 3 (Objective: 2) *Rationale:* Compassion is showing individuals that one cares. The nurse is sharing herself with the client. *Nursing Process:* Implementation *Client Need:* Psychosocial Integrity

3. *Answer:* 1, 2, 3, 4 (Objective: 3) *Rationale:* Caring for self is defined as helping oneself grow and actualize one's possibilities and it means taking the time to nurture oneself. All of the interventions listed above are correct except working 60 hours per week. *Nursing Process:* Assessment *Client Need:* Psychosocial Integrity

4. *Answer:* 1, 3, 4 (Objective: 5) *Rationale:* All of the responses are interventions to promote a healthier lifestyle, except for delaying exercise. *Nursing Process:* Implementation *Client Need:* Health Promotion and Maintenance

5. *Answer:* 1 (Objective: 6) *Rationale:* Personal knowing is developed through critical reflection on one's actions and feelings in practice. The other choices are examples of ethical knowing, empirical knowing, and aesthetic knowing. *Nursing Process:* Evaluation *Client Need:* Physiological Adaptation

6. *Answer:* 2 (Objective: 1) *Rationale:* Physical presence combined with the promise of availability, especially at a time of need, demonstrates caring in the form of nursing presence. *Nursing Process:* Implementation *Client Need:* Psychosocial Integrity

7. *Answer:* 3 (Objective: 4) *Rationale:* There are times when the nurse "enables" and "empowers" the client in order to enhance and encourage self-care. *Nursing Process:* Implementation *Client Need:* Psychosocial Integrity

8. *Answer:* 1, 4 (Objective: 4) *Rationale:* The nurse demonstrates both compassion and competence by providing the actions listed in the question. *Nursing Process:* Implementation *Client Need:* Safe, Effective Care Environment

9. *Answer:* 2 (Objective: 3) *Rationale:* Guided imagery uses the power of imagination as a therapeutic tool. Storytelling assists individuals to move toward wholeness. Music therapy involves listening, singing, rhythm, and body movement. *Nursing Process:* Implementation *Client Need:* Health Promotion and Maintenance

10. *Answer:* 1 (Objective: 1) *Rationale:* Caring means that people, relationships, and things matter. Caring is an integral part of nursing. *Nursing Process:* Implementation *Client Need:* Psychosocial Integrity

Chapter 26
Key Topic Review Answers

1. In nursing, communication is a dynamic process used to gather assessment data, to teach and persuade, and to express caring and comfort. It is an integral part of the helping relationship.

2. c, d, e, f

3. Failure to listen, improperly decoding the client's intended message, and placing the nurse's needs above the client's needs are major barriers to communication.

4. Face the person squarely in an open posture, lean into the person and maintain good eye contact, and try to be relatively relaxed.

5. a, c (Refer to Box 26–3 in the textbook.)

6. Elderspeak is a speech style similar to baby talk that the nurse is using in this situation by calling the client "Honey." This type of communication gives the elderly the message of being dependent and incompetent. It does not communicate respect. The characteristics of elderspeak include diminutives (inappropriate terms of endearment), inappropriate plural pronoun use, tag questions, and slow, loud speech.

7. Congruent communication

8. a

9. Teaching groups are to impart information to the participants, whereas self-help groups are voluntary organizations composed of people who share similar health, social, or daily living problems.

Case Study Answers

1. *What could the nurse do in order to create a more positive environment for the health interview?* The nurse could make sure the interview and exam take place in a private and non-threatening environment. Also, attentive listening could be used as well as open-ended questions.

2. *If the nurse shares a similar experience with the client, then what communication technique is the nurse using?* The nurse is using the therapeutic communication of offering self by empathetic listening and responding to the client and of being genuine in her desire to place the client at ease.

3. *What are three therapeutic responses the nurse could employ in this situation?* The nurse could use several therapeutic communication techniques such as offering self, giving information about procedures, acknowledging the client's apprehension, and using therapeutic touch.

4. *Using the information from the case study, supply the following information:*

   a. *Provide a nursing diagnosis for the client:* Alteration in urinary function as evidenced by reports pain with voiding, chills, fever, and back pain.

   b. *Identify the subjective and objective assessment information:* Subjective—client reporting back pain, chills, and burning when voiding. Objective—temperature of 101 degrees, grimaces with light palpation of lower abdomen.

NCLEX® Review Question Answers

1. *Answer:* 2, 3, 4 (Objective: 2) *Rationale:* The ability to communicate is related to the development of thought processes, the presence of intact sensory and motor systems, and the extent and nature of an individual's opportunities to practice communication skills. The nurse needs to develop a rapport with each group in order to effectively communicate. *Nursing Process:* Assessment *Client Need:* Health Promotion and Maintenance

2. *Answer:* 3 (Objective: 6) *Rationale:* The sender is a person or group who wishes to convey a message to another. The receiver is the listener. The second component is the message itself. Feedback is the message that the receiver returns to the sender. *Nursing Process:* Assessment *Client Need:* Physiological Integrity

3. *Answer:* 1 (Objective: 1) *Rationale:* Intimate-distance communication is characterized by body contact and heightened sensations of body heat and smell. Personal space is less overwhelming than intimate space. Social-distance and public-distance communication takes place with personal space greater than 4 feet. *Nursing Process:* Assessment *Client Need:* Physiological Integrity

4. *Answer:* 3 (Objective: 1) *Rationale:* Congruent communication is when the words and actions are focused in the same direction. Noncongruent communication is when actions and words do not match or focus in the same direction. Process recording is a word-for-word account of a conversation. Nonverbal communications are actions without verbal expression. *Nursing Process:* Implementation *Client Need:* Psychosocial and Physiological Integrity

5. *Answer:* 1 (Objective: 3) *Rationale:* A self-help group is small, voluntary organization. Giving information is a role of the nurse in a teaching group. Buffering stress is a nurse's role in work-related social groups. The "adding professionalism" choice is a random statement. *Nursing Process:* Implementation *Client Need:* Psychosocial Integrity

6. *Answer:* 1, 3 (Objective: 6) *Rationale:* Therapeutic communication techniques facilitate communication and focus on the client's concerns. The other choices are considered barriers to communication. *Nursing Process:* Application/

Implementation *Client Need:* Psychosocial Integrity

7. *Answer:* 3 (Objective: 6) *Rationale:* There are situations when appropriate use of touch reinforces caring feelings. However, the nurse must be sensitive to the differences in attitudes and practices of clients and self. The other answers are not acceptable uses of touch. *Nursing Process:* Implementation *Client Need:* Psychosocial Integrity

8. *Answer:* 1 (Objective: 8) *Rationale:* During the initial parts of the introductory phase, the client may display some resistant behaviors that inhibit involvement, cooperation, or change. It may be because of difficulty in asking for assistance. All of the other answers are untrue responses. *Nursing Process:* Assessment *Client Need:* Psychosocial Integrity

9. *Answer:* 2 (Objective: 6) *Rationale:* The preinteraction phase is similar to the planning stage before the interview. The three phases of the interview are opening the relationship, clarifying the problem, and structuring the contract. The introductory phase is when the client and nurse formulate the contract. *Nursing Process:* Planning *Client Need:* Safe, Effective Care Environment

10. *Answer:* 4 (Objective: 7) *Rationale:* Stereotyping negates the individual uniqueness of an individual. Being defensive prevents the client from expressing true concerns. Challenging responses indicate that the physician is not considering the client's feelings. *Nursing Process:* Implementation *Client Need:* Psychosocial Integrity

Chapter 27
Key Topic Review Answers

1. a   **2.** a   **3.** a   **4.** b   **5.** a

6. E-health

7. Anxiety

8. Concepts

9. Cultural

10. Avoid

11. g, a, i, b, f, j, h, e, d, c

12. c   **13.** a   **14.** b   **15.** d   **16.** a

Case Study Answers

1. *How will you be able to determine if Melba is ready to learn?* Readiness to learn is the demonstration of behaviors or cues that reflect the learner's motivation to learn at a specific time. Readiness reflects not only the desire or willingness to learn but also the ability to learn at a specific time. For example, a client may want to learn self-care during a dressing change, but if the client experiences pain or discomfort he or she may not be able to learn. The nurse can provide pain medication to make the client more comfortable and more able to learn. The nurse's role is often to encourage the development of readiness.

2. *Identify three ways you could facilitate learning.* A number of factors affect learning, including motivation, readiness, active involvement, relevance, feedback, nonjudgmental support, repetition, timing, environment, emotions, physiologic events, psychomotor ability, and cultural aspects.

3. *Discuss various teaching aids to help foster Melba's learning.*

- Keep language level at or below the fifth-grade level.
- Use active, not passive, voice.
- Use easy, common words of one or two syllables (e.g., *use* instead of *utilize* or *give* instead of *administer*).
- Use the second person (*you*) rather than the third person (*client*).
- Use a large type size (14 to 16 point).
- Write short sentences.
- Avoid using all capital letters.

NCLEX® Review Question Answers

1. *Answer:* 2 (Objective: 3) *Rationale:* Andragogy is the art and science of teaching adults. Geragogy is the term used to describe the process involved in stimulating and helping elders to learn. Pedagogy is the discipline concerned with helping children learn. Adherence is commitment or attachment to a regimen. *Nursing Process:* Planning *Client Need:* Health Promotion and Maintenance

2. *Answer:* 1 (Objective: 2) *Rationale:* Modeling is the process by which a person learns by observing the behavior of others. Imitation is the process by which individuals copy or reproduce what they have observed. Provide opportunities for learners to solve problems by trial and error. Positive reinforcement (e.g., a pleasant experience such as praise and encouragement) is fostering repetition of an action. *Nursing Process:* Planning *Client Need:* Health Promotion and Maintenance

3. *Answer:* 2 (Objective: 5) *Rationale:* Teaching a client how to self-administer insulin is in the psychomotor domain, one of Piaget's five major phases of cognitive development. The cognitive domain, the "thinking" domain, includes six

intellectual abilities and thinking processes beginning with knowing, comprehending, and applying to analysis, synthesis, and evaluation. The affective domain, known as the "feeling" domain, is divided into categories that specify the degree of a "person's depth of emotional response to tasks." *Nursing Process:* Planning *Client Need:* Health Promotion and Maintenance

4. *Answer:* 1 (Objective: 4) *Rationale:* The nurse is applying the humanistic theory by encouraging the learner to establish goals and promote self-directed learning. The nurse would be applying cognitive theory when encouraging a positive teacher–learner relationship. The nurse would be applying cognitive theory when providing a social, emotional, and physical environment conducive to learning. The nurse would be applying cognitive theory when selecting multisensory teaching strategies since perception is influenced by the senses. *Nursing Process:* Planning *Client Need:* Health Promotion and Maintenance

5. *Answer:* 3 (Objective: 1) *Rationale:* In teaching a client about heart disease who may need to know the effects of smoking before recognizing the need to stop smoking, motivation is the factor that can facilitate client learning. Readiness reflects not only the desire or willingness to learn but also the ability to learn at a specific time. Learning is more meaningful when the client is actively involved in the learning process. Motivation to learn is the desire to learn. It greatly influences how quickly and how much a person learns. Motivation is generally greatest when a person recognizes a need and believes the need will be met through learning. *Nursing Process:* Implementation *Client Need:* Health Promotion and Maintenance

6. *Answer:* 3 (Objective: 6) *Rationale:* A client experiencing an acute illness is a factor that inhibits learning. To facilitate learning it helps to have adequate family support for the client. To facilitate learning it helps if the client is emotionally ready. As the client stabilizes physically and emotionally, the nurse can provide opportunities to learn. *Nursing Process:* Planning *Client Need:* Health Promotion and Maintenance

7. *Answer:* 4 (Objective: 8) *Rationale:* If the client states a pattern of excuses for not reading the instructions, the nurse may have reason to suspect a literacy problem. A pattern of noncompliance in client behaviors may cause a nurse to suspect a literacy problem. A client reading the information slowly does not always indicate a literacy problem. A client insisting that he or she already knows the information could sometimes be an indication of a

literacy problem. *Nursing Process:* Planning *Client Need:* Health Promotion and Maintenance

8. *Answer:* 2 (Objective: 9) *Rationale:* "The client selects low-fat foods from a menu" is a learning outcome for a teaching plan. Avoid using words such as *knows, understands, believes*, and *appreciates* because they are neither observable nor measurable. State the client (learner) behavior or performance, not the nurse behavior. *Nursing Process:* Planning *Client Need:* Health Promotion and Maintenance

9. *Answer:* 4 (Objective: 7) *Rationale:* Sending a billing statement to the client's home address is not part of e-health. E-health includes many aspects, such as online appointment access, billing review, e-mail access between the client and health care provider, and online health information. *Nursing Process:* Planning *Client Need:* Health Promotion and Maintenance

10. *Answer:* 4 (Objective: 1) *Rationale:* The social factor is not an element in the nursing history that provides clues to learning needs. Several elements in the nursing history provide clues to learning needs: (a) age, (b) the client's understanding and perceptions of the health problem, (c) health beliefs and practices, (d) cultural factors, (e) economic factors, (f) learning style, and (g) the client's support systems. *Nursing Process:* Planning *Client Need:* Health Promotion and Maintenance

Chapter 28

Key Topic Review Answers

1. b   2. b   3. a   4. a   5. b
6. Democratic
7. Laissez-faire
8. Bureaucratic
9. Situational
10. Charismatic
11. h, c, e, j, a, i, g, d, f, b
12. a   13. c   14. d   15. a   16. b

Case Study Answers

1. *Is Nathaniel assuming the role of a leader or manager?* Nathaniel is assuming the role of a leader, as evidenced by the following: He influences others to work together to accomplish a specific goal. He also has the initiative, ability, and confidence to innovate change, motivate, facilitate, and mentor others.

2. *Compare and contrast the role of a leader and manager.* A leader influences others to work together

to accomplish a specific goal. Leaders are often visionary; they are informed, articulate, confident, and self-aware. Leaders also usually have outstanding interpersonal skills and are excellent listeners and communicators. They have initiative, ability, and confidence to innovate change, motivate, facilitate, and mentor others. Within their organizations, nurse leaders participate in and guide teams that assess the effectiveness of care, implement evidence-based practice, and construct process improvement strategies. They may be employed in a variety of positions—from shift team leader to institutional president. Leaders may also hold volunteer positions such as chairperson of a professional organization or community board of directors.

A manager is an employee of an organization who is given authority, power, and responsibility for planning, organizing, coordinating, and directing the work of others, and for establishing and evaluating standards. Managers understand organizational structure and culture. They control human, financial, and material resources. Managers set goals, make decisions, and solve problems. They initiate and implement change. The purposes of nursing leadership include (a) improving the health status of individuals or families, (b) increasing the effectiveness and level of satisfaction among professional colleagues, and (c) improving the attitudes of citizens and legislators toward the nursing profession and their expectations of it. As managers, nurses are responsible for managing client care, and some nurses assume a position within the organization as nurse manager, supervisor, or executive. As a manager, the nurse is responsible for (a) efficiently accomplishing the goals of the organization, (b) efficiently using the organization's resources, (c) ensuring effective client care, and (d) ensuring compliance with institutional, professional, regulatory, and governmental standards. Managers are also responsible for development of licensed and unlicensed personnel within their work group.

3. *What particular leadership style has Nathaniel developed?* A democratic (participative, consultative) leader encourages group discussion and decision making. This type of leader acts as a catalyst or facilitator, actively guiding the group toward achieving group goals. Group productivity and satisfaction are high as group members contribute to the work effort. The democratic leader assumes individuals are internally motivated (their driving force is intrinsic; they desire self-satisfaction), capable of making decisions, and value independence. Providing constructive feedback, offering information, making suggestions, and asking questions become the focus of the participative leader. This leadership style demands that the leader have faith in the group members to accomplish the goals. Although democratic leadership has been shown to be less efficient and more cumbersome than authoritarian leadership, it allows more self-motivation and more creativity among group members. It also calls for a great deal of cooperation and coordination among group members. This leadership style can be extremely effective in the health care setting.

NCLEX® Review Question Answers

1. *Answer:* 3 (Objective: 1) *Rationale:* The democratic leadership style demands that the leader have faith in the group members to accomplish the goals. In the laissez-faire leadership style, the leader assumes a "hands-off" approach. Under the autocratic leadership style, the group may feel secure because procedures are well defined and activities are predictable. The bureaucratic leader does not trust self or others to make decisions and instead relies on the organization's rules, policies, and procedures to direct the group's work efforts. *Nursing Process:* Assessment *Client Need:* Safe, Effective Care Environment

2. *Answer:* 3 (Objective: 3) *Rationale:* A transformational leader fosters creativity, risk taking, commitment, and collaboration by empowering the group to share in the organization's vision. A charismatic leader is rare and is characterized by an emotional relationship with group members. The charming personality of the leader evokes strong feelings of commitment to both the leader and the leader's cause and beliefs. The transactional leader has a relationship with followers based on an exchange for some resource valued by the follower. These incentives are used to promote loyalty and performance. Shared leadership recognizes that a professional workforce is made up of many leaders. No one person is considered to have knowledge or ability beyond that of other members of the work group. *Nursing Process:* Assessment *Client Need:* Safe, Effective Care Environment

3. *Answer:* 3 (Objective: 5) *Rationale:* Upper-level (top-level) managers are organizational executives who are primarily responsible for establishing goals and developing strategic plans. First-level managers are responsible for managing the work of nonmanagerial personnel and the day-to-day activities of a specific work group or groups. Middle-level managers supervise a number of first-level managers and are responsible for the activities in the departments they supervise. Middle-level managers serve as liaisons between first-level managers and upper-level managers. They may be called supervisors, nurse managers, or head nurses. *Nursing Process:* Assessment *Client Need:* Safe, Effective Care Environment

4. *Answer:* 1 (Objective: 4) *Rationale:* The management principle being demonstrated is accountability. Accountability is the ability and willingness to assume responsibility for one's actions and to accept the consequences of one's behavior. Authority is defined as the legitimate right to direct the work of others. It is an integral component of managing. Responsibility is an obligation to complete a task. Coordinating is the process of ensuring that plans are carried out and evaluating outcomes. *Nursing Process:* Assessment *Client Need:* Safe, Effective Care Environment

5. *Answer:* 4 (Objective: 11) *Rationale:* Planned change is an intended, purposeful attempt by an individual, group, organization, or larger social system to influence its own current status. Unplanned change is an alteration imposed by external events or persons; it occurs when unexpected events force a reaction. It is usually haphazard, and the results can be unpredictable. Drift is a type of unplanned change in which change occurs without effort on anyone's part. Situational, or natural, change also may be considered unplanned and occurs without any control by the person or group impacted. *Nursing Process:* Assessment *Client Need:* Safe, Effective Care Environment

6. *Answer:* 1 (Objective: 2) *Rationale:* The leader role influences others toward goal setting, either formally or informally. The manager role carries out predetermined policies, rules, and regulations; maintains an orderly, controlled, rational, and equitable structure; relates to people according to their roles; and feels rewarded when fulfilling the organizational mission or goals. *Nursing Process:* Planning *Client Need:* Safe, Effective Care Environment

7. *Answer:* 2 (Objective: 7) *Rationale:* Involve members in all decisions. Use a leadership style appropriate to the task and the members. Plan and organize activities of the group. Be open and encourage openness, so that real issues are confronted. *Nursing Process:* Assessment *Client Need:* Safe, Effective Care Environment

8. *Answer:* 3 (Objective: 11) *Rationale:* Perception that the change will improve the situation is considered a driving force. Restraining forces include: misunderstanding of the change and its implications; lack of time or energy;

and low tolerance for change related to intellectual or emotional insecurity. *Nursing Process:* Assessment *Client Need:* Safe, Effective Care Environment

9. *Answer:* 2 (Objective: 7) *Rationale:* Guidelines for dealing with resistance to change include: Emphasize the positive consequences of the change and how the individual or group will benefit. Clarify information and provide accurate information. Maintain a climate of trust, support, and confidence. Communicate with those who oppose the change. Get to the root of their reasons for opposition. *Nursing Process:* Planning *Client Need:* Safe, Effective Care Environment

10. *Answer:* 2 (Objective: 1) *Rationale:* The situational leader (a) flexes task and relationship behaviors, (b) considers the staff members' abilities, (c) knows the nature of the task to be done, and (d) is sensitive to the context or environment in which the task takes place. The task orientation focuses the leader on activities that encourage group productivity to get the work done. The relationship-orientation style is concerned with interpersonal relationships and focuses on activities that meet group members' needs. *Nursing Process:* Assessment *Client Need:* Safe, Effective Care Environment

Chapter 29
Key Topic Review Answers

1. b   **2.** a   **3.** a   **4.** b   **5.** b
6. Vital signs
7. Exhaustion
8. Compliance
9. Deficit
10. Hypothermia
11. j, f, c, a, d, i, h, g, e, b
12. d   **13.** b   **14.** c   **15.** a   **16.** c

Case Study Answers

1. *What are the normal vital signs for a 20-year-old male client?* A typical blood pressure for a healthy adult is 120/80 mm Hg (pulse pressure of 40).

> Oral Temperature Celsius (Fahrenheit) = 37 (98.6)
> Pulse average (range) = 80 (60–100)
> Respiration average (range) = 16 (12–20)

2. *What type of fever is the client most likely experiencing?* A temperature that rises to fever level rapidly following a normal temperature and then returns to normal within a few hours is called a fever spike.

3. *Why has the doctor ordered blood work?* A temperature that rises to fever level rapidly following a normal temperature and then returns to normal within a few hours is called a fever spike. Bacterial blood infections often cause fever spikes.

NCLEX® Review Question Answers

1. *Answer:* 1 (Objective: 1) *Rationale:* Conduction is the transfer of heat from one molecule to a molecule of lower temperature. Radiation is the transfer of heat from the surface of one object to the surface of another without contact between the two objects, mostly in the form of infrared rays. Vaporization is continuous evaporation of moisture from the respiratory tract and from the mucosa of the mouth and from the skin. Convection is the dispersion of heat by air currents. *Nursing Process:* Assessment *Client Need:* Physiological Integrity

2. *Answer:* 1 (Objective: 3) *Rationale:* With intermittent fever, the body temperature alternates at regular intervals between periods of fever and periods of normal or subnormal temperatures. During a remittent fever such as with a cold or influenza, a wide range of temperature fluctuations (more than 2°C [3.6°F]) occurs over the 24-hour period, all of which are above normal. In a relapsing fever, short febrile periods of a few days are interspersed with periods of 1 or 2 days of normal temperature. During a constant fever, the body temperature fluctuates minimally but always remains above normal. *Nursing Process:* Assessment *Client Need:* Physiological Integrity

3. *Answer:* 3 (Objective: 4) *Rationale:* Persons experiencing heatstroke generally have been exercising in hot weather, have warm, flushed skin, and often do not sweat. They usually have a temperature of 106°F or higher, and may be delirious, unconscious, or having seizures. Hypothermia is a core body temperature below the lower limit of normal. Heat exhaustion is a result of excessive heat and dehydration. Signs of heat exhaustion include paleness, dizziness, nausea, vomiting, fainting, and a moderately increased temperature (101–102°F). A blood pressure that is persistently above normal is a condition called hypertension. *Nursing Process:* Assessment *Client Need:* Physiological Integrity

4. *Answer:* 4 (Objective: 3) *Rationale:* When the Celsius reading is 40:

$$F = (40 \times 9/5) + 32 = (72) + 32 = 104$$

Nursing Process: Assessment *Client Need:* Physiological Integrity

5. Answer: 1 (Objective: 5) **Rationale:**
Pulse sites: The posterior tibial site is on the medial surface of the ankle where the posterior tibial artery passes behind the medial malleolus. The popliteal site is where the popliteal artery passes behind the knee. The pedal (dorsalis pedis) site is where the dorsalis pedis artery passes over the bones of the foot, on an imaginary line drawn from the middle of the ankle to the space between the big and second toes. The radial site is where the radial artery runs along the radial bone, on the thumb side of the inner aspect of the wrist. **Nursing Process:** Assessment **Client Need:** Physiological Integrity

6. Answer: 3 (Objective: 12) **Rationale:** Having the arm above the level of the heart can cause an erroneously low blood pressure result. Having the cuff wrapped too loosely or unevenly, having the bladder cuff too narrow, and assessing immediately after a meal or while the client smokes or has pain can cause an erroneously high blood pressure result. **Nursing Process:** Implementation **Client Need:** Physiological Integrity

7. Answer: 3 (Objective: 3) **Rationale:** Pull the pinna straight back and upward for children over age 3. Pull the pinna slightly upward and backward for an adult patient. Insert the probe slowly using a circular motion until snug. Point the probe slightly anteriorly, toward the eardrum. Presence of cerumen can affect the reading. **Nursing Process:** Implementation **Client Need:** Physiological Integrity

8. Answer: 4 (Objective: 9) **Rationale:** Dyspnea is difficult and labored breathing during which the individual has a persistent, unsatisfied need for air and feels distressed. Stridor is a shrill, harsh sound heard during inspiration with laryngeal obstruction. Stertor is a snoring or sonorous respiration, usually due to a partial obstruction of the upper airway. Wheeze is a continuous, high-pitched musical squeak or whistling sound occurring on expiration and sometimes on inspiration when air moves through a narrowed or partially obstructed airway. Bubbling is a gurgling sound heard as air passes through moist secretions in the respiratory tract. **Nursing Process:** Evaluation **Client Need:** Physiological Integrity

9. Answer: 1 (Objective: 9) **Rationale:** Hemoptysis is the presence of blood in the sputum. Productive cough is a cough accompanied by expectorated secretions. Nonproductive cough is a dry, harsh cough without secretions. Orthopnea is the ability to breathe only in upright sitting or standing positions. **Nursing Process:** Planning **Client Need:** Physiological Integrity

10. Answer: 4 (Objective: 11) **Rationale:** Phase 1—The pressure level at which the first faint, clear tapping or thumping sounds are heard. These sounds gradually become more intense. The first tapping sound heard during deflation of the cuff is the systolic blood pressure. Phase 2—The period during deflation when the sounds have a muffled, whooshing, or swishing quality. Phase 4—The time when the sounds become muffled and have a soft, blowing quality. Phase 5—The pressure level when the last sound is heard. **Nursing Process:** Evaluation **Client Need:** Physiological Integrity

Chapter 30
Key Topic Review Answers

1. a   **2.** b   **3.** a   **4.** a   **5.** b
6. Bruit
7. Aphasia
8. Reflex
9. Hernia
10. Discrimination
11. i, h, j, d, f, g, b, e, c, a
12. b   **13.** d   **14.** d   **15.** c   **16.** c

Case Study Answers

1. *Discuss the purposes of the physical examination.* Some of the purposes of the physical examination are to:

- Obtain baseline data about the client's functional abilities.
- Supplement, confirm, or refute data obtained in the nursing history.
- Obtain data that will help establish nursing diagnoses and plans of care.
- Evaluate the physiologic outcomes of health care and thus the progress of a client's health problem.
- Make clinical judgments about a client's health status.
- Identify areas for health promotion and disease prevention.

2. *Several positions are frequently required during the physical assessment. List client positions and provide a description of each one.*

Dorsal recumbent: Back-lying position with knees flexed and hips externally rotated; small pillow under the head; soles of feet on the surface.

Supine (horizontal recumbent): Back-lying position with legs extended; with or without pillow under the head.

Sitting: A seated position, back unsupported and legs hanging freely.

Lithotomy: Back-lying position with feet supported in stirrups; the hips should be in line with the edge of the table.

Sims: Side-lying position with lowermost arm behind the body, uppermost leg flexed at hip and knee, upper arm flexed at shoulder and elbow.

Prone: Lies on abdomen with head turned to the side, with or without a small pillow.

3. *List the equipment and supplies used for a health examination.*

Flashlight or penlight

Nasal speculum

Ophthalmoscope

Otoscope

Percussion (reflex) hammer

Tuning fork

Vaginal speculum

Cotton applicators

Gloves

Lubricant

Tongue blades (depressors)

NCLEX® Review Question Answers

1. *Answer:* 1 (Objective: 1) *Rationale:* The following statements would be correct responses by the nurse regarding purposes for a physical examination:

"To obtain baseline data about a client's functional abilities."

"To obtain data that will help establish nursing diagnoses and plans of care."

"To identify areas for health promotion and disease prevention."

"To supplement, confirm, or refute data obtained in the nursing history."

Nursing Process: Assessment *Client Need:* Physiological Integrity

2. *Answer:* 4 (Objective: 2) *Rationale:* Auscultation is the process of listening to sounds produced within the body. Inspection is the visual examination—that is, assessing by using the sense of sight. Palpation is the examination of the

body using the sense of touch. Percussion is the act of striking the body surface to elicit sounds that can be heard or vibrations that can be felt. *Nursing Process:* Assessment *Client Need:* Physiological Integrity

3. *Answer:* 3 (Objective: 3) *Rationale:* Jaundice (a yellowish tinge) may first be evident in the sclera of the eyes and then in the mucous membranes and the skin. Pallor is the result of inadequate circulating blood or hemoglobin and subsequent reduction in tissue oxygenation. Cyanosis (a bluish tinge) is most evident in the nail beds, lips, and buccal mucosa. Erythema is a redness associated with a variety of rashes. *Nursing Process:* Assessment *Client Need:* Physiological Integrity

4. *Answer:* 1 (Objective: 3) *Rationale:* Myopia means nearsightedness; hyperopia means farsightedness; presbyopia means loss of elasticity of the lens and thus loss of ability to see close objects; and stigmatism means an uneven curvature of the cornea that prevents horizontal and vertical rays from focusing on the retina. *Nursing Process:* Assessment *Client Need:* Physiological Integrity

5. *Answer:* 2 (Objective: 3) *Rationale:* Sound transmission and hearing are complex processes. In brief, sound can be transmitted by air conduction or bone conduction. Air-conducted transmission occurs by this process:

1. A sound stimulus enters the external canal and reaches the tympanic membrane.

2. The sound waves vibrate the tympanic membrane and reach the ossicles.

3. The sound waves travel from the ossicles to the opening in the inner ear (oval window).

4. The cochlea receives the sound vibrations.

5. The stimulus travels to the auditory nerve (the eighth cranial nerve) and the cerebral cortex.

Nursing Process: Assessment *Client Need:* Physiological Integrity

6. *Answer:* 4 (Objective: 3) *Rationale:* Organs in the Nine Abdominal Regions

The left hypochondriac region includes the stomach, the spleen, the tail of the pancreas, the splenic flexure of the colon, the upper half of the left kidney, and the suprarenal gland. The epigastric region includes the aorta, the pyloric end of the stomach, part of the duodenum, and the pancreas. The umbilical region includes the omentum, the mesentery, the lower part of the duodenum, and part of the jejunum and ileum. The right lumbar region includes the ascending colon, the lower half of the right kidney, and part of the duodenum and jejunum. *Nursing Process:* Assessment *Client Need:* Physiological Integrity

7. *Answer:* 2 (Objective: 5) *Rationale:* Cranial Nerve Functions and Assessment Methods

Cranial nerve II would be to ask the client to read a Snellen-type chart. Cranial nerve I would be to ask the client to close his/her eyes and identify different mild aromas, such as coffee, vanilla, peanut butter, orange/lemon, or chocolate. Cranial nerve VI would be to assess the client's directions of gaze.

Cranial nerve VII would be to ask the client to smile, raise the eyebrows, frown, puff out cheeks, close eyes tightly. *Nursing Process:* Assessment *Client Need:* Physiological Integrity

8. *Answer:* 1 (Objective: 3) *Rationale:* Adventitious Breath Sounds

Friction rub: Superficial grating or creaking sounds heard during inspiration and expiration. They are not relieved by coughing. Crackles (rales): Fine, short, interrupted crackling sounds; alveolar rales are high-pitched. Sound can be simulated by rolling a lock of hair near the ear. They are best heard on inspiration but can be heard on both inspiration and expiration. They may not be cleared by coughing. Gurgles (rhonchi): Continuous, low-pitched, coarse, gurgling, harsh, louder sounds with a moaning or snoring quality. They are best heard on expiration but can be heard on both inspiration and expiration. They may be altered by coughing. Wheeze: Continuous, high-pitched, squeaky musical sounds. This is best heard on expiration. It is not usually altered by coughing. *Nursing Process:* Assessment *Client Need:* Physiological Integrity

9. *Answer:* 3 (Objective: 4) *Rationale:* Client Positions and Body Areas Assessed

The lithotomy position is for assessing the female genitals, rectum, and female reproductive tract. The prone position is for assessing the posterior thorax and hip joint movement. The supine position is for assessing the head, neck, axillae, anterior thorax, lungs, breasts, heart, vital signs, heart, abdomen, extremities, and peripheral pulses. The sitting position is for assessing the head, neck, posterior and anterior thorax, lungs, breasts, axillae, heart, vital signs, upper and lower extremities, and reflexes. *Nursing Process:* Assessment *Client Need:* Physiological Integrity

10. *Answer:* 2 (Objective: 4) *Rationale:* Nursing Assessments Addressing Selected Client Situations

1. Client complains of abdominal pain: Inspect, auscultate, and palpate the abdomen; assess vital signs.
2. Client is admitted with a head injury: Assess level of consciousness using Glasgow Coma Scale (see Table 30–10 in the textbook); assess pupils for reaction to light and accommodation; assess vital signs.
3. The nurse prepares to administer a cardiotonic drug to a client: Assess apical pulse and compare with baseline data.
4. The client has just had a cast applied to the lower leg: Assess peripheral perfusion of toes, capillary blanch test, pedal pulse if able, and vital signs.
5. The client's fluid intake is minimal: Assess tissue turgor, fluid intake and output, and vital signs.

Nursing Process: Assessment *Client Need:* Physiological Integrity

Chapter 31
Key Topic Review Answers

1. b   **2.** a   **3.** a   **4.** b   **5.** a
6. Communicable
7. Opportunistic
8. Asepsis
9. Bacteria
10. Dirty
11. j, h, f, d, b, i, a, g, c, e
12. d   **13.** b   **14.** c   **15.** a   **16.** b

Case Study Answers

1. *What is the difference between asepsis and sepsis, and between medical asepsis and surgical asepsis?* Asepsis is the freedom from disease-causing microorganisms. To decrease the possibility of transferring microorganisms from one place to another, aseptic technique is used. There are two basic types of asepsis: medical and surgical. Medical asepsis includes all practices intended to confine a specific microorganism to a specific area, limiting the number, growth, and transmission of microorganisms. In medical asepsis, objects are referred to as clean, which means the absence of almost all microorganisms, or dirty (soiled, contaminated), which means likely to have microorganisms, some of which may be capable of causing infection. Surgical asepsis, or sterile technique, refers to those practices that keep an area or object free of all microorganisms; it includes practices that destroy all microorganisms and spores (microscopic dormant structures formed by some pathogens that are very hardy and often survive common cleaning techniques). Surgical asepsis is used for all procedures involving the sterile areas of the body. Sepsis is the state of infection and can take many forms, including septic shock.

2. *What four major categories of microorganisms cause infection in humans?* Four major categories of microorganisms cause infection in humans: bacteria, viruses, fungi, and parasites. Bacteria are by far the most common infection-causing microorganisms. Several hundred species can cause disease in humans and can live and be transported through air, water, food, soil, body tissues and fluids, and inanimate objects. Most of the microorganisms listed in Table 31–1 in the textbook are bacteria. Viruses consist primarily of nucleic acid and therefore must enter living cells in order to reproduce. Common virus families include the rhinovirus (causes the common cold), hepatitis, herpes, and human immunodeficiency virus. Fungi include yeasts and molds. *Candida albicans* is a yeast considered to be normal flora in the human vagina. Parasites live on other living organisms. They include protozoa such as the one that causes malaria, helminths (worms), and arthropods (mites, fleas, ticks).

3. *Explain the difference between standard precautions and transmission-based precautions.* Standard precautions: These precautions are used in the care of all hospitalized persons regardless of their diagnosis or possible infection status. They apply to blood, all body fluids, secretions, excretions except sweat (whether or not blood is present or visible), nonintact skin, and mucous membranes. Thus they combine the major features of UP and BSI.

Transmission-based precautions: These precautions are used in addition to standard precautions for clients with known or suspected infections that are spread in one of three ways: by airborne or droplet transmission, or by contact. The three types of transmission-based precautions may be used alone or in combination but always in addition to standard precautions. They encompass all of the conditions or diseases previously listed in the category-specific or disease-specific classifications developed by the CDC in 1983.

NCLEX® Review Question Answers

1. *Answer:* 2 (Objective: 1) *Rationale:* Asepsis is the freedom from disease-causing

microorganisms. Medical asepsis includes all practices intended to confine a specific microorganism to a specific area, limiting the number, growth, and transmission of microorganisms. Surgical asepsis, or sterile technique, refers to those practices that keep an area or object free of all microorganisms; it includes practices that destroy all microorganisms and spores (microscopic dormant structures formed by some pathogens that are very hardy and often survive common cleaning techniques). Sepsis is the state of infection and can take many forms, including septic shock. *Nursing Process:* Assessment *Client Need:* Physiological Integrity

2. *Answer:* 3 (Objective: 1) *Rationale:* Viruses consist primarily of nucleic acid and therefore must enter living cells in order to reproduce. Fungi include yeasts and molds. Bacteria are by far the most common infection-causing microorganisms. Parasites live on other living organisms. *Nursing Process:* Assessment *Client Need:* Physiological Integrity

3. *Answer:* 4 (Objective: 3) *Rationale:* Fatigue is not a sign of inflammation. Inflammation is a local and nonspecific defensive response of the tissues to an injurious or infectious agent. It is an adaptive mechanism that destroys or dilutes the injurious agent, prevents further spread of the injury, and promotes the repair of damaged tissue. It is characterized by five signs: (a) pain, (b) swelling, (c) redness, (d) heat, and (e) impaired function of the part, if the injury is severe. *Nursing Process:* Assessment *Client Need:* Physiological Integrity

4. *Answer:* 4 (Objective: 8) *Rationale:* Four commonly used methods of sterilization are moist heat, gas, boiling water, and radiation. Moist heat: To sterilize with moist heat (such as with an autoclave), steam under pressure is used because it attains temperatures higher than the boiling point. Gas: Ethylene oxide gas destroys microorganisms by interfering with their metabolic processes. It is also effective against spores. Its advantages are good penetration and effectiveness for heat-sensitive items. Its major disadvantage is its toxicity to humans. Boiling water: This is the most practical and inexpensive method for sterilizing in the home. The main disadvantage is that spores and some viruses are not killed by this method. Boiling a minimum of 15 minutes is advised for disinfection of articles in the home. Radiation: Both ionizing (such as alpha, beta, and x-rays) and nonionizing (ultraviolet light) radiation are used for disinfection and sterilization. The main drawback to ultraviolet light is that the rays do not penetrate deeply. Ionizing radiation is

used effectively in industry to sterilize foods, drugs, and other items that are sensitive to heat. Its main advantage is that it is effective for items difficult to sterilize; its chief disadvantage is that the equipment is very expensive. *Nursing Process:* Assessment *Client Need:* Physiological Integrity

5. *Answer:* 3 (Objective: 6) *Rationale:* Acute infections generally appear suddenly or last a short time. A chronic infection may occur slowly, over a very long period, and may last months or years. A local infection is limited to the specific part of the body where the microorganisms remain. If the microorganisms spread and damage different parts of the body, it is a systemic infection. Nosocomial infections are classified as infections that are associated with the delivery of health care services in a health care facility. *Nursing Process:* Assessment *Client Need:* Physiological Integrity

6. *Answer:* 3 (Objective: 9) *Rationale:* Six links make up the chain of infection: the etiologic agent, or microorganism; the place where the organism naturally resides (reservoir); a portal of exit from the reservoir; a method (mode) of transmission; a portal of entry into a host; and the susceptibility of the host. *Nursing Process:* Planning *Client Need:* Physiological Integrity

7. *Answer:* 2 (Objective: 4) *Rationale:* An antigen is a substance that induces a state of sensitivity or immune responsiveness (immunity). With active immunity, the host produces antibodies in response to natural antigens (e.g., infectious microorganisms) or artificial antigens (e.g., vaccines). With passive (or acquired) immunity, the host receives natural (e.g., from a nursing mother) or artificial (e.g., from an injection of immune serum) antibodies produced by another source. Antibodies, also called immunoglobulins, are part of the body's plasma proteins. *Nursing Process:* Assessment *Client Need:* Physiological Integrity

8. *Answer:* 1 (Objective: 11) *Rationale:* The CDC recommends antimicrobial hand cleansing agents in the following situations:

■ When there are known multiple resistant bacteria.

■ Before invasive procedures.

■ In special care units, such as nurseries and ICUs.

■ Before caring for severely immunocompromised clients.

Nursing Process: Assessment *Client Need:* Physiological Integrity

9. *Answer:* 3 (Objective: 11) *Rationale:* Disinfectants and antiseptics often have similar chemical components, but the disinfectant is a more concentrated solution. A disinfectant is a chemical preparation, such as phenol or iodine compounds, used on inanimate objects. Disinfectants are frequently caustic and toxic to tissues. An antiseptic is a chemical preparation used on skin or tissue. A disinfectant is an agent that destroys pathogens other than spores. *Nursing Process:* Assessment *Client Need:* Physiological Integrity

10. *Answer:* 2 (Objective: 10) *Rationale:* Airborne precautions are used for clients known to have or suspected of having serious illnesses transmitted by airborne droplet nuclei smaller than 5 microns. Droplet precautions are used for clients known or suspected to have serious illnesses transmitted by particle droplets larger than 5 microns. Contact precautions are used for clients known or suspected to have serious illnesses easily transmitted by direct client contact or by contact with items in the client's environment. Connection precautions do not exist. *Nursing Process:* Assessment *Client Need:* Physiological Integrity

Chapter 32
Key Topic Review Answers

1. a   **2.** b   **3.** a   **4.** b   **5.** a
6. Terrorism
7. Homicide
8. Scald
9. Radiation
10. Risk
11. h, f, a, i, j, b, g, e, c, d
12. c   **13.** b   **14.** d   **15.** d   **16.** c

Case Study Answers

1. *What preventive measures do you need to teach the couple?*

■ Keep emergency numbers near the telephone, or stored for speed dialing.

■ Be sure the smoke alarms are operable and appropriately located.

■ Teach clients to change the batteries in their smoke alarms annually on a special day such as a birthday or January 1.

■ Have a family "fire drill" plan. Every member needs to know the plan for the nearest exit from different locations of the home.

■ Keep fire extinguishers available and in working order.

■ Close windows and doors if possible; cover the mouth and nose with a damp cloth when exiting through a smoke-filled area; and avoid heavy smoke by assuming a bent position with the head as close to the floor as possible.

2. *Write a fire plan for the couple to follow.* Each fire plan will vary from student to student.

3. *Explain the three categories of fires.*

Class A: Paper, wood, upholstery, rags, ordinary rubbish

Class B: Flammable liquids and gases

Class C: Electrical

NCLEX® Review Question Answers

1. *Answer:* 4 (Objective: 4) *Rationale:* Lead poisoning (plumbism) is a risk for children exposed to lead paint chips, fumes from leaded gasoline, or any "leaded" substances. The ingestion of lead-based paint chips is the most common cause of lead poisoning in children. Common accidents during infancy include burns, suffocation or choking, automobile accidents, falls, and poisoning. *Nursing Process:* Planning *Client Need:* Safe, Effective Care Environment

2. *Answer:* 4 (Objective: 4) *Rationale:* A common accident during infancy is suffocation. Trash bags or any type of plastic bag must be kept out of an infant's reach. *Nursing Process:* Evaluation *Client Need:* Safe, Effective Care Environment

3. *Answer:* 2 (Objective: 4) *Rationale:* Obtaining a driver's license is an important event in the life of a U.S. adolescent, but the privilege is not always wisely handled. Teenagers may use driving as an outlet for stress, as a way to assert independence, or as a way to impress peers. When setting limits on automobile use, parents need to assess the teenager's level of responsibility, common sense, and ability to resist peer pressure. The age of the teenager alone does not determine readiness to handle this responsibility. Lead poisoning (plumbism) is a risk for children exposed to lead paint chips, fumes from leaded gasoline, or any "leaded" substances. The ingestion of lead-based paint chips is the most common cause of lead poisoning in children. Adolescents would need safety training about driving an automobile, not a tricycle. Adolescents have better coordination skills than toddlers. It is not necessary for an adolescent to sleep in a low bed. *Nursing Process:* Planning *Client Need:* Safe, Effective Care Environment

4. *Answer:* 2 (Objective: 4) *Rationale:* Suicide and homicide are two leading causes of death among teenagers. Adolescent males commit suicide at a higher rate than adolescent females, and African Americans commit homicide at a higher rate than European Americans. Suicides by firearms, drugs, and automobile exhaust gases are the most common. Factors influencing the high suicide and homicide rates include economic deprivation, family breakup, and the availability of firearms, which are the most frequently used weapons. *Nursing Process:* Planning *Client Need:* Psychosocial Integrity

5. *Answer:* 1 (Objective: 4) *Rationale:* Accidents are the leading cause of death in school-age children. The most frequent causes of fatalities, in descending order, are motor vehicle accidents, drownings, fires, and firearms. School-age children are also involved in many minor accidents, frequently resulting from outdoor activities and recreational equipment such as swings, bicycles, skateboards, and swimming pools. *Nursing Process:* Implementation *Client Need:* Health Promotion and Maintenance

6. *Answer:* 4 (Objective: 7) *Rationale:* Falls are the leading cause of accidents among older adults. They are also a major cause of hospital and nursing home admissions. Most falls occur in the home and are a major threat to the independence of older adults. Fear of falling is common in older adults, even in those who have not experienced a fall. This fear is of particular concern for those who live alone and who anticipate being helpless and unable to summon help after a fall. Suicide is a leading cause of death among teenagers. The incidence of suicide in older adults is increasing and often goes unnoticed when the causes are due to hidden self-destructive behaviors, such as starvation, overdosing with medications, and noncompliance with medical care, treatments, and medications. In older individuals, the suicide attempt is usually more serious, because it is truly intended to end the life, not just to get attention as is often seen in other age groups. Also, the method of suicide is generally more violent in the older person, such as a gunshot wound to the head, or hanging. Other accidental causes of death for middle-aged adults include falls, fires, burns, poisonings, and drownings. *Nursing Process:* Planning *Client Need:* Health Promotion and Maintenance

7. *Answer:* 2 (Objective: 2) *Rationale:* During the nursing assessment all of the following should be assessed: the behavior indicating the possible need for a restraint; underlying cause for assessed behavior; other protective measures that may be implemented before applying a restraint; status of skin to which restraint is to be applied; circulatory status distal to restraints and of extremities; effectiveness of other available safety precautions. *Nursing Process:* Assessment *Client Need:* Safe, Effective Care Environment

8. *Answer:* 1 (Objective: 6) *Rationale:* Avoid storing toxic liquids or solids in food containers, such as soft drink bottles, peanut butter jars, or milk cartons. Display the phone number of the poison control center near or on all telephones in the home so that it is available to baby-sitters, family, and friends. Teach children never to eat any part of an unknown plant or mushroom and not to put leaves, stems, bark, seeds, nuts, or berries from any plant into their mouths. Do not refer to medicine as candy or pretend false enjoyment when taking medications in front of children; allow them to see the necessity of the medicine without glamorizing it. *Nursing Process:* Evaluation *Client Need:* Safe, Effective Care Environment

9. *Answer:* 1 (Objective: 8) *Rationale:* If clients have frequent or recurrent seizures or take anticonvulsant medications, they should wear a medical identification tag (bracelet or necklace) and carry a card delineating any medications they take. Assist the client in determining which persons in the community should/must be informed of their seizure disorder (e.g., employers, health care providers such as dentists, motor vehicle department if driving, companions). Discuss safety precautions for inside and out of the home. If seizures are not well controlled, activities that may require restriction or direct supervision by others include tub bathing, swimming, cooking, using electric equipment or machinery, and driving. Discuss with the client and family factors that may precipitate a seizure. *Nursing Process:* Planning *Client Need:* Safe, Effective Care Environment

10. *Answer:* 3 (Objective: 6) *Rationale:* All of the following would be a preventive measure for an older client with poor vision: ensuring eyeglasses are functional, ensuring appropriate lighting, marking doorways and edges of steps as needed, and keeping the environment tidy. *Nursing Process:* Planning *Client Need:* Safe, Effective Care Environment

Chapter 33
Key Topic Review Answers

1. a **2.** b **3.** a **4.** a **5.** b

6. Pediculosis

7. Scabies

8. Hirsutism

9. Lanugo

10. Plaque

11. h, i, d, c, e, j, f, a, b, g

12. a **13.** b **14.** b **15.** c **16.** c

Case Study Answers

1. *What is the proper water temperature for the client's bath?* The temperature of the bath water should be between 43 and 46°C (110 to 115°F).

2. *List three reasons why a nurse would check the bath water.* The nurse must check the water temperature to avoid burning the client with water that is too hot. The water for a bath should be changed when it becomes dirty or cold.

3. *Why is it important to verify the temperature of the water for this client?* Clients with decreased cognitive problems will not be able to verify the temperature.

NCLEX® Review Question Answers

1. *Answer:* 1 (Objective: 10) *Rationale:* Hold soiled linen away from uniform. Do not shake soiled linen in the air because shaking can disseminate secretions and excretions and the microorganisms they contain. When stripping and making a bed, conserve time and energy by stripping and making up one side as much as possible before working on the other side. Linen for one client is never (even momentarily) placed on another client's bed. All of these methods prevent transmission of pathogens. *Nursing Process:* Implementation *Client Need:* Safe, Effective Care Environment

2. *Answer:* 3 (Objective: 6) *Rationale:* The water for a bath should feel comfortably warm to the client. People vary in their sensitivity to heat. The bath water temperature is generally included in the order; 37.7 to 46°C (100 to 115°F) may be ordered for adults. All other bath water temperatures listed are too cold or too hot. *Nursing Process:* Implementation *Client Need:* Physiological Integrity

3. *Answer:* 1 (Objective: 1) *Rationale:* Dental caries occur frequently during the toddler period, often as a result of the excessive intake of sweets or a prolonged use of the bottle during naps and at bedtime. The nurse should give parents the following instructions to promote and maintain dental health: Beginning at about 18 months of age, brush the child's teeth with a soft toothbrush. Use only a toothbrush moistened with water at first and introduce toothpaste later. Use one that contains fluoride. Give a fluoride supplement daily or as recommended by the physician or dentist, unless the drinking water is fluoridated.

Schedule an initial dental visit for the child at about 2 or 3 years of age, as soon as all 20 primary teeth have erupted. Some dentists recommend an inspection type of visit when the child is about 18 months old to provide an early pleasant introduction to the dental examination. Seek professional dental attention for any problems such as discoloring of the teeth, chipping, or signs of infection such as redness and swelling. *Nursing Process:* Evaluation *Client Need:* Health Promotion and Maintenance

4. *Answer:* 1 (Objective: 4) *Rationale:* During discharge planning for preventing dry skin the nurse should review the following with the client: Use cleansing creams to clean the skin rather than soap or detergent, which cause drying and, in some cases, allergic reactions. Use bath oils, but take precautions to prevent falls caused by slippery tub surfaces. Humidify the air with a humidifier or by keeping a tub or sink full of water. Use moisturizing or emollient creams that contain lanolin, petroleum jelly, or cocoa butter to retain skin moisture. *Nursing Process:* Implementation *Client Need:* Safe, Effective Care Environment

5. *Answer:* 1 (Objective: 4) *Rationale:* When providing foot care for a client, the nurse should check the water temperature before immersing the feet to prevent any burns. The nurse should wash the feet daily, and dry them well, especially between the toes. While washing the feet, the nurse should inspect the skin of the feet for breaks or red or swollen areas. Use a mirror if needed to visualize all areas. The nurse should cover the feet—except between the toes—with creams or lotions to moisten the skin. Lotion will also soften calluses. A lotion that reduces dryness effectively is a mixture of lanolin and mineral oil. *Nursing Process:* Implementation *Client Need:* Physiological Integrity

6. *Answer:* 4 (Objective: 4) *Rationale:* Healthy nail care practices are reflected in clean, short nails with smooth edges and intact cuticles. The client's nail should be cut or filed straight across beyond the end of the finger or toe. The client should avoid trimming or digging into nails at the lateral corners. This predisposes the client to ingrown toenails. *Nursing Process:* Evaluation *Client Need:* Physiological Integrity

7. *Answer:* 4 (Objective: 7) *Rationale:* The nurse must evaluate the client's understanding of measures to prevent tooth decay. Brushing the teeth thoroughly after meals and at bedtime, flossing the teeth daily, avoiding sweet foods and drinks between meals, and having a checkup by a dentist every 6 months are just some of the measures that must be understood by the client. *Nursing Process:* Evaluation *Client Need:* Physiological Integrity

8. *Answer:* 4 (Objective: 7) *Rationale:* The student nurse should perform all of the following when shaving a client with a safety razor: The student nurse holds the skin taut, particularly around creases, to prevent cutting the skin. The student nurse wears gloves in case facial nicks occur and she comes in contact with blood. The student nurse applies shaving cream or soap and water to soften the bristles and make the skin more pliable. The student nurse holds the razor so that the blade is at a 45-degree angle to the skin, and shaves in short, firm strokes in the direction of hair growth. *Nursing Process:* Implementation *Client Need:* Safe, Effective Care Environment

9. *Answer:* 1 (Objective: 6) *Rationale:* The appropriate actions must be followed by the nurse bathing a person with dementia. The following are just a few of the actions that must be followed. Move slowly and let the person know when you are going to move him or her. Use a supportive, calm approach and praise the person often. Gather everything that you will need for the bath (e.g., towels, washcloths, clothes) before approaching the person. Help the person feel in control. *Nursing Process:* Implementation *Client Need:* Physiological Integrity

10. *Answer:* 2 (Objective: 10) *Rationale:* Before a nurse inserts a hearing aid into a patient's ear it is very important to perform the following steps. Determine from the client if the earmold is for the left or the right ear. Gently press the earmold into the ear while rotating it backward. Inspect the earmold to identify the ear canal portion. Check that the earmold fits snugly by asking the client if it feels secure and comfortable. *Nursing Process:* Implementation *Client Need:* Physiological Integrity

Chapter 34
Key Topic Review Answers

1. a   2. a   3. b   4. a   5. a
6. Throat
7. Biopsy
8. Manometer
9. Aspiration
10. Blood
11. a, e, c, f, h, i, j, g, d, b
12. c   13. a   14. b   15. d   16. c

Case Study Answers

1. *Why did the physician order sputum specimens?*
The physician ordered an AFB to identify the presence of tuberculosis (TB).

2. *How will you collect the sputum specimens?* To collect a sputum specimen, the nurse follows these steps:

- Offer mouth care so that the specimen will not be contaminated with microorganisms from the mouth.
- Ask the client to breathe deeply and then cough up 1 to 2 tablespoons, or 15 to 30 mL (4 to 8 fluid drams), of sputum.
- Ask the client to expectorate (spit out) the sputum into the specimen container. Make sure the sputum does not contact the outside of the container. If the outside of the container does become contaminated, wash it with a disinfectant.
- Following sputum collection, offer mouthwash to remove any unpleasant taste.

3. *What PPE should you wear when you collect the sputum specimens?* Wear gloves and PPE to avoid direct contact with the sputum. Follow special precautions if tuberculosis is suspected, obtaining the specimen in a room equipped with a special airflow system or ultraviolet light, or outdoors. If these options are not available, wear a mask capable of filtering droplet nuclei.

4. *What information should you document in the client medical record after collecting the sputum specimens?* Document the collection of the sputum specimens on the client's chart. Include the amount, color, odor, and consistency (thick, tenacious, watery) of the sputum, the presence of hemoptysis (blood in the sputum), any measures needed to obtain the specimen (e.g., postural drainage), and any discomfort experienced by the client.

5. *How should the specimens be stored until they are transported to the laboratory?* Label and transport the specimens to the laboratory. Ensure that the specimen labels and the laboratory requisitions contain the correct information. Arrange for the specimens to be sent to the laboratory immediately or refrigerated. Bacterial cultures must be started immediately before any contaminating organisms can grow, multiply, and produce false results.

NCLEX® Review Question Answers

1. *Answer:* 3 (Objective: 2) *Rationale:* The normal hematocrit finding for an adult female is 36–46%. The normal hemoglobin finding for an adult female is 12–16 g/dL. The normal RBC finding for an adult female is 4.1–5.1 million/mm^3. The normal MCV finding for an adult female is 78–102 μm^3. *Nursing Process:* Assessment *Client Need:* Physiological Integrity

2. *Answer:* 2 (Objective: 2) *Rationale:* The normal sodium serum level is 135–145 mEq/L. The normal potassium serum level is 3.5–5.0 mEq/L. The normal chloride level is 95–105 mEq/L. The normal magnesium level is 1.5–2.5 mEq/L or 1.6–2.5 mg/dL. *Nursing Process:* Assessment *Client Need:* Physiological Integrity

3. *Answer:* 1 (Objective: 2) *Rationale:* The normal hematocrit level for an adult male is 37–49%. The normal hemoglobin level for an adult male is 13.8–18 g/dL. *Nursing Process:* Assessment *Client Need:* Physiological Integrity

4. *Answer:* 3 (Objective: 7) *Rationale:* For a male client using a circular motion to clean the urinary meatus is the correct technique. For a female client the perineal area should be cleaned from front to back. Always explain to the client that a urine specimen is required, give the reason, and explain the method to be used to collect it. A nurse should always perform hand hygiene and observe other appropriate infection control procedures. The nurse must ensure that the specimen label is attached to the specimen cup, not the lid, and that the laboratory requisition provides the correct information. *Nursing Process:* Implementation *Client Need:* Physiological Integrity

5. *Answer:* 2 (Objective: 11) *Rationale:* A bone marrow biopsy is the removal of a specimen of bone marrow for laboratory study. The biopsy is used to detect specific diseases of the blood, such as pernicious anemia and leukemia. The bones of the body commonly used for a bone marrow biopsy are the sternum, iliac crests, anterior or posterior iliac spines, and proximal tibia in children. The posterior superior iliac crest is the preferred site with the client placed prone or on the side. The knee-chest, lithotomy, and dorsal recumbent positions are incorrect positions for a bone marrow biopsy. *Nursing Process:* Implementation *Client Need:* Physiological Integrity

6. *Answer:* 4 (Objective: 11) *Rationale:* Assist the client to a dorsal recumbent position with only one head pillow. The client remains in this position for 1 to 12 hours, depending on the physician's orders. The knee-chest, lithotomy, and prone positions are incorrect positions for a lumbar puncture. *Nursing Process:* Implementation *Client Need:* Physiological Integrity

7. *Answer:* 3 (Objective: 11) *Rationale:* After a client returns from a lumbar puncture the nurse should have the client lie on the unaffected side with the head of the bed elevated 30 degrees for at least 30 minutes because this position facilitates expansion of the affected lung and eases respirations. If the head of bed is elevated at a position other than 30 degrees the client will not have ease of respiration and the client will not have proper expansion of the lungs. *Nursing Process:* Implementation *Client Need:* Physiological Integrity

8. Answer: 1 (Objective: 11) *Rationale:* An abdominal paracentesis is carried out to obtain a fluid specimen for laboratory study and to relieve pressure on the abdominal organs due to the presence of excess fluid. A physician performs the procedure with the assistance of a nurse. Strict sterile technique is followed. Normally about 1,500 mL is the maximum amount of fluid drained at one time to avoid hypovolemic shock. The fluid is drained very slowly for the same reason. *Nursing Process:* Implementation *Client Need:* Physiological Integrity

9. Answer: 1 (Objective: 4) *Rationale:* The nurse should state "Avoid collecting specimens during your menstrual period and for 3 days afterward, and while you have bleeding hemorrhoids or blood in your urine." Either of these situations would give a false positive to the fecal occult blood tests. Taking the sample from the center of a formed stool to ensure a uniform sample is a correct technique for a fecal occult blood test. Using a ballpoint pen to label the specimens with your name, address, age, and date of specimen is a correct technique for a fecal occult blood test. Avoiding contamination of the specimen with urine or toilet tissue is a correct technique for a fecal occult blood test. *Nursing Process:* Implementation *Client Need:* Physiological Integrity

10. Answer: 2 (Objective: 8) *Rationale:* Sterile gloves are not necessary for obtaining a throat culture. Wearing sterile gloves during this procedure is considered an unnecessary expense. To obtain a throat culture specimen, the nurse puts on clean gloves, then inserts the swab into the oropharynx and runs the swab along the tonsils and areas on the pharynx that are reddened or contain exudate. The gag reflex, active in some clients, may be decreased by having the client sit upright if health permits, open the mouth, extend the tongue, and say "ah," and by taking the specimen quickly. The sitting position and extension of the tongue help expose the pharynx; saying "ah" relaxes the throat muscles and helps minimize contraction of the constrictor muscle of the pharynx (the gag reflex). If the posterior pharynx cannot be seen, use a light and depress the tongue with a tongue blade. *Nursing Process:* Implementation *Client Need:* Physiological Integrity

Chapter 35
Key Topic Review Answers

1. b   2. a   3. a   4. b   5. b
6. Eyes
7. Intramuscular
8. Vial
9. Bevel
10. Plunger
11. a, d, e, g, i, j, h, f, c, b
12. b   13. d   14. d   15. a   16. c

Case Study Answers

1. *What are the 10 "rights" of medication administration?*
1. Right medication
2. Right dose
3. Right time
4. Right route
5. Right client
6. Right client education
7. Right documentation
8. Right to refuse
9. Right assessment
10. Right evaluation

2. *The Compazine is available in an ampule. How will you properly prepare the Compazine from the ampule?*

Preparation
1. Check the medication administration record (MAR).
2. Organize the equipment.

Performance
1. Perform hand hygiene and observe other appropriate infection control procedures (e.g., clean gloves).
2. Prepare the medication from the ampule for drug withdrawal.
3. Provide for client privacy.
4. Prepare the client.
5. Explain the purpose of the medication and how it will help, using language that the client can understand. Include relevant information about effects of the medication.
6. Select, locate, and clean the site.
7. Prepare the syringe for injection.
8. Withdraw the needle.

9. Activate the needle safety device or discard the uncapped needle and attached syringe into the proper receptacle.

10. Document all relevant information.

11. Assess effectiveness of the medication at the time it is expected to act.

NCLEX® Review Question Answers

1. Answer: 1 (Objective: 16) **Rationale:** The type of syringe used for subcutaneous injections depends on the medication to be given. Generally a 2-mL syringe is used for most subcutaneous injections. Needle sizes and lengths are selected based on the client's body mass, the intended angle of insertion, and the planned site. Generally a #25-gauge, 5/8-inch needle is used for adults of normal weight and the needle is inserted at a 45-degree angle; a 3/8-inch needle is used at a 90-degree angle. A child may need a 1/2-inch needle inserted at a 45-degree angle. One method nurses use to determine length of needle is to pinch the tissue at the site and select a needle length that is half the width of the skinfold. To determine the angle of insertion, a general rule to follow relates to the amount of tissue that can be bunched or grasped at the site. A 45-degree angle is used when 1 inch of tissue can be grasped at the site; a 90-degree angle is used when 2 inches of tissue can be grasped. **Nursing Process:** Implementation **Client Need:** Physiological Integrity

2. Answer: 1 (Objective: 1) **Rationale:** A drug that produces the same type of response as the physiologic or endogenous substance is called an agonist. Conversely, a drug that inhibits cell function by occupying receptor sites is called an antagonist. The antagonist prevents natural body substances or other drugs from activating the functions of the cell by occupying the receptor sites. A receptor, usually a protein, is located on the surface of a cell membrane or within the cell. A cell membrane contains receptors for physiologic or endogenous substances such as hormones and neurotransmitters. Biotransformation, also called detoxification or metabolism, is a process by which a drug is converted to a less active form. Most biotransformation takes place in the liver, where many drug-metabolizing enzymes in the cells detoxify the drugs. **Nursing Process:** Assessment **Client Need:** Physiological Integrity

3. Answer: 2 (Objective: 3) **Rationale:** Drug habituation denotes a mild form of psychologic dependence. The individual develops the habit of taking the substance and feels better after taking it. The habituated individual tends to continue the habit even though it may be injurious to health. Drug dependence is a person's reliance on or need to take a drug or substance. The two types of dependence, physiologic and psychologic, may occur separately or together. Physiologic dependence is due to biochemical changes in body tissues, especially the nervous system. These tissues come to require the substance for normal functioning. A dependent person who stops using the drug experiences withdrawal symptoms. Psychologic dependence is emotional reliance on a drug to maintain a sense of well-being, accompanied by feelings of need or cravings for that drug. There are varying degrees of psychologic dependence, ranging from mild desire to craving and compulsive use of the drug. **Nursing Process:** Planning **Client Need:** Psychosocial Integrity

4. Answer: 2 (Objective: 7) **Rationale:** When converting pounds to kilograms: The pound is a smaller unit than the kilogram, and the nurse converts by dividing or multiplying by 2.2:

$$2.2 \text{ lb} = 1 \text{ kg}$$
$$110 \text{ lb} = x \text{ kg}$$
$$x = \frac{110 \times 1}{2.2}$$
$$= 50 \text{ kg}$$

Any other amount listed is incorrect. **Nursing Process:** Implementation **Client Need:** Physiological Integrity

5. Answer: 1 (Objective: 7) **Rationale:** Erythromycin 500 mg is ordered. It is supplied in a liquid form containing 250 mg in 5 mL. To calculate the dosage, the nurse uses the formula

$$\frac{\text{Dose on hand (250 mg)}}{\text{Quantity on hand (5 mL)}} = \frac{\text{desired dose (500 mg)}}{\text{quantity desired } (x)}$$

Then the nurse cross multiplies:

$$250 \, x = 5 \text{ mL} \times 500 \text{ mg}$$
$$x = \frac{5 \text{ mL} \times 500 \text{ mg}}{250 \text{ mg}}$$
$$x = 10 \text{ mL}$$

Therefore, the dose ordered is 10 mL. The nurse can also use this formula to calculate dosages:

$$\text{Amount to administer } (x) = \frac{\text{desired dose}}{\text{dose on hand}} \times \text{quantity on hand}$$

Nursing Process: Implementation **Client Need:** Physiological Integrity

6. Answer: 1 (Objective: 14) **Rationale:** When handling a syringe, the nurse may touch the outside of the barrel and the handle of the plunger; however, the nurse must avoid letting any unsterile object touch the tip or inside of the barrel, the shaft of the plunger, or the shaft or tip of the needle. *Nursing Process:* Implementation *Client Need:* Physiological Integrity

7. *Answer:* 4 (Objective: 17) *Rationale:* The client should remain in the left lateral or supine position for at least 5 minutes to help retain the suppository. Assist the client to a left lateral or left Sims position, with the upper leg flexed. Unwrap the suppository and lubricate the smooth, rounded end, or see manufacturer's instructions. The rounded end is usually inserted first and lubricant reduces irritation of the mucosa. Press the client's buttocks together for a few minutes. *Nursing Process:* Implementation *Client Need:* Physiological Integrity

8. *Answer:* 1 (Objective: 17) *Rationale:* Explain that the client may experience a feeling of fullness, warmth, and, occasionally, discomfort when the fluid comes in contact with the tympanic membrane. Insert the tip of the syringe into the auditory meatus, and direct the solution gently upward against the top of the canal. The solution will flow around the entire canal and out at the bottom. The solution is instilled gently because strong pressure from the fluid can cause discomfort and damage the tympanic membrane. Straighten the ear canal prior to inserting the tip of the syringe and during the procedure. After the procedure the nurse should place a cotton fluff in the auditory meatus to absorb the excess fluid. *Nursing Process:* Implementation *Client Need:* Physiological Integrity

9. *Answer:* 2 (Objective: 17) *Rationale:* The client needs to remain lying in the supine position for 5 to 10 minutes following the insertion. Gently insert the applicator into the vagina about 5 cm (2 in.). Slowly push the plunger until the applicator is empty. Remove the applicator and place it on the towel. The applicator is put on the towel to prevent the spread of microorganisms. Discard the applicator if disposable or clean it according to the manufacturer's directions. *Nursing Process:* Implementation *Client Need:* Physiological Integrity

10. *Answer:* 3 (Objective: 17) *Rationale:* When applying a transdermal patch the nurse must select a clean, dry area that is free of hair and matches the manufacturer's recommendations. The nurse should then remove the patch from its protective covering, holding it without touching the adhesive edges, and apply it by pressing firmly with the palm of the hand for about 10 seconds. *Nursing Process:* Implementation *Client Need:* Physiological Integrity

Chapter 36
Key Topic Review Answers

1. a   2. b   3. a   4. b   5. a
6. Health
7. Maceration
8. Cleaning
9. Piston
10. Skin
11. i, j, a, b, h, c, f, d, g, e
12. b   13. a   14. b   15. a   16. c

Case Study Answers

1. *Explain the local effects of cold.* The physiologic effects of cold are opposite to the effects of heat. Cold lowers the temperature of the skin and underlying tissues and causes vasoconstriction. Vasoconstriction reduces blood flow to the affected area and thus reduces the supply of oxygen and metabolites, decreases the removal of wastes, and produces skin pallor and coolness. Prolonged exposure to cold results in impaired circulation, cell deprivation, and subsequent damage to the tissues from lack of oxygen and nourishment. The signs of tissue damage due to cold are a bluish-purple mottled appearance of the skin, numbness, and sometimes blisters and pain. Cold is most often used for sports injuries (e.g., sprains, strains, fractures) to limit postinjury swelling and bleeding.

2. *Explain the systemic effects of cold.* With extensive cold applications and vasoconstriction, a client's blood pressure can increase because blood is shunted from the cutaneous circulation to the internal blood vessels. Shivering, a generalized effect of prolonged cold, is a normal response as the body attempts to warm itself.

3. *List some indications for applying ice to the injured ankle.* Indicators include muscle spasms, inflammation, pain, and traumatic injury.

4. *Summarize the guidelines a nurse should follow for all local cold applications.*
- Determine the client's ability to tolerate the therapy.
- Identify conditions that might contraindicate treatment (e.g., bleeding, circulatory impairment).
- Explain the application to the client.
- Assess the skin area to which the cold will be applied.
- Ask the client to report any discomfort.
- Return to the client 15 minutes after starting the cold application and observe the local skin

area for any untoward signs (e.g., redness). Stop the application if any problems occur.

■ Remove the equipment at the designated time, and dispose of it appropriately.

■ Examine the area to which the heat or cold was applied, and record the client's response.

NCLEX® Review Question Answers

1. Answer: 1 (Objective: 6) **Rationale:** A purulent exudate is thicker than serous exudate because of the presence of pus, which consists of leukocytes, liquefied dead tissue debris, and dead and living bacteria. A serosanguineous (consisting of clear and blood-tinged drainage) exudate is commonly seen in surgical incisions. A serous exudate consists chiefly of serum (the clear portion of the blood) derived from blood and the serous membranes of the body, such as the peritoneum. It looks watery and has few cells. A sanguineous (hemorrhagic) exudate consists of large amounts of red blood cells, indicating damage to capillaries that is severe enough to allow the escape of red blood cells from plasma. This type of exudate is frequently seen in open wounds. **Nursing Process:** Assessment **Client Need:** Physiological Integrity

2. Answer: 3 (Objective: 16) **Rationale:** In applying electric pads, the nurse needs to teach the client the following guidelines:

■ Do not insert sharp objects (e.g., pins) into the pad. The pin could damage a wire and cause an electric shock.

■ Ensure that the body area is dry unless there is a waterproof cover on the pad. Electricity in the presence of water can cause a shock.

■ Use pads with a preset heating switch so a client cannot increase the heat.

■ Do not place the pad under the client. Heat will not dissipate, and the client may be burned. **Nursing Process:** Implementation **Client Need:** Safe, Effective Care Environment

3. Answer: 4 (Objective: 16) **Rationale:** The following temperatures of the water in the bag are considered safe in most situations and provide the desired effect: normal adult and child over 2 years, 46 to 52°C (115 to 125°F); debilitated or unconscious adult, or child under 2 years, 40.5 to 46°C (105 to 115°F). The client fills the bag two-thirds full with water. After filling the bag with water the client dries the bag and holds it upside down to test it for leakage. The client expels the remaining air out of the bag before securing the top. **Nursing Process:** Implementation **Client Need:** Safe, Effective Care Environment

4. Answer: 4 (Objective: 13) **Rationale:** The bandage should be firm, but not too tight. Ask the client if the bandage feels comfortable. A tight bandage can interfere with blood circulation, whereas a loose bandage does not provide adequate protection. Bandages can be used to support a wound (e.g., a fractured bone). Bandages can also be used to immobilize a wound (e.g., a strained shoulder). Bandages can be used to apply pressure (e.g., elastic bandages on the lower extremities to improve venous blood flow). **Nursing Process:** Evaluation **Client Need:** Physiological Integrity

5. Answer: 3 (Objective: 13) **Rationale:** Dressings are applied for the following purposes: to protect the wound from mechanical injury, to protect the wound from microbial contamination, to provide thermal insulation, and to prevent hemorrhage (when applied as a pressure dressing or with elastic bandages). **Nursing Process:** Planning **Client Need:** Physiological Integrity

6. Answer: 3 (Objective: 13) **Rationale:** Transparent dressings are often applied to wounds including ulcerated or burned skin areas. These dressings offer several advantages: they are elastic; they can be placed over a joint without disrupting the client's mobility; they act as temporary skin; and they are nonporous, nonabsorbent, self-adhesive dressings that do not require changing as other dressings do. They are often left in place until healing has occurred or as long as they remain intact, and adhere only to the skin area around the wound and not to the wound itself because they keep the wound moist. **Nursing Process:** Implementation **Client Need:** Physiological Integrity

7. Answer: 3 (Objective: 14) **Rationale:** Black wounds are covered with thick necrotic tissue, or eschar. Black wounds require debridement (removal of the necrotic material). Removal of nonviable tissue from a wound must occur before the wound can be staged or heal. Wounds that are red are usually in the late regeneration phase of tissue repair (i.e., developing granulation tissue). They need to be protected to avoid disturbance to regenerating tissue. Yellow wounds are characterized primarily by liquid to semiliquid "slough" that is often accompanied by purulent drainage or previous infection. The nurse cleanses yellow wounds to remove nonviable tissue. Blue is not part of the RYB color code of wounds. **Nursing Process:** Assessment **Client Need:** Physiological Integrity

8. Answer: 2 (Objective: 10) **Rationale:** Any at-risk client confined to bed—even when a special support mattress is used—should be repositioned at least every 2 hours, depending on the client's need, to allow another body surface to bear the weight. Six body positions can usually be used: prone, supine, right and left lateral (side-lying), and right and left Sims positions. When a lateral position is used, the nurse should avoid positioning the client directly on the trochanter and instead position the client on a 30-degree angle. A written schedule should be established for turning and repositioning. A knee-chest position would not be appropriate. *Nursing Process:* Implementation *Client Need:* Physiological Integrity

9. *Answer:* 1 (Objective: 8) *Rationale:* Albumin is an important indicator of nutritional status. A value below 3.5 g/dL indicates poor nutrition and may increase the risk of poor healing and infection. *Nursing Process:* Assessment *Client Need:* Physiological Integrity

10. *Answer:* 2 (Objective: 8) *Rationale:* Administering an analgesic 15 minutes before the procedure if the client is complaining of pain at the wound site does not give enough time for the analgesic to be effective. Check the medical orders to determine if the specimen is to be collected for an aerobic (growing only in the presence of oxygen) or anaerobic (growing only in the absence of oxygen) culture. Aerobic organisms are generally found on the surface of the wound, whereas anaerobic organisms would be found in deep wounds, tunnels, and cavities. Administer an analgesic 30 minutes before the procedure if the client is complaining of pain at the wound site. *Nursing Process:* Assessment *Client Need:* Physiological Integrity

Chapter 37
Key Topic Review Answers

1. b   2. a   3. b   4. a   5. a
6. Circulatory
7. Suture
8. Sedation
9. Clot
10. Closed
11. c, i, g, h, f, a, e, j, d, b
12. d   13. c   14. b   15. a   16. c

Case Study Answers

1. *Define major surgery and minor surgery.* Major surgery involves a high degree of risk, for a variety of reasons: It may be complicated or prolonged, large losses of blood may occur, vital organs may be involved, or postoperative complications may be likely. Minor surgery normally involves little risk, produces few complications, and is often performed in an outpatient setting.

2. *Give two examples of major surgery and two examples of minor surgery.* Major surgery examples are organ transplant, open heart surgery, and removal of a kidney. Minor surgery examples are breast biopsy, removal of tonsils, and knee surgery.

3. *Why would you need to remove the hair on the client's abdomen before surgery?* Remove hair from the surgical site only when necessary or according to the primary care practitioner's orders or institutional policies and procedures. Personnel skilled in hair removal should remove hair using techniques that preserve skin integrity. Electric clippers or a depilatory cream should be used to reduce the risk of traumatizing the skin during hair removal. If a depilatory is used, hypersensitivity testing is performed prior to applying it to the surgical site. Skin trauma and abrasions increase the risk of microorganisms colonizing the surgical site. If hair is to be removed, it is done as close to the time of surgery as possible and not in the vicinity of the sterile field to avoid dispersal of loose hair and potential contamination of the sterile field.

NCLEX® Review Question Answers

1. *Answer:* 2 (Objective: 2) *Rationale:* The intraoperative phase begins when the client is transferred to the operating table and ends when the client is admitted to the postanesthesia care unit (PACU), also called the postanesthetic room or recovery room. The preoperative phase begins when the decision to have surgery is made and ends when the client is transferred to the operating table. The postoperative phase begins with the admission of the client to the postanesthesia area and ends when healing is complete. Surgery is a unique experience of a planned physical alteration encompassing three phases: preoperative, intraoperative, and postoperative. These three phases are together referred to as the perioperative period. *Nursing Process:* Planning *Client Need:* Safe, Effective Care Environment

2. *Answer:* 4 (Objective: 10) *Rationale:* Antibiotics would not be as much of a risk as the other medications listed. The regular use of certain medications can increase surgical risk. Consider these examples:

- Anticoagulants increase blood coagulation time.

- Tranquilizers may interact with anesthetics, increasing the risk of respiratory depression.

■ Corticosteroids may interfere with wound healing and increase the risk of infection.

■ Diuretics may affect fluid and electrolyte balance.

Clients may be unaware of the potential adverse interactions of medications and may fail to report the use of medications for conditions unrelated to the indication for surgery. The astute nurse interviewer should question the client and family about the use of commonly prescribed medications, over-the-counter preparations, and any herbal remedies for specific conditions mentioned during the nursing history. *Nursing Process:* Assessment *Client Need:* Safe, Effective Care Environment

3. *Answer:* 1 (Objective: 7) *Rationale:* Clean the surgical site and surrounding areas. This can be accomplished before the surgical prep by having the client shower and shampoo or wash the surgical site before arriving in the surgical setting, or by washing the surgical site in the surgical setting immediately before applying an antimicrobial agent. Prepare the surgical site and surrounding area with an antimicrobial agent when indicated. A nontoxic antimicrobial agent with a broad range of germicidal action is used to inhibit the growth of microorganisms during and following the surgical procedure. The agent selected depends on the client's history of hypersensitivity reactions, the location of the surgical site, and the skin condition. The area prepared needs to be large enough to accommodate an extension of the incision and any potential drain sites or additional incisions if needed. Remove hair from the surgical site only when necessary or according to the primary care practitioner's orders or institutional policies and procedures. Document surgical skin preparation in the client's record. Documentation should include the skin condition, including any growths, abrasions, or rashes; hair removal and the techniques used, if performed; the skin preparation, including cleansing and antimicrobial agent applied; who performed the preoperative skin preparation; and any adverse or hypersensitivity responses noted. *Nursing Process:* Assessment *Client Need:* Safe, Effective Care Environment

4. *Answer:* 1 (Objective: 11) *Rationale:* The nurse wears sterile gloves, not exam gloves. Before removing skin sutures, the nurse needs to verify the orders for suture removal (in many instances, only alternate interrupted sutures are removed one day, and the remaining sutures are removed a day or two later) and whether a dressing is to be applied following the suture removal. The nurse will grasp the suture at the knot with a pair of forceps. Sutures are cut as close to the skin as possible on one side of the visible part because the suture material that is visible to the eye is in contact with resident bacteria of the skin and must not be pulled beneath the skin during removal. Suture material that is beneath the skin is considered free from bacteria. *Nursing Process:* Implementation *Client Need:* Physiological Integrity

5. *Answer:* 3 (Objective: 9) *Rationale:* Instruct the client to report promptly to the primary care practitioner any increasing redness, swelling, pain, or discharge from the incision or drain sites. Instruct the client to use pain medications as ordered, not allowing pain to become severe before taking the prescribed dose. Teach the client to avoid using alcohol or other central nervous system depressants while taking narcotic analgesics. Emphasize the importance of adequate rest for healing and immune function. *Nursing Process:* Planning *Client Need:* Health Promotion and Maintenance

6. *Answer:* 2 (Objective: 10) *Rationale:* The proper technique is to place the bulk of the dressing over the drain area and below the drain, depending on the client's usual position. Sterile gloves must be worn during the procedure. The dressing should be secured with tape or ties. The sterile dressings are applied one at a time over the drain and the incision. *Nursing Process:* Evaluation *Client Need:* Physiological Integrity

7. *Answer:* 1 (Objective: 9) *Rationale:* The client should hold his or her breath for 2 to 3 seconds. The client should be in a sitting position. The client should inhale slowly and evenly through the nose until the greatest chest expansion is achieved. The client should exhale slowly through the mouth. *Nursing Process:* Evaluation *Client Need:* Physiological Integrity

8. *Answer:* 3 (Objective: 12) *Rationale:* Draw up the ordered volume of irrigating solution in the syringe; 30 mL of solution per instillation is usual, but up to 60 mL may be given per instillation if ordered. Attach the syringe to the nasogastric tube and slowly inject the solution. Gently aspirate the solution. Forceful withdrawal could damage the gastric mucosa. *Nursing Process:* Implementation *Client Need:* Physiological Integrity

9. *Answer:* 1 (Objective: 6) *Rationale:* The student nurse should assist the client to a lying position in bed. Reach inside the stocking from the top and, grasping the heel, turn the upper portion of the stocking inside out so the foot portion is inside the stocking leg. Have the client point his or her toes, then position the stocking on the client's foot. Ease the stocking over the toes, taking care to place the toe and heel portions of the stocking appropriately. *Nursing Process:* Evaluation *Client Need:* Physiological Integrity

   10. *Answer:* 4 (Objective: 6) *Rationale:* Atelectasis is a condition in which alveoli collapse and are not ventilated. Thrombophlebitis is inflammation of the veins, usually of the legs and associated with a blood clot. Pulmonary embolism is a blood clot that has moved to the lungs and blocks a pulmonary artery, thus obstructing blood flow to a portion of the lung. Pneumonia is inflammation of the alveoli. *Nursing Process:* Planning *Client Need:* Physiological Integrity

Chapter 38
Key Topic Review Answers

   1. a   **2.** b   **3.** a   **4.** a   **5.** b
   6. Perception
   7. Stress
   8. Culture
   9. Attention
   10. Overload
   11. h, f, e, j, d, c, g, i, b, a
   12. d   **13.** b   **14.** a   **15.** c   **16.** c

Case Study Answers

   1. *What actions should you take to help with her visual impairment?*

   ■ Orient the client to the arrangement of room furnishings and maintain an uncluttered environment.

   ■ Keep pathways clear and do not rearrange furniture without orienting the client. Ensure that housekeeping personnel are informed about this.

   ■ Organize self-care articles within the client's reach and orient the client to her location.

   ■ Keep the call light within easy reach and place the bed in the low position.

   ■ Assist with ambulation by standing at the client's side, walking about 1 foot ahead, and allowing her to grasp your arm. Confirm whether the client prefers grasping your arm with the dominant or nondominant hand.

   2. *What actions should you take to help with her hearing impairments?* Clients with hearing impairments who are unable to hear the alarms of IV

pumps and cardiac monitors need to be assessed frequently. They can be taught to use their visual sense to identify kinks in the IV tubing or a loose ECG lead, and so on. For home safety, clients with impaired hearing need to obtain devices that either amplify sounds or respond with flashing lights to sounds such as a doorbell or smoke detector, a baby crying, or a burglar alarm. The sounds of doorbells and alarm clocks may be amplified or changed to a lower frequency or buzzerlike sound. These devices can be obtained from hearing aid dealers, telephone companies, and appliance stores. An important consequence of a decline in hearing as a person ages is difficulty understanding speech. Factors that influence this difficulty are the environment, rate of speech, and presence of an accent. Environments that are noisy and reverberant (echoing, hollow sounds) cause difficulty for elderly listeners. Elderly clients with a hearing loss have difficulty understanding fast speech. Research indicates that the older adult's ability to process the fast verbal information is slower and that rapid speech allows for less time for the older adult to recognize the acoustic or auditory cues of the speech. A person who speaks with an accent can also affect speech understanding by the older person. Non-native English speakers may vary their pronunciation of syllables and/or words, making it challenging for the older adult.

   3. *How can environmental stimuli be adjusted for this client?* The client functions best when the environment is somewhat similar to that of the individual's ordinary daily life. Sometimes nurses need to take steps to adjust the client's environment to prevent either sensory overload or sensory deprivation.

NCLEX® Review Question Answers

   1. *Answer:* 2 (Objective: 8) *Rationale:* The following guidelines should be adhered to by nurses:

   ■ Always announce your presence when entering the client's room and identify yourself by name.

   ■ Stay in the client's field of vision if the client has a partial vision loss.

   ■ Speak in a warm and pleasant tone of voice. Some people tend to speak louder than necessary when talking to a blind person.

   ■ Always explain what you are about to do before touching the person.

   ■ Explain the sounds in the environment.

   ■ Indicate when the conversation has ended and when you are leaving the room.

Nursing Process: Evaluation *Client Need:* Physiological Integrity

2. *Answer:* 2 (Objective: 5) ***Rationale:*** Delirium alertness fluctuates. The client may be alert and oriented during the day but become confused and disoriented at night. The dementia client's level of alertness is generally normal. ***Nursing Process:*** Planning ***Client Need:*** Physiological Integrity

3. *Answer:* 1 (Objective: 7) ***Rationale:*** The nurse should teach the client the following: wear protective eye goggles when using power tools, riding motorcycles, spraying chemicals, and so on. Wear ear protectors when working in an environment with high noise levels or brief loud impulse noises (e.g., blasting). Wear dark glasses with UV protection to avoid damage from ultraviolet rays and never look directly into the sun. Have regular health examinations. ***Nursing Process:*** Planning ***Client Need:*** Health Promotion and Maintenance

4. *Answer:* 4 (Objectives: 7, 8) ***Rationale:*** Eliminate unnecessary noise. Reinforce reality by interpreting unfamiliar sounds, sights, and smells; correct any misconceptions of events or situations. Address the person by name and introduce yourself frequently: "Good morning, Mr. Richards. I am Betty Brown. I will be your nurse today." Identify time and place as indicated: "Today is December 5, and it is 8:00 in the morning." Ask the client, "Where are you?" and orient the client to place (e.g., nursing home) if indicated. ***Nursing Process:*** Implementation ***Client Need:*** Psychosocial Integrity

5. *Answer:* 2 (Objective: 7) ***Rationale:*** The spouse should get the following: a phone dialer with large numbers, reading material with large print, an amplified telephone, and a magnifying glass. ***Nursing Process:*** Evaluation ***Client Need:*** Physiological Integrity

6. *Answer:* 2 (Objective: 3) ***Rationale:*** The nurse should inform the client beforehand of the care to be provided, not during the care. The nurse should also provide mouth care, perform range-of-motion exercises, and provide aromatic stimuli. Too much environmental stimuli can be very distressing to a client. ***Nursing Process:*** Planning ***Client Need:*** Physiological Integrity

7. *Answer:* 2 (Objective: 1) ***Rationale:*** Stereognosis is the ability to perceive and understand an object through touch by its size, shape, and texture. Sensory reception is the process of receiving stimuli or data. Sensory perception involves the conscious organization and translation of the data or stimuli into meaningful information. Sensoristasis is the term used to describe when a person is in

optimal arousal. ***Nursing Process:*** Assessment ***Client Need:*** Physiological Integrity

8. *Answer:* 1 (Objectives: 7, 8) ***Rationale:*** Encourage the client to use eyeglasses and hearing aids during waking hours. Address the client by name and touch the client while speaking if this is not culturally offensive. Provide a telephone, radio and/or TV, clock, and calendar. Encourage the use of self-stimulation techniques such as singing, humming, whistling, or reciting. ***Nursing Process:*** Planning ***Client Need:*** Safe, Effective Care Environment

9. *Answer:* 3 (Objective: 4) ***Rationale:*** Gustatory—"Have you experienced any changes in taste?" Visual—"When did you last visit an eye doctor?" Auditory—"Do you experience any dizziness or vertigo?" Olfactory—"Can you distinguish foods by their odors and tell when something is burning?" ***Nursing Process:*** Assessment ***Client Need:*** Physiological Integrity

10. *Answer:* 2 (Objective: 1) ***Rationale:*** Specific sensory tests include:

- Visual acuity—use a Snellen chart or other reading material such as a newspaper, and visual fields.

- Hearing acuity—observe the client's conversation with others and perform the whisper test and the Weber and Rinne tuning fork tests.

- Olfactory sense— identification of specific aromas.

- Gustatory sense—identification of three tastes such as lemon, salt, and sugar.

- Tactile sense—test light touch, sharp and dull sensation, two-point discrimination, hot and cold sensation, vibration sense, position sense, and stereognosis.

Nursing Process: Assessment ***Client Need:*** Physiological Integrity

Chapter 39
Key Topic Review Answers

1. a   **2.** b   **3.** a   **4.** a   **5.** a
6. Positive
7. Self
8. Specific
9. Strength
10. Ideal
11. f, d, c, h, i, b, j, a, g, e
12. a   **13.** d   **14.** a   **15.** d   **16.** d

Case Study Answers

1. *What nursing techniques may help clients analyze the problem and enhance self-concept?*

- Encourage clients to appraise the situation and express their feelings.
- Encourage clients to ask questions.
- Provide accurate information.
- Become aware of distortions, inappropriate or unrealistic standards, and faulty labels in clients' speech.
- Explore clients' positive qualities and strengths.
- Encourage clients to express positive self-evaluation more than negative self-evaluation.
- Avoid criticism.
- Teach clients to substitute negative self-talk ("I can't walk to the store anymore") with positive self-talk ("I can walk half a block each morning"). Negative self-talk reinforces a negative self-concept.

2. *List five stressors that affect self-concept.*

- Change in physical appearance (e.g., facial wrinkles)
- Declining physical, mental, or sensory abilities
- Inability to achieve goals
- Relationship concerns
- Sexuality concerns
- Unrealistic ideal self

3. *During your assessment, what questions should you ask the client?*

- How would you describe your personal characteristics? *or,* How do you see yourself as a person?
- How do others describe you as a person?
- What do you like about yourself?
- What do you do well?
- What are your personal strengths, talents, and abilities?
- What would you change about yourself if you could?
- Does it bother you a great deal if you think someone doesn't like you?

NCLEX® Review Question Answers

1. *Answer:* 1 (Objective: 1) *Rationale:* Nurses can employ the following specific strategies to reinforce strengths:

- Stress positive thinking rather than self-negation.
- Notice and verbally reinforce client strengths.
- Provide honest, positive feedback.
- Encourage the setting of attainable goals.

Nursing Process: Planning *Client Need:* Psychosocial Integrity

2. *Answer:* 1 (Objective: 2) *Rationale:* Guidelines for conducting a psychosocial assessment include the following:

- Create a quiet, private environment.
- Minimize interruptions if possible.
- Maintain appropriate eye contact.
- Sit at eye level with the client.

Nursing Process: Assessment *Client Need:* Psychosocial Integrity

3. *Answer:* 1 (Objective: 4) *Rationale:* Guidelines for conducting a psychosocial assessment include the following:

- Indicate acceptance of the client by not criticizing, frowning, or demonstrating shock.
- Ask open-ended questions to encourage the client to talk rather than close-ended questions that tend to block free sharing.
- Avoid asking more personal questions than are actually needed.
- Minimize the writing of detailed notes during the interview because this can create client concern that confidential material is being "recorded" as well as interfere with your ability to focus on what the client is saying.

Nursing Process: Assessment *Client Need:* Psychosocial Integrity

4. *Answer:* 4 (Objective: 5) *Rationale:* The question "What are your responsibilities in the family?" is used to assess role performance and family relationships.

The following are questions to determine a client's self-esteem:

- Are you satisfied with your life?
- How do you feel about yourself?
- Are you accomplishing what you want?

Nursing Process: Assessment *Client Need:* Psychosocial Integrity

5. *Answer:* 1 (Objective: 5) *Rationale:* To enhance her son's self-esteem she would take the following actions:

- Give him opportunities to "practice" who he is.
- Allow him to explore and experiment with the world around him.
- Allow him to express himself as a unique individual.

■ Encouraging him to stay connected with all memories would not be the best answer. This would be more appropriate for an elderly patient.

Nursing Process: Evaluation *Client Need:* Psychosocial Integrity

6. *Answer:* 2 (Objective: 5) *Rationale:* The question "What are your relationships like with your other relatives?" is used to assess family relationships. The following questions are appropriate to ask a client when assessing body image:

■ Is there any part of your body you would like to change?

■ Are you comfortable discussing your surgery?

■ How do you feel about your appearance?

Nursing Process: Assessment *Client Need:* Psychosocial Integrity

7. *Answer:* 3 (Objective: 3) *Rationale:* The ideal self is the individual's perception of how one should behave based on certain personal standards, aspirations, goals, and values. Body image is how a person perceives the size, appearance, and functioning of the body and its parts. Global self refers to the collective beliefs and images one holds about oneself. Self-concept is one's mental image of oneself. *Nursing Process:* Assessment *Client Need:* Psychosocial Integrity

8. *Answer:* 4 (Objective: 2) *Rationale:* Erikson's stages of psychosocial development are as follows:

■ Middle adulthood stage: generativity vs. stagnation

■ Adolescence: identity vs. role confusion

■ Early adulthood: intimacy vs. isolation

■ Older adults: integrity vs. despair

Nursing Process: Assessment *Client Need:* Psychosocial Integrity

9. *Answer:* 2 (Objective: 4) *Rationale:* People undergoing role strain are frustrated because they feel or are made to feel inadequate or unsuited to a role. Role strain is often associated with sex-role stereotypes. Role conflicts arise from opposing or incompatible expectations. Role development involves socialization into a particular role. Role ambiguity occurs when expectations are unclear, and people do not know what to do or how to do it and are unable to predict the reactions of others to their behavior. *Nursing Process:* Assessment *Client Need:* Psychosocial Integrity

10. *Answer:* 1 (Objective: 4) *Rationale:* Change or loss of job or other significant role, loss of financial security, abusive relationship, and unrealistic expectations are considered stressors affecting self-concept. *Nursing Process:* Assessment *Client Need:* Psychosocial Integrity

Chapter 40
Key Topic Review Answers

1. b   2. a   3. b   4. a   5. a
6. Responsibilities
7. Condom
8. Brain
9. Arousal
10. Frigid
11. g, a, j, b, i, h, c, e, f, d
12. b   13. d   14. b   15. c   16. d

Case Study Answers

1. *Explain how to provide client teaching for testicular self-examination.*

■ Choose one day of each month (e.g., the first or last day of each month) to examine yourself.

■ Examine yourself when you are taking a warm shower or bath.

■ Support the testicle underneath with one hand. Place the fingers of the other hand under the testicle and the thumb on top (this may be easier to do if the leg on that side is raised).

■ Roll each testicle between the thumb and fingers of your hand, feeling for lumps, thickening, or a hardening in consistency.

■ The testes should feel smooth. Palpate the epididymis, a cordlike structure on the top and back of the testicle. The epididymis feels soft and not as smooth as a testicle.

■ Locate the spermatic cord, or vas deferens, which extends upward from the scrotum toward the base of the penis. It should feel firm and smooth.

■ Using a mirror, inspect your testicles for swelling, any enlargement, or lumps in the skin of the testicle.

■ Promptly report any lumps or other changes to your health care provider.

2. *Explain how to prevent the transmission of STIs and HIV.*

■ Limit the number of sexual partners.

■ Use condoms in nonmonogamous and homosexual relationships or other relationships that have the potential for STI transmission.

■ Follow safe sex practices during oral sex, including the use of a latex dental dam during cunnilingus to prevent STI transmission.

■ Talk openly with sexual partners about how to have "safer sex" and be honest about any history of an STI.

■ Abstain from high-risk sexual activity with a partner known to have or suspected of having an STI.

■ Report to a health care facility for examination whenever in doubt about possible exposure or when signs of an STI are evident.

■ When an STI is diagnosed, notify all partners and encourage them to seek treatment.

■ Avoid transfusions of banked blood or blood products. Use autologous transfusions (donation of own blood before surgery) for elective surgery whenever possible.

3. *Summarize the nursing strategies to deal with the client's inappropriate sexual behavior.*

■ Communicate that the behavior is not acceptable by saying, for example, "I really do not like the things you are saying," or "I see you are not dressed. I will be back in 10 minutes and will help you with breakfast when you get your clothes on."

■ Tell the client how the behavior makes you feel: "When you act like that toward me, I am very uncomfortable. It embarrasses me and makes it hard for me to give you the kind of nursing care you need."

■ Identify the behavior you expect: "Please call me by my name, not 'Honey,'" or "I expect you to keep yourself covered when I am in the room. If you are feeling hot or something is uncomfortable, let me know, and I will try to make you more comfortable."

■ Set firm limits: Take the client's hand and move it away, use direct eye contact, and say, "Don't do that!"

■ Try to refocus clients from the inappropriate behavior to their real concerns and fears; offer to discuss sexuality concerns: "All morning you have been making very personal sexual comments about yourself. Sometimes people talk like that when they are concerned about the sexual part of their life and how their illness will affect them. Are there things that you have questions about or would like to talk about?"

■ Report the incident to your nursing instructor, charge nurse, or clinical nurse specialist. Discuss the incident, your feelings, and possible interventions.

■ Assign a nurse who will confront the behavior and relate to the client in a consistent manner.

■ Clarify the consequences of continued inappropriate behavior (avoidance, withdrawal of services, no chance to help resolve underlying concerns of client).

NCLEX® Review Question Answers

1. *Answer:* 4 (Objective: 8) *Rationale:* When an STI is diagnosed, notify all partners and encourage them to seek treatment. Use condoms in nonmonogamous and homosexual relationships or other relationships that have the potential for STI transmission. Follow safe sex practices during oral sex including the use of a latex dental dam during cunnilingus to prevent STI transmission. Report to a health care facility for examination whenever in doubt about possible exposure or when signs of an STI are evident. *Nursing Process:* Planning *Client Need:* Health Promotion and Maintenance

2. *Answer:* 2 (Objective: 9) *Rationale:* Press the breast tissue against the chest wall firmly enough to know how your breast feels. A ridge of firm tissue in the lower curve of each breast is normal. Use the finger pads (tips) of the three middle fingers (held together) on your left hand to feel for lumps. Use small circular motions systematically all the way around the breast as many times as necessary until the entire breast is covered. Look for any change in size or shape; lumps or thickenings; any rashes or other skin irritations; dimpled or puckered skin; any discharge or change in the nipples. *Nursing Process:* Evaluation *Client Need:* Health Promotion and Maintenance

3. *Answer:* 4 (Objective: 8) *Rationale:* The correct statements should have been: "I will report the incident to my nursing instructor, charge nurse, or clinical nurse specialist." "I will communicate that the behavior is not acceptable." "I will identify the behavior I expect." "I will set firm limits with the client." *Nursing Process:* Evaluation *Client Need:* Psychosocial Integrity

4. *Answer:* 1 (Objective: 9) *Rationale:* Methods of contraception include: chemical barriers—insertion of spermicidal foams, creams, jellies, or suppositories into the vagina before intercourse; mechanical barriers—vaginal diaphragm, cervical cap, condom; abstinence; surgical sterilization—tubal ligation and vasectomy; intrauterine devices (IUDs). *Nursing Process:* Planning *Client Need:* Physiological Integrity

5. *Answer:* 2 (Objective: 9) *Rationale:* The following statements by the nurse would be correct: "Diuretics decrease vaginal lubrication." "Antipsychotics decrease sexual desire." "Narcotics inhibit sexual desire and response." "Barbiturates in large amounts decrease sexual desire." ***Nursing Process:*** Planning ***Client Need:*** Physiological Integrity

6. ***Answer:*** 4 (Objective: 9) ***Rationale:*** "Alcohol is a sexual stimulant" is an incorrect statement. Alcohol is a relaxant and central nervous system depressant. The following statements would be correct conceptions: "Sexual ability is not lost due to age." "There is no evidence that sexual activity weakens a person." "Chronic alcoholism is associated with erectile dysfunction." ***Nursing Process:*** Evaluation ***Client Need:*** Physiological Integrity

7. ***Answer:*** 1 (Objective: 1) ***Rationale:*** The orgasmic phase is the involuntary climax of sexual tension, accompanied by physiologic and psychologic release. The response cycle starts in the brain, with conscious sexual desires called the desire phase. The resolution phase, the period of return to the unaroused state, may last 10 to 15 minutes after orgasm, or longer if there is no orgasm. Myotonia, an increase of tension in muscles, may increase until released by orgasm, or it may also simply fade away. ***Nursing Process:*** Assessment ***Client Need:*** Physiological Integrity

8. ***Answer:*** 1 (Objective: 1) ***Rationale:*** Body image, a central part of the sense of self, is constantly changing. Gender identity is one's self-image as a female or male. Gender-role behavior is the outward expression of a person's sense of maleness or femaleness as well as the expression of what is perceived as gender-appropriate behavior. Androgyny, or flexibility in gender roles, is the belief that most characteristics and behaviors are human qualities that should not be limited to one specific gender or the other. ***Nursing Process:*** Assessment ***Client Need:*** Physiological Integrity

9. ***Answer:*** 2 (Objective: 9) ***Rationale:*** The following statements would not need any further education: "*Preorgasmic* women have never experienced an orgasm." "*Rapid ejaculation* is one of the most common sexual dysfunctions among men." "*Vulvodynia* is constant, unremitting burning that is localized to the vulva with an acute onset." "*Vestibulitis* causes severe pain only on touch or attempted vaginal entry." ***Nursing Process:*** Evaluation ***Client Need:*** Health Promotion and Maintenance

10. ***Answer:*** 1 (Objective: 3) ***Rationale:*** One technique nurses can use to help clients with altered sexual function is the PLISSIT model, developed by Annon (1974) for this purpose. The model involves

four progressive levels represented by the acronym PLISSIT:

P	Permission giving
LI	Limited information
SS	Specific suggestions
IT	Intensive therapy

The following are incorrect choices: PLIISIT, PLLISSIT, PLISIT. ***Nursing Process:*** Assessment ***Client Need:*** Physiological Integrity

Chapter 41
Key Topic Review Answers

1. b   2. a   3. a   4. a   5. a
6. Kosher
7. Presencing
8. Planning
9. Sacred
10. Forgiveness
11. f, g, d, h, c, i, b, a, j, e
12. d   13. a   14. c   15. b   16. b

Case Study Answers

1. *The client asks you to pray with him. Describe some of the guidelines you should follow.*

- When assessing whether a client would like you to pray, ask to pray in a way that allows both of you to feel comfortable if the answer is no.
- Personalize the prayer.
- Prayer may be the springboard to further discussion or catharsis.
- Remember that some clients would like to pray aloud with you, just as you may with them.
- Facilitate the clients' prayer practices.

2. *Summarize the practice guidelines you should follow to support the client's religious practices.*

- Create a trusting relationship with the client so that any religious concerns or practices can be openly discussed and addressed.
- If unsure of client religious needs, ask how nurses can assist in having these needs met. Avoid relying on personal assumptions when caring for clients.
- Do not discuss personal spiritual beliefs with a client unless the client requests it.
- Inform clients and family caregivers about spiritual support available at your institution (e.g., chapel or meditation room, chaplain services).

■ Remember the difference between facilitating/supporting a client's religious practice and participating in it yourself.

■ All spiritual interventions must be done within agency guidelines.

3. *Give some examples of spiritual needs that would be related to others.*

■ Need to forgive others

■ Need to cope with loss of loved ones

NCLEX® Review Question Answers

1. Answer: 4 (Objective: 5) *Rationale:* It is important for nurses to understand health-related information about specific religions. Seventh-Day Adventists—Avoid unnecessary treatments on Saturday (Sabbath). Sabbath begins Friday sundown, ends Saturday sundown. Adventists prefer restful, spirit-nurturing, family activities on Sabbaths. They are likely to be vegetarian and abstain from caffeinated beverages. They do not smoke or drink alcohol. Buddhist—May be vegetarian. Facilitate meditation (may desire incense, visual focal point, use breathing or chanting, etc.). Jehovah's Witnesses—Abstain from most blood products; need to discuss alternative treatments such as blood conservation strategies, autologous techniques, hematopoietic agents, nonblood volume expanders, and so on; contact local Jehovah's Witness hospital liaison committee. Latter-Day Saints (LDS or Mormons)—Avoid alcohol, caffeine, smoking. Prefer to wear temple undergarments. Arrange for priestly blessing if requested. *Nursing Process:* Assessment *Client Need:* Psychosocial Integrity

2. Answer: 1 (Objective: 2) *Rationale:* Religion is an organized system of beliefs and practices. It offers a way of spiritual expression that provides guidance for believers in responding to life's questions and challenges. Spiritual distress refers to a challenge to the spiritual well-being or to the belief system that provides strength, hope, and meaning to life. Spiritual health, or spiritual well-being, is manifested by a feeling of being "generally alive, purposeful, and fulfilled." Spirituality refers to that part of being human that seeks meaningfulness through intra-, inter-, and transpersonal connection. *Nursing Process:* Assessment *Client Need:* Psychosocial Integrity

3. Answer: 2 (Objective: 1) *Rationale:* An atheist is one without belief in a God. An agnostic is a person who doubts the existence of God or a supreme being or believes the existence of God has not been proved. Monotheism is the belief in the existence of one God, while polytheism is the belief in more than

one god. *Nursing Process:* Assessment *Client Need:* Psychosocial Integrity

4. Answer: 2 (Objective: 5) *Rationale:* Orthodox Jews are not to eat shellfish or pork. Members of the Church of Jesus Christ of Latter-Day Saints (Mormons) are not to drink caffeinated or alcoholic beverages. Buddhists and Hindus are generally vegetarian, not wanting to take life to support life. *Nursing Process:* Assessment *Client Need:* Psychosocial Integrity

5. Answer: 2 (Objective: 1) *Rationale:* The correct statements would be:

"Being there in a way that is meaningful to another person."

"Giving of self in the present moment."

"Listening, with full awareness of the privilege of doing so."

"Being available with all of the self."

Nursing Process: Implementation *Client Need:* Psychosocial Integrity

6. Answer: 3 (Objective: 1) *Rationale:* The following statements would demonstrate practice guidelines supporting religious practices: "Do not discuss personal spiritual beliefs with a client unless the client requests it." "Create a trusting relationship with the client so that any religious concerns or practices can be openly discussed and addressed." "If unsure of client religious needs, ask how nurses can assist in having these needs met." "Acquaint yourself with the religions, spiritual practices, and cultures of the area in which you are working." *Nursing Process:* Evaluation *Client Need:* Psychosocial Integrity

7. Answer: 4 (Objective: 1) *Rationale:* Personalizing the prayer is an appropriate practice guideline for praying with clients. The following statements are also appropriate practice guidelines for praying with clients: "Clients' preferences for prayer reflect their personalities." "Before praying, assess what they would like for you to pray." "Prayer may be the springboard to further discussion or catharsis." *Nursing Process:* Implementation *Client Need:* Psychosocial Integrity

8. Answer: 3 (Objective: 5) *Rationale:* Muslims follow the practice of prayer fives times a day, and the Muslim client may need assistance to maintain this commitment. *Nursing Process:* Assessment *Client Need:* Psychosocial Integrity

9. Answer: 4 (Objective: 1) *Rationale:* Planning in relation to spiritual needs should be designed to do one or more of the following:

■ Promote a sense of hope.

■ Help the client fulfill religious obligations.

- Help the client draw on and use inner resources more effectively to meet the present situation.
- Help the client find meaning in existence and the present situation.

Nursing Process: Planning ***Client Need:*** Psychosocial Integrity

10. ***Answer:*** 4 (Objective: 3) ***Rationale:*** The need to cope with loss of loved ones is a need related to others. Needs related to the self include:

- Need for meaning and purpose
- Need to express creativity
- Need for hope

Nursing Process: Planning ***Client Need:*** Psychosocial Integrity

Chapter 42
Key Topic Review Answers

1. b **2.** a **3.** a **4.** b **5.** b
6. Suppression
7. Fantasy
8. Coping
9. Intervention
10. Strategy
11. e, f, c, j, h, b, i, a, g, d
12. c **13.** d **14.** d **15.** a **16.** c

Case Study Answers

1. *What level of anxiety is the client most likely experiencing?* The client is most likely experiencing severe anxiety—see Table 42–2 in the textbook.

2. *Describe various methods you could teach the client to minimize stress and anxiety.*

- Listen attentively; try to understand the client's perspective on the situation.
- Provide an atmosphere of warmth and trust; convey a sense of caring and empathy.
- Determine if it is appropriate to encourage the client's participation in the plan of care; give the client choices about some aspects of care but do not overwhelm the client with choices.
- Stay with the client as needed to promote safety and feelings of security and to reduce fear.
- Control the environment to minimize additional stressors, such as by reducing noise, limiting the number of persons in the room, and providing care by the same nurse as much as possible.
- Implement suicide precautions if indicated.

- Communicate in short, clear sentences.
- Help clients to
  a. Determine situations that precipitate anxiety and identify signs of anxiety.
  b. Verbalize feelings, perceptions, and fears as appropriate. Some cultures discourage the expression of feelings.
  c. Identify personal strengths.
  d. Recognize usual coping patterns and differentiate positive from negative coping mechanisms.
  e. Identify new strategies for managing stress (e.g., exercise, massage, progressive relaxation).
  f. Identify available support systems.
- Teach clients about
  a. The importance of adequate exercise, a balanced diet, and rest and sleep to energize the body and enhance coping abilities.
  b. Support groups available such as Alcoholics Anonymous, Weight Watchers or Overeaters Anonymous, and parenting and child abuse support groups.
  c. Educational programs available such as time management, assertiveness training, and meditation groups.

3. *Explain the difference between anxiety and fear.* The source of anxiety may not be identifiable; the source of fear is identifiable. Anxiety is related to the future, that is, to an anticipated event. Fear is related to the present. Anxiety is vague, whereas fear is definite. Anxiety is the result of psychologic or emotional conflict; fear is the result of a discrete physical or psychologic entity.

Review Question Answers

1. ***Answer:*** 2 (Objective: 3) ***Rationale:*** The client is experiencing moderate anxiety as evidenced by voice tremors and pitch changes, facial twitches, shakiness, and slightly elevated respiratory and heart rates, and she told you "I feel like I have butterflies in my stomach." Mild anxiety would be characterized by mild restlessness, sleeplessness, increased verbalization, feelings of increased arousal and alertness, and no changes in respiratory and heart rates. Severe anxiety is characterized by communication difficulties; increased motor activity; inability to relax, focus, and concentrate; ease of distractibility; tachycardia; and hyperventilation. Panic anxiety is characterized by increased motor activity, agitation, unpredictable responses, distorted or exaggerated perception, dyspnea, palpitations, choking, chest pain, and feeling of impending doom.

Nursing Process: Assessment *Client Need:*
Psychosocial Integrity

   2. *Answer:* 1 (Objective: 3) *Rationale:* The source
of anxiety may not be identifiable; the source of fear
is identifiable. Anxiety is related to the future, that is,
to an anticipated event. Fear is related to the present.
Anxiety is vague, whereas fear is definite. Anxiety is
the result of psychologic or emotional conflict; fear is
the result of a discrete physical or psychologic entity.
Nursing Process: Evaluation *Client Need:*
Psychosocial Integrity

   3. *Answer:* 1 (Objective: 7) *Rationale:* Try to
understand the meaning of the client's anger. After
the interaction is completed, take time to process
your feelings and your responses to the client with
your colleagues. Let clients talk about their anger.
Listen to the client, and act as calmly as possible.
Nursing Process: Implementation *Client Need:*
Psychosocial Integrity

   4. *Answer:* 3 (Objective: 9) *Rationale:* Nurses
can prevent burnout by using the techniques to
manage stress discussed for clients. Nurses must first
recognize their stress and become attuned to such
responses as feelings of being overwhelmed, fatigue,
angry outbursts, physical illness, and increases in
coffee drinking, smoking, or substance abuse. Once
attuned to stress and personal reactions, it is
necessary to identify which situations produce the
most pronounced reactions so that steps may be taken
to reduce the stress. Suggestions include:

■ Get involved in constructive change efforts if
organizational policies and procedures cause
stress.

■ Develop collegial support groups to deal with
feelings and anxieties generated in the work
setting.

■ Learn to say no.

■ Establish a regular exercise program to direct
energy outward.

Nursing Process: Implementation *Client Need:*
Psychosocial Integrity

   5. *Answer:* 2 (Objective: 8) *Rationale:*

■ The adolescent is characterized by: changing
physique, relationships involving sexual
attraction, exploring independence, choosing a
career.

■ The young adult is characterized by:
marriage, leaving home, managing a home,
getting started in an occupation, continuing one's
education, having children.

■ The middle adult is characterized by:
physical changes of aging, maintaining social
status and standard of living, helping

teenage children to become independent, aging
parents.

■ The older adult is characterized by:
decreasing physical abilities and health, changes
in residence, retirement and reduced income,
death of spouse and friends.

Nursing Process: Assessment *Client Need:*
Psychosocial Integrity

   6. *Answer:* 1 (Objective: 5) *Rationale:*
Displacement is the transferring or discharging of
emotional reactions from one object or person to
another object or person. An example would be when
a husband and wife are fighting, and the husband
becomes so angry he hits a door instead of his wife.
Denial is an attempt to screen or ignore unacceptable
realities by refusing to acknowledge them. An
example would be a woman who, though told her
father has metastatic cancer, continues to plan a
family reunion 18 months in advance. Projection is a
process in which blame is attached to others or the
environment for unacceptable desires, thoughts,
shortcomings, and mistakes. An example would be a
mother who is told that her child must repeat a grade
in school, and she blames this on the teacher's poor
instruction. Substitution is the replacement of a
highly valued, unacceptable, or unavailable object by
a less valuable, acceptable, or available object. An
example would be a woman who wants to marry a
man exactly like her dead father and settles for
someone who looks a little bit like him. *Nursing
Process:* Assessment *Client Need:* Psychosocial
Integrity

   7. *Answer:* 2 (Objective: 5) *Rationale:*
Regression is resorting to an earlier, more
comfortable level of functioning that is
characteristically less demanding and responsible. An
example would be an adult who throws a temper
tantrum when he does not get his own way.
Rationalization is justification of certain behaviors by
faulty logic and ascribing motives that are socially
acceptable but did not in fact inspire the behavior. An
example would be a mother who spanks her toddler
too hard and says it was all right because he couldn't
feel it through the diaper anyway. Reaction formation
is a mechanism that causes people to act exactly
opposite to the way they feel. An example would be
an executive who resents his bosses for calling in a
consulting firm to make recommendations for change
in his department, but verbalizes complete support of
the idea and is exceedingly polite and cooperative.
Repression is an unconscious mechanism by which
threatening thoughts, feelings, and desires are kept
from becoming conscious; the repressed material is
denied entry into consciousness. An example would

be a teenager who, having seen his best friend killed in a car accident, becomes amnesic about the circumstances surrounding the accident.

Nursing Process: Assessment *Client Need:* Psychosocial Integrity

8. *Answer:* 4 (Objective: 9) *Rationale:* To minimize stress and anxiety the nurse should communicate in short, clear sentences; provide an atmosphere of warmth and trust; convey a sense of caring and empathy; listen attentively; try to understand the client's perspective on the situation; and control the environment to minimize additional stressors, such as by reducing noise, limiting the number of persons in the room, and providing care by the same nurse as much as possible. *Nursing Process:* Planning *Client Need:* Psychosocial Integrity

9. *Answer:* 2 (Objective: 7) *Rationale:* Common characteristics of crises include:

- All crises are experienced as sudden. The person is usually not aware of a warning signal, even if others could "see it coming." The individual or family may feel that they had little or no preparation for the event or trauma.

- The crisis is often experienced as ultimately life threatening, whether this perception is realistic or not.

- Communication with significant others is often decreased or cut off.

- There may be perceived or real displacement from familiar surroundings or loved ones.

- All crises have an aspect of loss, whether actual or perceived. The losses can include an object, a person, a hope, a dream, or any significant factor for that individual.

Nursing Process: Planning *Client Need:* Psychosocial Integrity

10. *Answer:* 1 (Objective: 3) *Rationale:* The clinical manifestations of stress include:

- Pupils dilate to increase visual perception when serious threats to the body arise.

- Sweat production (diaphoresis) increases to control elevated body heat due to increased metabolism.

- Heart rate and cardiac output increase to transport nutrients and by-products of metabolism more efficiently.

- Skin is pallid because of constriction of peripheral blood vessels, an effect of norepinephrine.

Nursing Process: Evaluation *Client Need:* Psychosocial Integrity

Chapter 43

Key Topic Review Answers

1. a   2. b   3. a   4. a   5. a
6. Mortis
7. Algor
8. Mortician/Undertaker
9. Shroud
10. Hopelessness
11. d, j, a, b, c, i, e, g, h, f
12. c   13. a   14. d   15. c   16. b

Case Study Answers

1. *Which type of loss is the client experiencing?* An actual loss can be recognized by others. An anticipatory loss is experienced before the loss actually occurs.

2. *Explain grief, bereavement, and mourning.* Grief is the total response to the emotional experience related to loss. Grief is manifested in thoughts, feelings, and behaviors associated with overwhelming distress or sorrow. Bereavement is the subjective response experienced by the surviving loved ones after the death of a person with whom they have shared a significant relationship. Mourning is the behavioral process through which grief is eventually resolved or altered; it is often influenced by culture, spiritual beliefs, and custom. Grief and mourning are experienced not only by the person who faces the death of a loved one but also by the person who suffers other kinds of loses. Grieving is essential for good mental and physical health. It permits the individual to cope with the loss gradually and to accept it as part of reality. Grief is a social process; it is best shared and carried out with the assistance of others.

3. *List four appropriate questions to ask during the assessment.*

- Are you having trouble sleeping? Eating? Concentrating? Breathing?

- Do you have any pain or other new physical problems?

- What are you doing to help you deal with this loss?

- Are you taking any drugs or medications to help you cope with this loss?

NCLEX® Review Question Answers

1. *Answer:* 2 (Objective: 1) *Rationale:* Bereavement is the subjective response experienced

by the surviving loved ones after the death of a person with whom they have shared a significant relationship. Grief is the total response to the emotional experience related to loss. Grief is manifested in thoughts, feelings, and behaviors associated with overwhelming distress or sorrow. Mourning is the behavioral process through which grief is eventually resolved or altered; it is often influenced by culture, spiritual beliefs, and custom. Loss is an actual or potential situation in which something that is valued is changed or no longer available. ***Nursing Process:*** Assessment ***Client Need:*** Psychosocial Integrity

2. ***Answer:*** 1 (Objective: 9) ***Rationale:*** Rigor mortis is the stiffening of the body that occurs about 2 to 4 hours after death. It results from a lack of adenosine triphosphate (ATP), which causes the muscles to contract, which in turn immobilizes the joints. Rigor mortis starts in the involuntary muscles (heart, bladder, and so on), then progresses to the head, neck, and trunk, and finally reaches the extremities. All other times are incorrect. ***Nursing Process:*** Assessment ***Client Need:*** Physiological Integrity

3. ***Answer:*** 1 (Objective: 2) ***Rationale:*** Denial occurs when one refuses to believe that loss is happening, or is unready to deal with practical problems, such as a prosthesis after loss of leg. A client in denial may assume artificial cheerfulness to prolong denial. Anger is when a client or family may direct anger at nurse or staff about matters that normally would not bother them. Bargaining occurs when one seeks to bargain to avoid loss. The bargaining client may express feelings of guilt or fear of punishment for past sins, real or imagined. Depression occurs when one grieves over what has happened and what cannot be. The depressed client may talk freely (e.g., reviewing past losses such as money or job), or may withdraw. ***Nursing Process:*** Assessment ***Client Need:*** Psychosocial Integrity

4. ***Answer:*** 1 (Objective: 2) ***Rationale:*** During the shock and disbelief stage the client refuses to accept loss, has stunned feelings, and accepts the situation intellectually but denies it emotionally. During the developing awareness stage, reality of loss begins to penetrate consciousness, and anger may be directed at the agency, nurses, or others. During the restitution stage the client conducts rituals of mourning (e.g., funeral). During the stage of resolving the loss the client attempts to deal with the painful void, is still unable to accept a new love object to replace the lost person or object, may accept a more dependent relationship with a support person, and thinks over and talks about

memories of the lost person or object. ***Nursing Process:*** Assessment ***Client Need:*** Psychosocial Integrity

5. ***Answer:*** 2 (Objective: 2) ***Rationale:*** Conservation/withdrawal—during this phase, survivors feel a need to be alone to conserve and replenish both physical and emotional energy. The social support available to the bereaved has decreased, and they may experience despair and helplessness. Shock—during this phase the survivors are left with feelings of confusion, unreality, and disbelief that the loss has occurred. They are often unable to process the normal thought sequences. This phase may last from a few minutes to many days. Awareness of loss—during this phase the friends and family resume normal activities. The bereaved experience the full significance of their loss. The healing phase is the turning point. During this phase, the bereaved move from distress about living without their loved one to learning to live more independently. ***Nursing Process:*** Assessment ***Client Need:*** Psychosocial Integrity

6. ***Answer:*** 1 (Objective: 7) ***Rationale:*** For an unconscious client experiencing airway clearance problems the nursing student would put the client in a lateral position. For a conscious client with an airway clearance problem the nursing student would place him in a Fowler's position. If the client is diaphoretic the nursing student would give the client frequent baths, change the linen, and regularly change the client's position. The nursing student would provide skin care to the client in response to incontinence of urine or feces. ***Nursing Process:*** Implementation ***Client Need:*** Physiological Integrity

7. ***Answer:*** 4 (Objective: 6) ***Rationale:*** The dying person's bill of rights includes:

■ I have the right not to die alone.

■ I have the right to express my feelings and emotions about my approaching death in my own way.

■ I have the right to expect continuing medical and nursing attention even though cure goals must be changed to comfort goals.

■ I have the right to be free from pain.

Nursing Process: Planning ***Client Need:*** Psychosocial Integrity

8. ***Answer:*** 4 (Objective: 6) ***Rationale:*** Clinical manifestations of impending clinical death include:

■ Slower and weaker pulse.

■ Difficulty swallowing and gradual loss of the gag reflex.

- Mottling and cyanosis of the extremities.

- Rapid, shallow, irregular, or abnormally slow respirations. *Nursing Process:* Implementation *Client Need:* Physiological Integrity

9. *Answer:* 2 (Objective: 4) *Rationale:*

- Infancy to 5 years—Does not understand concept of death. Infant's sense of separation forms basis for later understanding of loss and death. Believes death is reversible, a temporary departure, or sleep. Emphasizes immobility and inactivity as attributes of death.

- 5 to 9 years—Understands that death is final. Believes own death can be avoided. Associates death with aggression or violence. Believes wishes or unrelated actions can be responsible for death.

- 9 to 12 years—Understands death as the inevitable end of life. Begins to understand own mortality, expressed as interest in afterlife or as fear of death.

- 12 to 18 years—Fears a lingering death.

Nursing Process: Assessment *Client Need:* Psychosocial Integrity

10. *Answer:* 3 (Objective: 9) *Rationale:* Nursing personnel may be responsible for care of a body after death. Normally the body is placed in a supine position with the arms either at the sides, palms down, or across the abdomen. Dentures are usually inserted to help give the face a natural appearance. The mouth is then closed. One pillow is placed under the head and shoulders to prevent blood from discoloring the face by settling in it. The eyelids are closed and held in place for a few seconds so they remain closed. All jewelry is removed, except a wedding band in some instances, which is taped to the finger. *Nursing Process:* Implementation *Client Need:* Physiological Integrity

Chapter 44

Key Topic Review Answers

1. a   2. b   3. a   4. a   5. a
6. Hypertrophy
7. Osteoporosis
8. Atrophy
9. Contracture
10. Ankylosed
11. e, a, b, c, j, g, d, f, i, h
12. d   13. d   14. a   15. a   16. a

Case Study Answers

1. *Provide the client and his family education about the following topics:*

Maintaining Musculoskeletal Function

- Teach the systematic performance of passive or assistive ROM exercises to maintain joint mobility.

- Demonstrate, as appropriate, the proper way to perform isotonic, isometric, or isokinetic exercises to maintain muscle mass and tone (collaborate with the physical therapist about these). Incorporate ADLs into exercise program if appropriate.

- Provide a written schedule for the type, frequency, and duration of exercises; encourage the use of a progress graph or chart to facilitate adherence with the therapy.

- Offer an ambulation schedule.

- Instruct in the availability of assistive ambulatory devices and correct use of them.

- Discuss pain control measures required before exercise.

Preventing Injury

- Provide assistive devices for moving and transferring, whenever possible, and teach safe transfer and ambulation techniques.

- Discuss safety measures to avoid falls (e.g., locking wheelchairs, wearing appropriate footwear, using rubber tips on crutches, keeping the environment safe, and using mechanical aids such as raised toilet seat, grab bars, urinal, and bedpan or commode to facilitate toileting).

- Teach the use of proper body mechanics, especially for those times when assistive equipment is not used.

- Teach ways to prevent postural hypotension.

Managing Energy to Prevent Fatigue

- Discuss activity and rest patterns and develop a plan as indicated; intersperse rest periods with activity periods.

- Discuss ways to minimize fatigue such as performing activities more slowly and for shorter periods, resting more often, and using more assistance as required.

- Provide information about available resources to help with ADLs and home maintenance management.

- Teach ways to increase energy (e.g., increasing intake of high-energy foods, ensuring adequate rest and sleep, controlling pain, sharing feelings with a trusted listener).

- Teach techniques to monitor activity tolerance as appropriate.

Preventing Back Injuries

■ Understand that the use of body mechanics will not necessarily prevent injury if manually handling a load greater than 51 pounds without the use of assistive devices.

■ Avoid lifting anything greater than 51 pounds—use assistive equipment, get help from co-workers, and participate in the purchasing/ordering process of appropriate assistive equipment for your work setting.

■ Become consciously aware of your posture and body mechanics.

■ When standing for a period of time, periodically move legs and hips, and flex one hip and knee and rest your foot on an object if possible.

■ When sitting, keep your knees slightly higher than your hips.

■ Use a firm mattress and soft pillow that provide good body support at natural body curvatures.

■ Exercise regularly to maintain overall physical condition and regulate weight; include exercises that strengthen the pelvic, abdominal, and spinal muscles.

■ Avoid movements that cause pain or require spinal flexion with straight legs (e.g., toe-touching and sit-ups) or spinal rotation (twisting).

■ When moving an object, spread your feet apart to provide a wide base of support.

■ When lifting an object, distribute the weight between the large muscles of the legs and arms, limiting the load to 15 to 25 pounds held at elbow height.

■ Wear comfortable low-heeled shoes that provide good foot support and reduce the risk of slipping, stumbling, or turning your ankle.

NCLEX® Review Question Answers

1. *Answer:* 4 (Objective: 3) *Rationale:* The following statements would be correct when providing client teaching about preventing back injuries:

■ When sitting, keep your knees slightly higher than your hips.

■ When standing for a period of time, periodically move legs and hips, and flex one hip and knee and rest your foot on an object if possible.

■ Use a firm mattress and soft pillow that provide good body support at natural body curvatures.

■ Exercise regularly to maintain overall physical condition and regulate weight; include exercises that strengthen the pelvic, abdominal, and spinal muscles.

Nursing Process: Planning *Client Need:* Physiological Integrity

2. *Answer:* 1 (Objective: 7) *Rationale:* Practice guidelines for wheelchair safety include:

■ Raise the footplates before transferring the client into the wheelchair.

■ Always lock the brakes on both wheels of the wheelchair when the client transfers in or out of it.

■ Lower the footplates after the transfer, and place the client's feet on them.

■ Ensure the client is positioned well back in the seat of the wheelchair.

Nursing Process: Evaluation *Client Need:* Safe, Effective Care Environment

3. *Answer:* 3 (Objective: 7) *Rationale:* The following are correct statements that indicate understanding of stretcher safety:

■ Never leave a client unattended on a stretcher unless the wheels are locked and the side rails are raised on both sides and/or the safety straps are securely fastened across the client.

■ Always push a stretcher from the end where the client's head is positioned. This position protects the client's head in the event of a collision.

■ Maneuver the stretcher when entering the elevator so that the client's head goes in first.

■ Fasten safety straps across the client on a stretcher, and raise the side rails.

Nursing Process: Evaluation *Client Need:* Safe, Effective Care Environment

4. *Answer:* 1 (Objective: 2) *Rationale:* Active ROM exercises guidelines include:

■ Perform each ROM exercise as taught to the point of slight resistance, but not beyond, and never to the point of discomfort.

■ Perform the movements systematically, using the same sequence during each session.

■ Perform each exercise three times.

■ Perform each series of exercises twice daily.

Nursing Process: Implementation *Client Need:* Safe, Effective Care Environment

5. *Answer:* 3 (Objective: 5) *Rationale:* During client teaching about controlling postural hypotension, the client should verbalize the following:

■ Wear elastic stockings at night to inhibit venous pooling in the legs.

■ Never bend down all the way to the floor or stand up too quickly after stooping.

- Use a rocking chair to improve circulation in the lower extremities.
- Get out of a hot bath very slowly, because high temperatures can lead to venous pooling.

Nursing Process: Planning *Client Need:* Safe, Effective Care Environment

6. Answer: 1 (Objective: 2) *Rationale:* Isotonic (dynamic) exercises are those in which the muscle shortens to produce muscle contraction and active movement. Isometric (static or setting) exercises are those in which there is muscle contraction without moving the joint (muscle length does not change). Isokinetic (resistive) exercises involve muscle contraction or tension against resistance; thus, they can be either isotonic or isometric. Aerobic exercise is activity during which the amount of oxygen taken in the body is greater than that used to perform the activity. *Nursing Process:* Implementation *Client Need:* Physiological Integrity

7. Answer: 1 (Objective: 7) *Rationale:* Positioning a client in good body alignment and changing the position regularly (every 2 hours) and systematically are essential aspects of nursing practice. For all clients, it is important to assess the skin and provide skin care before and after a position change. Any position, correct or incorrect, can be detrimental if maintained for a prolonged period. Frequent change of position helps to prevent muscle discomfort, undue pressure resulting in pressure ulcers, damage to superficial nerves and blood vessels, and contractures. *Nursing Process:* Evaluation *Client Need:* Physiological Integrity

8. Answer: 1 (Objective: 4) *Rationale:* Fowler's position, or a semisitting position, is a bed position in which the head and trunk are raised 45 to 90 degrees. In the dorsal recumbent (back-lying) position, the client's head and shoulders are slightly elevated on a small pillow. In the prone position, the client lies on the abdomen with the head turned to one side. In the lateral (side-lying) position, the person lies on one side of the body. Flexing the top hip and knee and placing this leg in front of the body creates a wider, triangular base of support and achieves greater stability. *Nursing Process:* Implementation *Client Need:* Safe, Effective Care Environment

9. Answer: 2 (Objective: 7) *Rationale:* Always support or hold the client rather than the equipment and ensure their safety and dignity. Obtain essential equipment before starting (e.g., transfer belt, wheelchair), and check its function. Remove obstacles from the area used for the transfer. Explain the transfer to the nursing personnel who are helping; specify who will give directions (one person needs to be in charge). Nursing

Process: Implementation *Client Need:* Safe, Effective Care Environment

10. Answer: 2 (Objective: 7) *Rationale:* When nurses measure clients for axillary crutches, it is most important to obtain the correct length for the crutches and the correct placement of the hand piece. The nurse must measure for the crutches and determine the correct placement of the hand bar. The nurse measures the angle of elbow flexion. It should be about 30 degrees. The client lies in a supine position and the nurse measures from the anterior fold of the axilla to the heel of the foot and adds 2.5 cm (1 in.). The client stands erect and positions the crutch. The nurse makes sure the shoulder rest of the crutch is at least three finger widths, that is, 2.5 to 5 cm (1 to 2 in.), below the axilla. The client stands upright and supports the body weight by the hand grips of the crutches. *Nursing Process:* Implementation *Client Need:* Safe, Effective Care Environment

Chapter 45
Key Topic Review Answers

1. a   2. b   3. a   4. a   5. b
6. Sleep
7. Rhythms
8. Wet dreams
9. Insomnia
10. Narcolepsy
11. j, i, a, d, g, b, c, h, f, e
12. d   13. a   14. a   15. b   16. c

Case Study Answers

1. *Explain the two types of sleep.* There are two types of sleep: NREM (non-rapid eye movement) sleep and REM (rapid eye movement) sleep. During sleep, NREM and REM sleep alternate in cycles. NREM sleep occurs when activity in the RAS is inhibited. About 75% to 80% of sleep during a night is NREM sleep. NREM sleep is divided into four stages, each associated with distinct brain activity and physiology. Stage I is the stage of very light sleep and lasts only a few minutes. During this stage, the person feels drowsy and relaxed, the eyes roll from side to side, and the heart and respiratory rates drop slightly. The sleeper can be readily awakened and may deny that he or she was sleeping. Stage II is the stage of light sleep during which body processes continue to slow down. The eyes are generally still, the heart and respiratory rates decrease slightly, and body temperature falls. Stage II lasts only about 10 to 15 minutes but constitutes 44% to 55% of total sleep.

An individual in stage II requires more intense stimuli than in stage I to awaken. Stages III and IV are the deepest stages of sleep, differing only in the percentage of delta waves recorded during a 30-second period. During deep sleep or delta sleep, the sleeper's heart and respiratory rates drop 20% to 30% below those exhibited during waking hours. The sleeper is difficult to arouse. The person is not disturbed by sensory stimuli, the skeletal muscles are very relaxed, reflexes are diminished, and snoring is most likely to occur. Even swallowing and saliva production are reduced during delta sleep. These stages are essential for restoring energy and releasing important growth hormones. REM sleep usually recurs about every 90 minutes and lasts 5 to 30 minutes. Most dreams take place during REM sleep, but usually will not be remembered unless the person arouses briefly at the end of the REM period. During REM sleep, the brain is highly active, and brain metabolism may increase as much as 20%. For example, during REM sleep, levels of acetylcholine and dopamine increase, with the highest levels of acetylcholine release occurring during REM sleep. Since both of these neurotransmitters are associated with cortical activation, it makes sense that their levels would be high during dreaming sleep. This type of sleep is also called paradoxical sleep because EEG activity resembles that of wakefulness. Distinctive eye movements occur, voluntary muscle tone is dramatically decreased, and deep tendon reflexes are absent. In this phase, the sleeper may be difficult to arouse or may wake spontaneously, gastric secretions increase, and heart and respiratory rates often are irregular. It is thought that the regions of the brain that are used in learning, thinking, and organizing information are stimulated during REM sleep.

2. *Describe factors that affect sleep.* Both the quality and the quantity of sleep are affected by a number of factors. Sleep quality is a subjective characteristic and is often determined by whether or not a person wakes up feeling energetic or not. Quantity of sleep is the total time the individual sleeps. Illness, environment, lifestyle, emotional stress, stimulants and alcohol, diet, smoking, motivation, and medications are some of the factors that affect sleep.

3. *Explain the information that should be included in a sleep diary.* A sleep diary may include all or selected aspects of the following information that pertain to the client's specific problem:

■ Time of (a) going to bed, (b) trying to fall asleep, (c) falling asleep (approximate time), (d) any instances of waking up and duration of these periods, (e) waking up in the morning, and (f) time and duration of any naps

■ Activities performed 2 to 3 hours before going to bed (type, duration, and time)

■ Consumption of caffeinated beverages and alcohol and amounts of those beverages

■ Any prescribed and over-the-counter medications, and herbal remedies, taken during the day

■ Bedtime rituals before bed

■ Any difficulties remaining awake during the day and times when difficulties occurred

■ Any worries that the client believes may affect sleep

■ Factors that the client believes have a positive or negative effect on sleep

NCLEX® Review Question Answers

1. *Answer:* 2 (Objective: 7) *Rationale:* A sleep specialist may ask clients to keep a sleep diary or log for 1 to 2 weeks in order to get a more complete picture of their sleep complaints. A sleep diary may include all or selected aspects of the following information that pertain to the client's specific problem: activities performed 2 to 3 hours before going to bed (type, duration, and time); consumption of caffeinated beverages and alcohol and amounts of those beverages; bedtime rituals before bed; any prescribed and over-the-counter medications, and herbal remedies taken during the day. *Nursing Process:* Planning *Client Need:* Physiological Integrity

2. *Answer:* 4 (Objective: 7) *Rationale:* "When I'm in pain, I will take the prescribed analgesics 30 minutes before I go to sleep" would have been a correct statement. The following statements by the client would be correct: "I should wear loose-fitting nightwear." "I will void before bedtime." "I will perform hygienic routines prior to bedtime." *Nursing Process:* Evaluation *Client Need:* Physiological Integrity

3. *Answer:* 3 (Objective: 8) *Rationale:* Sleep medications often prescribed on a prn (as-needed) basis for clients include the sedative-hypnotics, which induce sleep, and antianxiety drugs or tranquilizers, which decrease anxiety and tension. When prn sleep medications are ordered in institutional settings, the nurse is responsible for making decisions with the client about when to administer them. These medications should be administered only with complete knowledge of their actions and effects and only when indicated. Sleep medications affect REM sleep more than NREM sleep. Antianxiety medications decrease levels of arousal by facilitating the action of neurons in the CNS that suppress responsiveness to stimulation. Sleep medications vary in their onset and duration of action and will impair waking function as long as they are chemically active. Initial doses of medications should be low and increases added gradually, depending on the client's response. *Nursing Process:* Evaluation *Client Need:* Physiological Integrity

4. *Answer:* 1 (Objective: 5) *Rationale:* Hypersomnia refers to conditions where the affected individual obtains sufficient sleep at night but still cannot stay awake during the day. Narcolepsy is a disorder of excessive daytime sleepiness caused by the lack of the chemical hypocretin in the area of the central nervous system that regulates sleep. Sleep apnea is characterized by frequent short breathing pauses during sleep. A parasomnia is behavior that may interfere with sleep and/or occurs during sleep. *Nursing Process:* Assessment *Client Need:* Physiological Integrity

5. *Answer:* 2 (Objective: 2) *Rationale:* NREM sleep is divided into four stages, each associated with distinct brain activity and physiology. Stage I is the stage of very light sleep and lasts only a few minutes. During this stage, the person feels drowsy and relaxed, the eyes roll from side to side, and the heart and respiratory rates drop slightly. The sleeper can be readily awakened and may deny that he or she was sleeping. Stage II is the stage of light sleep during which body processes continue to slow down. The eyes are generally still, the heart and respiratory rates decrease slightly, and body temperature falls. Stage II lasts only about 10 to 15 minutes but constitutes 44% to 55% of total sleep. An individual in stage II requires more intense stimuli than in stage I to awaken. Stages III and IV are the deepest stages of sleep, differing only in the percentage of delta waves recorded during a 30-second period. During deep sleep or delta sleep, the sleeper's heart and respiratory rates drop 20% to 30% below those exhibited during waking hours. The sleeper is difficult to arouse. The person is not disturbed by sensory stimuli, the skeletal muscles are very relaxed, reflexes are diminished, and snoring is most likely to occur. Even swallowing and saliva production are reduced during delta sleep. These stages are essential for restoring energy and releasing important growth hormones. *Nursing Process:* Assessment *Client Need:* Physiological Integrity

6. *Answer:* 3 (Objective: 2) *Rationale:* Physiologic changes during NREM sleep include:

- Arterial blood pressure falls.

- Pulse rate decreases.
- Peripheral blood vessels dilate.
- Cardiac output decreases.

Nursing Process: Evaluation *Client Need:* Physiological Integrity

7. *Answer:* 4 (Objective: 8) *Rationale:* To reduce environmental distractions in hospitals the following should be practiced: Lower the ring tone of nearby telephones; discontinue use of the paging system after a certain hour (e.g., 2100 hours) or reduce its volume; keep required staff conversations at low levels; conduct nursing reports or other discussions in a separate area away from client rooms; perform only essential noisy activities during sleeping hours. *Nursing Process:* Assessment *Client Need:* Physiological Integrity

8. *Answer:* 1 (Objective: 8) *Rationale:* The following are suggestions to promote sleep: Get adequate exercise during the day to reduce stress, but avoid excessive physical exertion at least 3 hours before bedtime. Establish a regular bedtime and wake-up time for all days of the week to enhance biological rhythm. Avoid dealing with office work or family problems before bedtime. Establish a regular, relaxing bedtime routine before sleep such as reading, listening to soft music, or taking a warm bath. *Nursing Process:* Planning *Client Need:* Physiological Integrity

9. *Answer:* 1 (Objective: 8) *Rationale:* Interventions to promote sleep can include the following: If a bedtime snack is necessary, give only low-carbohydrate snack or a milk drink. Create a sleep-conducive environment that is dark, quiet, comfortable, and cool. Give analgesics before bedtime to relieve aches and pains. Avoid giving the client heavy meals 2 to 3 hours before bedtime. *Nursing Process:* Planning *Client Need:* Physiological Integrity

10. *Answer:* 4 (Objective: 1) *Rationale:* Night terrors are partial awakenings from non-REM, stage III or IV sleep. They are usually seen in children 3 to 6 years of age. The child may sleepwalk, or may sit up in bed screaming and thrashing about. Children experiencing night terrors usually cannot be wakened, but should be protected from injury, helped back to bed, and soothed back to sleep. Baby-sitters should be alerted to the possibility of a night terror occurring. Children do not remember the incident the next day, and there is no indication of a neurological or emotional problem. Excessive fatigue and a full bladder may contribute to the problem. Having the child take an afternoon nap and empty the bladder before going to sleep at night may be helpful. *Nursing Process:* Evaluation *Client Need:* Physiological Integrity

Chapter 46

Key Topic Review Answers

1. b   2. b   3. a   4. a   5. b
6. Analgesic
7. Ceiling
8. Equianalgesia
9. Placebo
10. Transdermal
11. f, h, j, a, b, c, g, e, d, i
12. a   13. d   14. c   15. b   16. d

Case Study Answers

1. *As the fifth vital sign, pain should be screened for every time vital signs are evaluated. Define pain.* Pain is an unpleasant and highly personal experience that may be imperceptible to others, while consuming all parts of the person's life. The widely agreed-upon definition of pain is, "Pain is an unpleasant sensory and emotional experience associated with actual or potential tissue damage, or described in terms of such damage." Three parts of this definition have important implications for nurses. First, pain is a physical *and* emotional experience, not all in the body or all in the mind. Second, it is in response to actual *or* potential tissue damage, so there may not be abnormal lab or radiographic reports despite real pain. Finally, pain is described in terms of such damage. This final component is aligned with McCaffery's often-quoted definition of pain, "Pain is whatever the experiencing person says it is, existing whenever he says it does." Given that some clients are reluctant to disclose the presence of pain unless prompted, nurses will not know of the client's pain until they assess for it. Additionally, it is clear that even nonverbal clients (e.g., preverbal children, intubated clients, the cognitively impaired) experience pain that demands nursing assessment and treatment even if clients are unable to "describe in terms" the nature of their discomfort.

2. *Identify the two major components of a pain assessment.* Pain assessments consist of two major components: (a) a pain history to obtain facts from the client and (b) direct observation of behaviors, physical signs of tissue damage, and secondary physiologic responses of the client.

3. *Explain the pain intensity scale.* The use of pain intensity scales is an easy and reliable method of determining the client's pain intensity. Such scales provide consistency for nurses to communicate with the client and other health care providers. To avoid confusion, scales used should use a 0 to 10 range with 0 indicating "no pain" and the highest number indicating the "worst pain possible" for that individual.

Review Question Answers

1. *Answer:* 3 (Objective: 1) *Rationale:* Pain is more than a symptom of a problem; it is a high-priority problem in itself. Pain presents both physiologic and psychologic dangers to health and recovery. Severe pain is viewed as an emergency situation deserving attention and prompt professional treatment. *Nursing Process:* Assessment *Client Need:* Physiological Integrity

2. *Answer:* 2 (Objective: 1) *Rationale:* When pain lasts only through the expected recovery period, it is described as acute pain, whether it has a sudden or slow onset and regardless of the intensity. Chronic pain, on the other hand, is prolonged, usually recurring or persisting over 6 months or longer, and interferes with functioning. Pain may be referred (appear to arise in different areas) to other parts of the body. Visceral pain (pain arising from organs or hollow viscera) often presents this way, being perceived in an area remote from the organ causing the pain. *Nursing Process:* Assessment *Client Need:* Physiological Integrity

3. *Answer:* 2 (Objective: 1) *Rationale:* Pain tolerance is the maximum amount of painful stimuli that a person is willing to withstand without seeking avoidance of the pain or relief. Pain threshold is the least amount of stimuli that is needed for a person to feel a sensation he or she labels as pain. Dysesthesia is an unpleasant abnormal sensation. Allodynia is where nonpainful stimuli (e.g., contact with linen, water, or wind) produce pain. *Nursing Process:* Assessment *Client Need:* Physiological Integrity

4. *Answer:* 1 (Objective: 1) *Rationale:* Linking the rating to health and functioning scores, pain in the 1 to 3 range is deemed mild pain, a rating of 4 to 6 is moderate pain, and pain reaching 7 to 10 is ranked severe pain and is associated with the worst outcomes. *Nursing Process:* Assessment *Client Need:* Physiological Integrity

5. *Answer:* 3 (Objective: 1) *Rationale:*

Acute Pain

Mild to severe

Sympathetic nervous system responses:

■ Increased pulse rate

■ Increased respiratory rate

■ Elevated blood pressure

■ Diaphoresis

■ Dilated pupils

Related to tissue injury; resolves with healing

Client appears restless and anxious

Client reports pain

Client exhibits behavior indicative of pain: crying, rubbing area, holding area

Chronic Pain

Mild to severe

Parasympathetic nervous system responses:

- Vital signs normal
- Dry, warm skin
- Pupils normal or dilated

Continues beyond healing

Client appears depressed and withdrawn

Client often does not mention pain unless asked

Pain behavior often absent

Nursing Process: Assessment *Client Need:* Physiological Integrity

6. *Answer:* 4 (Objective: 5) *Rationale:* That the amount of tissue damage is directly related to the amount of pain is a misconception about pain. The following are correct statements about pain: The person who experiences the pain is the only authority about its existence and nature. Pain is a subjective experience, and the intensity and duration of pain vary considerably among individuals. Even with severe pain, periods of physiologic and behavioral adaptation can occur.

Nursing Process: Assessment *Client Need:* Physiological Integrity

7. *Answer:* 4 (Objective: 10) *Rationale:* "A nonopioid should not be given at the same time as an opioid" is a false statement. It is safe to administer a nonopioid and opioid at the same time. Giving a dose of nonopioid at the same time as a dose of opioid poses no more danger than giving the doses at different times. In fact, many opioids are compounded with a nonopioid (e.g., Percocet [oxycodone and acetaminophen]). The following statements are true about nonopioids: Nonopioids alone are rarely sufficient to relieve severe pain, but they are an important part in the total analgesic plan. Side effects from long-term use of NSAIDs are considerably more severe and life threatening than the side effects from daily doses of oral morphine or other opioids. Giving a dose of nonopioid at the same time as a dose of opioid poses no more danger than giving the doses at different times.

Nursing Process: Assessment *Client Need:* Physiological Integrity

8. *Answer:* 4 (Objective: 7) *Rationale:* Mnemonic for Pain Assessment: COLDERR

Character:	describe the sensation (e.g., sharp, aching, burning)
Onset:	when it started, how it has changed
Location:	where it hurts (all locations)
Duration:	constant versus intermittent in nature
Exacerbation:	factors that make it worse
Relief:	factors that make it better (medications and other factors)
Radiation:	pattern of shooting/spreading/location of pain away from its origin

Nursing Process: Planning *Client Need:* Physiological Integrity

9. *Answer:* 3 (Objective: 3) *Rationale:* The Puerto Rican culture tends to be loud and outspoken in their expressions of pain. Do not judge or disapprove. This is a socially learned way to cope with the pain. The Asian American culture values silence. Some clients may be quiet when in pain. Becoming verbally loud may be viewed as causing dishonor to themselves and their family. The African American culture believes pain and suffering is a part of life and is to be endured. The Mexican American culture believes that enduring pain is a sign of strength. Native Americans are quiet, less expressive verbally and nonverbally, and may tolerate a high level of pain.

Nursing Process: Assessment *Client Need:* Psychosocial Integrity

10. *Answer:* 4 (Objective: 8) *Rationale:* Maintain an unbiased attitude (open mind) about what may relieve the pain. New ways to relieve pain are continually being developed. It is not always possible to explain the effectiveness of particular pain relief measures; however, the use of approaches the patient believes will work should be considered. Provide measures to relieve pain before it becomes severe. Consider the client's ability and willingness to participate actively in pain relief measures. Clients who are excessively fatigued, sedated, or have altered levels of consciousness are less able to participate actively. Establish a trusting relationship. Convey your concern, and acknowledge that you believe that the client is experiencing pain. A trusting relationship promotes expression of the client's thoughts and feelings and enhances effectiveness of planned pain therapies.

Nursing Process: Assessment *Client Need:* Physiological Integrity

Chapter 47

Key Topic Review Answers

1. a   2. a   3. a   4. b   5. b
6. Nutrition
7. Nutrients
8. Starches
9. Fiber
10. Enzymes
11. c, j, f, a, b, i, g, d, h, e
12. d   13. a   14. d   15. a   16. a

Case Study Answers

1. *Explain the combinations of plant proteins that provide complete proteins*. The combinations of plant proteins that provide complete proteins are grains plus legumes; legumes plus nuts or seeds; and grains, legumes, nuts or seeds plus milk or milk products.

2. *Identify ways the client can improve his appetite*.

   ■ Provide familiar food that the person likes. Often the relatives of clients are pleased to bring food from home but may need some guidance about special diet requirements.

   ■ Select small portions so as not to discourage the anorexic client.

   ■ Avoid unpleasant or uncomfortable treatments immediately before or after a meal.

   ■ Provide a tidy, clean environment that is free of unpleasant sights and odors. A soiled dressing, a used bedpan, an uncovered irrigation set, or even used dishes can negatively affect the appetite.

   ■ Encourage or provide oral hygiene before mealtime. This improves the client's ability to taste.

   ■ Relieve illness symptoms that depress appetite before mealtime; for example, give an analgesic for pain or an antipyretic for a fever or allow rest for fatigue.

   ■ Reduce psychologic stress. A lack of understanding of therapy, the anticipation of an operation, and fear of the unknown can cause anorexia. Often, the nurse can help by discussing feelings with the client, giving information and assistance, and allaying fears.

3. *Discuss variations in nutritional practices and preferences among the client's culture*.

   ■ Gifts of food are common and should never be rejected.

   ■ Diets are often high in fat, cholesterol, and sodium.

   ■ Being overweight is viewed as positive.

   ■ Most persons are lactose intolerant.

Review Question Answers

1. *Answer:* 4 (Objective: 1) *Rationale:* Carbohydrates, fats, and protein are referred to as macronutrients, because they are needed in large amounts (e.g., hundreds of grams) to provide energy. Micronutrients—vitamins and minerals—are those required in small amounts (e.g., milligrams or micrograms) to metabolize the energy-providing nutrients. *Nursing Process:* Assessment *Client Need:* Physiological Integrity

2. *Answer:* 4 (Objective: 1) *Rationale:* Fiber is present in the outer layer of grains and bran, and in the skin, seeds, and pulp of many vegetables and fruits. Starches are the insoluble, nonsweet forms of carbohydrate. Most sugars are produced naturally by plants, especially fruits, sugar cane, and sugar beets. Fiber, a complex carbohydrate derived from plants, supplies roughage, or bulk, to the diet. *Nursing Process:* Assessment *Client Need:* Physiological Integrity

3. *Answer:* 2 (Objective: 2) *Rationale:* Nonessential amino acids include alanine, aspartic acid, cystine, glutamic acid, glycine, hydroxyproline, proline, serine, and tyrosine. The nine essential amino acids are histidine, isoleucine, leucine, lysine, methionine, phenylalanine, tryptophan, threonine, and valine. Essential amino acids are those that cannot be manufactured in the body and must be supplied as part of the protein ingested in the diet. Nonessential amino acids are those that the body can manufacture. Most animal proteins, including meats, poultry, fish, dairy products, and eggs, are complete proteins. *Nursing Process:* Assessment *Client Need:* Physiological Integrity

4. *Answer:* 2 (Objective: 2) *Rationale:* Lipids are organic substances that are greasy and insoluble in water but soluble in alcohol or ether. In common use, the terms *fats* and *lipids* are used interchangeably. Fats are lipids that are solid at room temperature. Oils are lipids that are liquid at room temperature. *Nursing Process:* Assessment *Client Need:* Physiological Integrity

5. *Answer:* 1 (Objective: 4) *Rationale:* To calculate the BMI use the following formula:

$$BMI = \frac{Weight\ in\ kilograms}{(Height\ in\ meters)^2}$$

or

$$\frac{70\ kilograms}{1.5 \times 1.5\ (meters)^2} = 31.11$$

Nursing Process: Assessment *Client Need:* Physiological Integrity

6. *Answer:* 2 (Objective: 5) *Rationale:* The following suggestions may help parents meet the child's nutritional needs and promote effective parent–child interactions: (a) Make mealtime a pleasant time by avoiding tensions at the table and discussions of bad behavior; (b) offer a variety of simple, attractive foods in small portions, and avoid meals that combine foods into one dish, such as a stew; (c) do not use food as a reward or punish a child who does not eat; (d) schedule meals, sleep, and snack times that will allow for optimum appetite and behavior; and (e) avoid the routine use of sweet desserts. *Nursing Process:* Implementation *Client Need:* Physiological Integrity

7. *Answer:* 2 (Objective: 8) *Rationale:* A food diary is a detailed record of measured amounts (portion sizes) of all food and fluids a client consumes during a specified period, usually 3 to 7 days. A diet history is a comprehensive, time-consuming assessment of a client's food intake that involves an extensive interview by a nutritionist or dietitian. A food frequency record is a checklist that indicates how often general food groups or specific foods are eaten. For a 24-hour food recall, the nurse asks the client to recall all the food and beverages the client consumes during a typical 24-hour period when at home. *Nursing Process:* Implementation *Client Need:* Physiological Integrity

8. *Answer:* 4 (Objective: 11) *Rationale:* Note that the word "clear" in clear diet means "colorless." A clear liquid diet is limited to water, tea, coffee, clear broths, ginger ale, or other carbonated beverages, strained and clear juices, and plain gelatin. A full liquid diet contains only liquids or foods that turn to liquid at body temperature, such as ice cream. The soft diet is easily chewed and digested. *Nursing Process:* Evaluation *Client Need:* Physiological Integrity

9. *Answer:* 3 (Objective: 12) *Rationale:* Enteral feedings can be given intermittently or continuously. Intermittent feedings are the administration of 300 to 500 mL of enteral formula several times per day. The stomach is the preferred site for these feedings, which are usually administered over at least 30 minutes. *Nursing Process:* Implementation *Client Need:* Physiological Integrity

10. *Answer:* 4 (Objective: 13) *Rationale:* Avoid unpleasant or uncomfortable treatments immediately before or after a meal. Provide familiar food that the client likes. Encourage or provide oral hygiene before mealtime. Provide a tidy, clean environment that is free of unpleasant sights and odors. *Nursing Process:* Planning *Client Need:* Physiological Integrity

Chapter 48
Key Topic Review Answers

1. a   **2.** b   **3.** a   **4.** a   **5.** a
6. Diuretics
7. Flaccid
8. Irrigation
9. Nephrostomy
10. Vesicostomy
11. c, b, i, a, j, g, d, f, e, h
12. a   **13.** d   **14.** a   **15.** b   **16.** d

Case Study Answers

1. *List the steps a nurse must follow to measure fluid output.*

- Wear clean gloves to prevent contact with microorganisms or blood in urine.
- Ask the client to void in a clean urinal, bedpan, commode, or toilet collection device ("hat").
- Instruct the client to keep urine separate from feces and to avoid putting toilet paper in the urine collection container.
- Pour the voided urine into a calibrated container.
- Holding the container at eye level, read the amount in the container. Containers usually have a measuring scale on the inside.
- Record the amount on the fluid intake and output sheet, which may be at the bedside or in the bathroom.
- Rinse the urine collection and measuring containers with cool water and store appropriately.
- Remove gloves and perform hand hygiene.
- Calculate and document the total output on the client's chart at the end of each shift and at the end of 24 hours.

2. *Identify various goals for clients with urinary elimination problems.* The goals established will vary according to the diagnosis and defining characteristics. Examples of overall goals for clients with urinary elimination problems may include the following:

- Maintain or restore a normal voiding pattern.
- Regain normal urine output.
- Prevent associated risks such as infection, skin breakdown, fluid and electrolyte imbalance, and lowered self-esteem.

- Perform toilet activities independently with or without assistive devices.
- Contain urine with the appropriate device, catheter, ostomy appliance, or absorbent product.

3. *Explain how this client can maintain normal urinary elimination.* Most interventions to maintain normal urinary elimination are independent nursing functions. These include promoting adequate fluid intake, maintaining normal voiding habits, and assisting with toileting.

NCLEX® Review Question Answers

1. *Answer:* 1 (Objective: 2) *Rationale:* Oliguria is low urine output, usually less than 500 mL a day or 30 mL an hour for an adult. Polyuria (or diuresis) refers to the production of abnormally large amounts of urine by the kidneys, often several liters more than the client's usual daily output. Polydipsia is excessive fluid intake. Anuria refers to a lack of urine production. *Nursing Process:* Assessment *Client Need:* Physiological Integrity

2. *Answer:* 2 (Objective: 2) *Rationale:* Urinary frequency is voiding at frequent intervals, that is, more than four to six times per day. Nocturia is voiding two or more times at night. Urgency is the sudden strong desire to void. Dysuria means voiding that is either painful or difficult. *Nursing Process:* Assessment *Client Need:* Physiological Integrity

3. *Answer:* 4 (Objective: 7) *Rationale:* Ways to prevent a recurrence of a UTI include: Girls and women should always wipe the perineal area from front to back following urination or defecation in order to prevent introduction of gastrointestinal bacteria into the urethra. Drink eight 8-ounce glasses of water per day to flush bacteria out of the urinary system. Wear cotton rather than nylon underclothes. Avoid tight-fitting pants or other clothing that creates irritation to the urethra and prevents ventilation of the perineal area. *Nursing Process:* Planning *Client Need:* Physiological Integrity

4. *Answer:* 4 (Objective: 8) *Rationale:* Intermittent self-catheterization protects the upper urinary tract from reflux, reduces incidence of urinary tract infection, enables the client to retain independence and gain control of the bladder, and allows normal sexual relations without incontinence. *Nursing Process:* Evaluation *Client Need:* Physiological Integrity

5. *Answer:* 3 (Objective: 4) *Rationale:* The normal color or clarity of urine is straw, amber, or transparent. Abnormal color or clarity of urine is dark amber, dark orange, red, dark brown, cloudy, mucous plugs, viscid, thick. *Nursing Process:* Assessment *Client Need:* Physiological Integrity

6. *Answer:* 3 (Objective: 6) *Rationale:* Normal results for a urine specific gravity should be in the range of 1.010 to 1.025. All other results not in this range are considered abnormal. *Nursing Process:* Assessment *Client Need:* Physiological Integrity

7. *Answer:* 3 (Objective: 8) *Rationale:* Lubricate the catheter 6 to 7 inches for males. If not the entire part of the catheter that is inserted into the male penis will not be lubricated. This will make the procedure very uncomfortable for the client as well as cause harm to the client. The following statements are correct steps: Pick up a cleansing ball with the forceps in your dominant hand and wipe from the center of the meatus in a circular motion around the glans. Grasp the catheter firmly 2 to 3 in. from the tip. Ask the client to take a slow deep breath and insert the catheter as the client exhales. *Nursing Process:* Implementation *Client Need:* Physiological Integrity

8. *Answer:* 3 (Objective: 6) *Rationale:* Facilitating and promoting urinary elimination includes the following: Advise the client and family to install grab bars and elevated toilet seats as needed. Teach the client to empty the bladder completely at each voiding. Emphasize the importance of drinking eight to ten 8-ounce glasses of water daily. Suggest clothing that is easily removed for toileting, such as elastic-waist pants or pants with Velcro closures. *Nursing Process:* Evaluation *Client Need:* Physiological Integrity

9. *Answer:* 3 (Objective: 7) *Rationale:* Initially perform each contraction 10 times, three times daily. Gradually increase the count to a full 10 seconds for both contraction and relaxation. To control episodes of stress incontinence, perform a pelvic muscle contraction when initiating any activity that increases intra-abdominal pressure, such as coughing, laughing, sneezing, or lifting. Develop a schedule that will help remind you to do these exercises, for example, before getting out of bed in the morning. Contract your pelvic muscles whereby you pull your rectum, urethra, and vagina up inside, and hold for a count of 3 to 5 seconds. Then relax the same muscles for a count of 3 to 5 seconds. *Nursing Process:* Planning *Client Need:* Health Promotion and Maintenance

10. *Answer:* 2 (Objective: 8) *Rationale:* For preventing catheter-associated urinary infections the following guidelines should be practiced: Maintain a sterile closed-drainage system. Do not disconnect the catheter and drainage tubing unless absolutely necessary. Provide routine perineal hygiene, including cleansing with soap and water after defecation. Prevent contamination of the catheter with feces. *Nursing Process:* Evaluation *Client Need:* Preventing Catheter-Associated Urinary Infections

Chapter 49
Key Topic Review Answers

1. a   **2.** b   **3.** b   **4.** a   **5.** a

6. Flatulence

7. Ostomy

8. Bedpan

9. Enema

10. Cathartics

11. h, j, a, f, i, b, d, g, e, c

12. c   **13.** b   **14.** b   **15.** d   **16.** d

Case Study Answers

1. *Identify ways for the client to manage diarrhea.*

■ Drink at least 8 glasses of water per day to prevent dehydration. Consider drinking a few glasses of electrolyte replacement fluids each day.

■ Eat foods with sodium and potassium. Most foods contain sodium. Potassium is found in meats and many vegetables and fruits, especially purple grape juice, tomatoes, potatoes, bananas, cooked peaches, and apricots.

■ Increase foods containing soluble fiber, such as rice, oatmeal, and skinless fruits and potatoes.

■ Avoid alcohol and beverages with caffeine, which aggravate the problem.

■ Limit foods containing insoluble fiber, such as high-fiber whole-wheat and whole-grain breads and cereals, and raw fruits and vegetables.

■ Limit fatty foods.

■ Thoroughly clean and dry the perianal area after passing stool to prevent skin irritation and breakdown. Use soft toilet tissue to clean and dry the area. Apply a Dimethicone-based cream or alcohol-free barrier film as needed.

■ If possible, discontinue medications that cause diarrhea.

■ When diarrhea has stopped, reestablish normal bowel flora by eating fermented dairy products, such as yogurt or buttermilk.

■ Seek a physican consultation right away if weakness, dizziness, or loose stools persist for more than 48 hours.

2. *Provide the client with information about healthy defecation.*

■ Establish a regular exercise regimen.

■ Include high-fiber foods, such as vegetables, fruits, and whole grains, in the diet.

■ Maintain fluid intake of 2,000 to 3,000 mL a day.

■ Do not ignore the urge to defecate.

■ Allow time to defecate, preferably at the same time each day.

■ Avoid over-the-counter medications to treat constipation and diarrhea.

3. *Identify three major causes of diarrhea.* Some causes of diarrhea include: psychologic stress (e.g., anxiety); medications; antibiotics; cathartics; allergy to food, fluid, or drugs; intolerance of food or fluid.

NCLEX® Review Question Answers

1. *Answer:* 1 (Objective: 1) *Rationale:* A gastrostomy is an opening through the abdominal wall into the stomach. A jejunostomy opens through the abdominal wall into the jejunum. A colostomy opens into the colon (large bowel). An ileostomy opens into the ileum (small bowel). *Nursing Process:* Assessment *Client Need:* Physiological Integrity

2. *Answer:* 2 (Objective: 8) *Rationale:* A carminative enema is given primarily to expel flatus. A retention enema introduces oil or medication into the rectum and sigmoid colon. A return-flow enema is used occasionally to expel flatus. Cleansing enemas may also be described as high or low. *Nursing Process:* Assessment *Client Need:* Physiological Integrity

3. *Answer:* 2 (Objective: 6) *Rationale:* Ask the client to assume a left side-lying position, with the knees flexed and the back toward the nurse. Place a bedpad under the client's buttocks and a bedpan nearby to receive stool. Drape the client for comfort and to avoid unnecessary exposure of the body. Gently insert the index finger into the rectum and move the finger along the length of the rectum. *Nursing Process:* Implementation *Client Need:* Physiological Integrity

4. *Answer:* 2 (Objectives: 2, 7) *Rationale:* Client teaching for healthy defecation: Include high-fiber foods, such as vegetables, fruits, and whole grains, in the diet. Maintain fluid intake of 2,000 to 3,000 mL a day. Allow time to defecate, preferably at the same time each day. Avoid over-the-counter medications to treat constipation and diarrhea. *Nursing Process:* Evaluation *Client Need:* Physiological Integrity

5. *Answer:* 3 (Objectives: 2, 7) *Rationale:* Limit foods containing insoluble fiber, such as high-fiber whole-wheat and whole-grain breads and cereals, and raw fruits and vegetables. Increase foods containing soluble fiber, such as rice, oatmeal, and skinless fruits and potatoes. Drink at least 8 glasses of water per day to prevent dehydration. Eat foods with sodium and potassium. Limit fatty foods. *Nursing Process:* Planning *Client Need:* Physiological Integrity

6. *Answer:* 2 (Objective: 9) *Rationale:* Ostomy appliances can be applied for up to 7 days. The pouch is emptied when it is 1/3 to 1/2 full. Most pouches contain odor barrier material. If the pouch overfills, it can cause separation of the skin barrier from the skin and stool can come in contact with the skin. *Nursing Process:* Evaluation *Client Need:* Physiological Integrity

7. *Answer:* 4 (Objective: 9) *Rationale:* The divided colostomy is often used in situations where spillage of feces into the distal end of the bowel needs to be avoided. The single stoma is created when one end of bowel is brought out through an opening onto the anterior abdominal wall. In the loop colostomy, a loop of bowel is brought out onto the abdominal wall and supported by a plastic bridge, or a piece of rubber tubing. The divided colostomy consists of two edges of bowel brought out onto the abdomen but separated from each other. *Nursing Process:* Evaluation *Client Need:* Physiological Integrity

8. *Answer:* 3 (Objective: 2) *Rationale:* Although the squatting position best facilitates defecation, on a toilet seat the best position for most people seems to be leaning forward. A client should be encouraged to defecate when the urge is recognized. Regular exercise helps clients develop a regular defecation pattern. For clients who have difficulty sitting down and getting up from the toilet, an elevated toilet seat can be attached to a regular toilet. *Nursing Process:* Implementation *Client Need:* Physiological Integrity

9. *Answer:* 2 (Objective: 3) *Rationale:*

Adult: brown Clay or white, absence of bile pigment (bile obstruction); diagnostic study using barium

Infant: yellow Black or tarry, drug (e.g., iron); bleeding from upper gastrointestinal tract (e.g., stomach, small intestine); diet high in red meat and dark green vegetables (e.g., spinach)

Red, bleeding from lower gastrointestinal tract (e.g., rectum); some foods (e.g., beets)

Pale, malabsorption of fats; diet high in milk and milk products and low in meat

Orange or green, intestinal infection

Nursing Process: Assessment *Client Need:* Physiological Integrity

10. *Answer:* 3 (Objective: 8) *Rationale:* Oil solutions lubricate the feces and the colonic mucosa. Isotonic solutions distend the colon, stimulate peristalsis, and soften feces. Hypertonic solutions draw water into the colon. Hypotonic solutions distend the colon, stimulate peristalsis, and soften feces. Soapsud solutions irritate the mucosa and distend the colon. Nursing Process: Evaluation *Client Need:* Physiological Integrity

Chapter 50
Key Topic Review Answers

1. a   **2.** a   **3.** b   **4.** b   **5.** b
6. Oxygen
7. Intrapulmonary
8. Atelectasis
9. Diffusion
10. Apnea
11. a, e, j, h, c, f, i, b, d, g
12. d   **13.** b   **14.** a   **15.** c   **16.** d

Case Study Answers

1. *Which factors does adequate ventilation depend on?*
Adequate ventilation depends on several factors:
- Clear airways
- An intact central nervous system and respiratory center
- An intact thoracic cavity capable of expanding and contracting
- Adequate pulmonary compliance and recoil

2. *Which factors affect the rate of oxygen transport from the lungs to the tissues?*
The following factors can affect the rate of oxygen transport from the lungs to the tissues:
- Cardiac output
- Number of erythrocytes and blood hematocrit
- Exercise

3. *Which factors influencing oxygenation affect the cardiovascular system as well as the respiratory system?* Factors that influence oxygenation affect the cardiovascular system as well as the respiratory system. These factors include age, environment, lifestyle, health status, medications, and stress.

4. *What are oxygen therapy safety precautions?*

■ For home oxygen use or when the facility permits smoking, teach family members and roommates to smoke only outside or in provided smoking rooms away from the client and oxygen equipment.

■ Place cautionary signs reading "No Smoking: Oxygen in Use" on the client's door, at the foot or head of the bed, and on the oxygen equipment.

■ Instruct the client and visitors about the hazard of smoking with oxygen in use.

■ Make sure that electric devices (such as razors, hearing aids, radios, televisions, and heating pads) are in good working order to prevent the occurrence of short-circuit sparks.

■ Avoid materials that generate static electricity, such as woolen blankets and synthetic fabrics. Cotton blankets should be used, and clients and caregivers should be advised to wear cotton fabrics.

■ Avoid the use of volatile, flammable materials, such as oils, greases, alcohol, ether, and acetone (e.g., nail polish remover), near clients receiving oxygen.

■ Be sure that electric monitoring equipment, suction machines, and portable diagnostic machines are all electrically grounded.

■ Make known the location of fire extinguishers, and make sure personnel are trained in their use.

NCLEX® Review Question Answers

1. *Answer:* 3 (Objective: 1) *Rationale:* Adequate ventilation depends on several factors:

■ Clear airways

■ An intact central nervous system and respiratory center

■ An intact thoracic cavity capable of expanding and contracting

■ Adequate pulmonary compliance and recoil

Nursing Process: Assessment *Client Need:* Physiological Integrity

2. *Answer:* 1 (Objective: 5) *Rationale:* Normal respiration (eupnea) is quiet, rhythmic, and effortless. Tachypnea (rapid rate) is seen with fevers, metabolic acidosis, pain, and with hypercapnia or hypoxemia. Bradypnea is an abnormally slow respiratory rate, which may be seen in clients who have taken drugs such as morphine, who have metabolic alkalosis, or who have increased intracranial pressure (e.g., from brain injuries). Apnea is the cessation of breathing. *Nursing Process:* Assessment *Client Need:* Physiological Integrity

3. *Answer:* 3 (Objective: 5) *Rationale:* Cheyne-Stokes respirations are the marked rhythmic waxing and waning of respirations from very deep to very shallow breathing and temporary apnea; common causes include congestive heart failure, increased intracranial pressure, and overdose of certain drugs. Biot's (cluster) respirations are shallow breaths interrupted by apnea; may be seen in clients with central nervous system disorders. Orthopnea is the inability to breathe except in an upright or standing position. Difficult or uncomfortable breathing is called dyspnea. *Nursing Process:* Assessment *Client Need:* Physiological Integrity

4. *Answer:* 4 (Objective: 7) *Rationale:* The nonrebreather mask delivers the highest oxygen concentration possible—95% to 100%—by means other than intubation or mechanical ventilation, at liter flows of 10 to 15 L per minute. *Nursing Process:* Assessment *Client Need:* Physiological Integrity

5. *Answer:* 2 (Objective: 7) *Rationale:* The Venturi mask delivers oxygen concentrations varying from 24% to 40% or 50% at liter flows of 4 to 10 L per minute. The nonrebreather mask delivers the highest oxygen concentration possible—95% to 100%—by means other than intubation or mechanical ventilation, at liter flows of 10 to 15 L per minute. One-way valves on the mask and between the reservoir bag and the mask prevent the room air and the client's exhaled air from entering the bag so only the oxygen in the bag is inspired. The simple face mask delivers oxygen concentrations from 40% to 60% at liter flows of 5 to 8 L per minute, respectively. The partial rebreather mask delivers oxygen concentrations of 60% to 90% at liter flows of 6 to 10 L per minute, respectively. The oxygen reservoir bag that is attached allows the client to rebreathe about the first third of the exhaled air in conjunction with oxygen. *Nursing Process:* Assessment *Client Need:* Physiological Integrity

6. *Answer:* 4 (Objective: 7) *Rationale:* Because an endotracheal tube passes through the epiglottis and glottis, the client is unable to speak while it is in place. Endotracheal tubes are most commonly inserted for clients who have had general anesthetics or for those in emergency situations where mechanical ventilation is required. An endotracheal tube is inserted by the primary care provider, nurse, or respiratory therapist with specialized education. It is inserted through the mouth or the nose and into the trachea with the guide of a laryngoscope. The tube terminates just superior to the bifurcation of the trachea into the bronchi. The tube may have an air-filled cuff to prevent air leakage around it. *Nursing Process:* Assessment *Client Need:* Physiological Integrity

7. *Answer:* 2 (Objective: 6) *Rationale:*

Residual volume (RV): The amount of air remaining in the lungs after maximal exhalation

Total lung capacity (TLC): The total volume of the lungs at maximum inflation; calculated by adding the V_T, IRV, ERV, and RV

Vital capacity (VC): Total amount of air that can be exhaled after a maximal inspiration; calculated by adding the V_T, IRV, and ERV

Expiratory reserve volume (ERV): Maximum amount of air that can be exhaled following a normal exhalation

Nursing Process: Assessment *Client Need:* Physiological Integrity

8. *Answer:* 2 (Objective: 1) *Rationale:* The cough reflex consists of the following:

- Nerve impulses are sent through the vagus nerve to the medulla.

- A large inspiration of approximately 2.5 L occurs.

- The epiglottis and glottis (vocal cords) close.

- A strong contraction of abdominal and internal intercostal muscles dramatically raises the pressure in the lungs.

- The epiglottis and glottis open suddenly.

- Air rushes outward with great velocity.

- Mucus and any foreign particles are dislodged from the lower respiratory tract and are propelled up and out.

Nursing Process: Assessment *Client Need:* Physiological Integrity

9. *Answer:* 4 (Objective: 7) *Rationale:* Oxygen therapy safety precautions include:

- For home oxygen use or when the facility permits smoking, teach family members and roommates to smoke only outside or in provided smoking rooms away from the client and oxygen equipment.

- Place cautionary signs reading "No Smoking: Oxygen in Use" on the client's door, at the foot or head of the bed, and on the oxygen equipment.

- Instruct the client and visitors about the hazard of smoking with oxygen in use.

- Make sure that electric devices (such as razors, hearing aids, radios, televisions, and heating pads) are in good working order to prevent the occurrence of short-circuit sparks.

- Avoid materials that generate static electricity, such as woolen blankets and synthetic fabrics. Cotton blankets should be used, and clients and caregivers should be advised to wear cotton fabrics.

- Avoid the use of volatile, flammable materials, such as oils, greases, alcohol, ether, and acetone (e.g., nail polish remover), near clients receiving oxygen.

- Be sure that electric monitoring equipment, suction machines, and portable diagnostic machines are all electrically grounded.

- Make known the location of fire extinguishers, and make sure personnel are trained in their use.

Nursing Process: Assessment *Client Need:* Physiological Integrity

10. *Answer:* 4 (Objective: 7) *Rationale:* Put on sterile gloves. Keep your dominant hand sterile during the procedure. Clean the lumen and entire inner cannula thoroughly using a brush or pipe cleaners moistened with sterile normal saline. Rinse the inner cannula thoroughly in the sterile normal saline. After rinsing, gently tap the cannula against the inside edge of the sterile saline container. *Nursing Process:* Implementation *Client Need:* Physiological Integrity

Chapter 51

Key Topic Review Answers

1. a   2. b   3. a   4. b   5. a
6. Ischemia
7. Heart
8. Multiplying
9. Preload
10. Afterload
11. b, d, c, j, g, i, h, f, e, a
12. d   13. a   14. a   15. d   16. d

Case Study Answers

1. *Why is the physician concerned about my lipid levels being elevated?* A strong link exists between elevated serum lipid levels and the development of coronary heart disease. Lipoproteins circulate in the blood and are made up of cholesterol, triglycerides, and phospholipids. A high dietary intake of saturated fats is the most critical factor for the development of elevated serum lipids. The average American diet often contains more than 40% of its calories in fats. The American Heart Association recommends that less than 30% of total calories come from fats.

2. *What is hypertension?* Hypertension (or increased blood pressure) increases the risk of coronary heart disease in several ways. First, it increases the workload of the heart, increasing

oxygen demand and coronary blood flow. The increased workload also causes hypertrophy of the ventricles. Over time this can contribute to heart failure. Second, hypertension causes endothelial damage to the blood vessels, which stimulates the development of atherosclerosis.

3. *What are the risk factors for coronary heart disease?* Nonmodifiable risk factors are heredity, age, and gender (women's risk increases postmenopause); modifiable risk factors are elevated serum lipid level, hypertension, cigarette smoking, diabetes, obesity, and sedentary lifestyle; other risk factors are heat and cold, previous health status, stress and coping, dietary factors, alcohol intake, and elevated homocysteine level.

NCLEX® Review Question Answers

1. *Answer:* 1 (Objective: 2) *Rationale:* Modifiable risk factors for coronary heart disease include: elevated serum lipid level; hypertension; cigarette smoking; diabetes; obesity; sedentary lifestyle. Nonmodifiable risk factors include: heredity; age; gender (women's risk increases postmenopause). Other risk factors include: heat and cold; previous health status; stress and coping; dietary factors; alcohol intake; elevated homocysteine level. *Nursing Process:* Assessment *Client Need:* Physiological Integrity

2. *Answer:* 1 (Objective: 4) *Rationale:* The condition that increases afterload is hypertension; the conditions that increase preload are hypervolemia, valvular disorders such as mitral regurgitation, and congenital defects such as patent ductus arteriosus; and the conditions that affect myocardial function are myocardial infarction, cardiomyopathy, and coronary artery disease. *Nursing Process:* Assessment *Client Need:* Physiological Integrity

3. *Answer:* 4 (Objective: 2) *Rationale:* Normal changes of aging may contribute to problems of circulation in elders, even when there is no actual pathology:

- Blood vessels become less elastic and have an increase in calcification. This results in a restricted blood flow and a decrease of oxygen and nutrients to tissues (heart, peripheral, and cerebral).

- Impaired valve function in the heart is often the result of increased stiffness and calcification and results in a decrease in cardiac output.

- A decrease of muscle tone in the heart results in a decrease in cardiac output.

- There is a decrease in baroreceptor response to blood pressure changes, making the heart and blood vessels less responsive to exercise and

stress. This often results in dizziness, falls, orthostatic hypotension, and mental changes.

- A decrease in conduction ability in the heart also makes the heart less responsive to changes and stresses. This can also result in dizziness, falls, orthostatic hypotension, and mental changes.

Nursing Process: Assessment *Client Need:* Physiological Integrity

4. *Answer:* 2 (Objective: 7) *Rationale:* Promoting a Healthy Heart: Exercise regularly, participating in at least 20 minutes (40 minutes is preferred) of vigorous exercise four to five times a week, do not smoke, eat a diet low in total fat, saturated fats, and cholesterol, reduce stress, and manage anger. *Nursing Process:* Planning *Client Need:* Physiological Integrity

5. *Answer:* 4 (Objective: 1) *Rationale:* Deoxygenated blood from the veins enters the right side of the heart through the superior and inferior venae cavae. Four hollow chambers within the heart, two upper atria and two lower ventricles, are separated longitudinally by the interventricular septum, forming two parallel pumps. The heart is a hollow, cone-shaped organ about the size of a fist. The heart is located in the mediastinum, between the lungs and underlying the sternum. *Nursing Process:* Evaluation *Client Need:* Physiological Integrity

6. *Answer:* 2 (Objective: 1) *Rationale:* With each heartbeat, the myocardium goes through a cycle of contraction (systole) and relaxation (diastole). Systole is when the heart ejects (propels) the blood into the pulmonary and systemic circulations. Diastole is when the ventricles fill with blood. The diastolic phase of the cardiac cycle is twice as long as the systolic phase. This is important because diastole (or ventricular filling) is largely a passive process. The longer diastolic phase allows this filling to occur. At the end of the diastolic phase the atria contract, adding an additional volume to the ventricles. This volume is sometimes called atrial kick. *Nursing Process:* Assessment *Client Need:* Physiological Integrity

7. *Answer:* 1 (Objective: 1) *Rationale:* The primary pacemaker of the heart is the sinoatrial (SA or sinus) node, located where the superior venae cavae enters the right atrium. The SA node normally initiates electrical impulses that are conducted throughout the heart and result in ventricular contraction. In adults, it usually discharges impulses at a regular rate of 60 to 100 times per minute, the "normal" heart rate. The impulse then spreads throughout the atria via the interatrial pathways. These conduction pathways converge and narrow through the atrioventricular (AV) node, slightly delaying transmission of the impulse to the ventricles. This delay allows the atria to contract slightly before ventricular contraction occurs. From the AV node, the impulse then progresses down through the intraventricular septum to the ventricular conduction pathways: the bundle of His, the right and left bundle branches, and the Purkinje fibers. *Nursing Process:* Assessment *Client Need:* Physiological Integrity

8. *Answer:* 4 (Objective: 1) *Rationale:* Resistance is opposition to flow; peripheral vascular resistance impedes or opposes blood flow to the tissues. PVR is determined by:

- The viscosity, or thickness, of the blood
- Blood vessel length
- Blood vessel diameter

Nursing Process: Assessment *Client Need:* Physiological Integrity

9. *Answer:* 3 (Objective: 6) *Rationale:* Lipoproteins circulate in the blood and are made up of cholesterol, triglycerides, and phospholipids. Homocysteine is an amino acid that has been shown to be increased in many people with atherosclerosis. Clients with elevated homocysteine levels may have an increased risk of myocardial infarction, coronary artery disease, cerebrovascular accidents (stroke), and peripheral vascular disease. Clients can reduce their homocysteine level by taking a multivitamin that provides folate, vitamin B_6, vitamin B_{12}, and riboflavin. *Nursing Process:* Planning *Client Need:* Physiological Integrity

10. *Answer:* 1 (Objective: 9) *Rationale:* Signs of heart failure may include:

- Pulmonary congestion; adventitious lung sounds
- Shortness of breath
- Increased heart rate
- Increased respiratory rate
- Peripheral vasoconstriction; cold, pale extremities
- Distended neck veins

Nursing Process: Assessment *Client Need:* Physiological Integrity

Chapter 52
Key Topic Review Answers

1. b   **2.** a   **3.** a   **4.** b   **5.** a
6. Calcium
7. Hyper
8. Blood
9. Drip
10. Butterfly
11. c, j, a, i, h, f, g, e, d, b
12. a   **13.** b   **14.** c   **15.** d   **16.** d

Case Study Answers

1. *Why is water vital to health and normal cellular function?* Water is vital to health and normal cellular function because it serves as a medium for metabolic reactions within cells; a transporter for nutrients, waste products, and other substances; a lubricant; an insulator and shock absorber; and one means of regulating and maintaining body temperature.

2. *Explain the thirst mechanism.* The thirst mechanism is the primary regulator of fluid intake. The thirst center is located in the hypothalamus of the brain. A number of stimuli trigger this center, including the osmotic pressure of body fluids, vascular volume, and angiotensin (a hormone released in response to decreased blood flow to the kidneys). For example, a long-distance runner loses significant amounts of water through perspiration and rapid breathing during a race, increasing the concentration of solutes and the osmotic pressure of body fluids. This increased osmotic pressure stimulates the thirst center, causing the runner to experience the sensation of thirst and the desire to drink to replace lost fluids. Thirst is normally relieved immediately after drinking a small amount of fluid, even before it is absorbed from the gastrointestinal tract. However, this relief is only temporary, and the thirst returns in about 15 minutes. The thirst is again temporarily relieved after the ingested fluid distends the upper gastrointestinal tract. These mechanisms protect the individual from drinking too much, because it takes from 30 minutes to 1 hour for the fluid to be absorbed and distributed throughout the body.

3. *List the four routes of fluid output.* The four routes of fluid output are (1) urine, (2) insensible loss through the skin as perspiration and through the lungs as water vapor in the expired air, (3) noticeable loss through the skin, and (4) loss through the intestines in feces.

NCLEX® Review Question Answers

1. *Answer:* 3 (Objective: 1) *Rationale:* Women have a lower percentage of body water than men. Approximately 60% of the average healthy adult's weight is water, the primary body fluid. In good health this volume remains relatively constant and the person's weight varies by less than 0.2 kg (0.5 lb) in 24 hours, regardless of the amount of fluid ingested. Infants have the highest proportion of water, accounting for 70% to 80% of their body weight. Water makes up a greater percentage of a lean person's body weight than an obese person's. *Nursing Process:* Assessment *Client Need:* Physiological Integrity

2. *Answer:* 1 (Objective: 1) *Rationale:* Diffusion is the continual intermingling of molecules in liquids, gases, or solids brought about by the random movement of the molecules. Osmosis is the movement of water across cell membranes, from the less concentrated solution to the more concentrated solution. Osmosis occurs when the concentration of solutes on one side of a selectively permeable membrane, such as the capillary membrane, is higher than on the other side. Osmosis is an important mechanism for maintaining homeostasis and fluid balance. Osmolality is determined by the total solute concentration within a fluid compartment and is measured as parts of solute per kilogram of water. *Nursing Process:* Assessment *Client Need:* Physiological Integrity

3. *Answer:* 3 (Objective: 3) *Rationale:* Hyponatremia is a sodium deficit, or serum sodium level of less than 135 mEq/L, and is, in acute care settings, a common electrolyte imbalance. Hypernatremia is excess sodium in ECF, or a serum sodium of greater than 145 mEq/L. Hypokalemia is a potassium deficit or a serum potassium level of less than 3.5 mEq/L. Hyperkalemia is a potassium excess or a serum potassium level greater than 5.0 mEq/L. *Nursing Process:* Assessment *Client Need:* Physiological Integrity

4. *Answer:* 3 (Objective: 5) *Rationale:* When a person hyperventilates, more carbon dioxide than normal is exhaled (not oxygen), carbonic acid levels fall, and the pH rises to greater than 7.45. *Nursing Process:* Assessment *Client Need:* Physiological Integrity

5. *Answer:* 1 (Objective: 5) *Rationale:* The normal values of arterial blood gases are:

pH	7.35–7.45
PaO_2	80–100 mm Hg
$PaCO_2$	35–45 mm Hg
HCO_3^-	22–26 mEq/L
Base excess	−2 to +2 mEq/L
O_2 saturation	95–98%

Nursing Process: Assessment *Client Need:* Physiological Integrity

6. *Answer:* 2 (Objective: 7) *Rationale:* The following steps are appropriate for the nurse who is starting an intravenous infusion: Partially fill the drip chamber with solution. Adjust the pole so that the container is suspended about 1 m (3 ft) above the client's head. Use the client's nondominant arm, unless contraindicated. Clean the skin at the site of entry with a topical antiseptic swab. *Nursing Process:* Implementation *Client Need:* Physiological Integrity

7. *Answer:* 3 (Objective: 6) *Rationale:* The following pertain to wellness care and promoting fluid and electrolyte balance: Consume six to eight glasses of water daily, avoid excess amounts of foods or fluids high in salt, sugar, and caffeine, limit alcohol intake because it has a diuretic effect, increase fluid intake before, during, and after strenuous exercise, particularly when the environmental temperature is high, and replace lost electrolytes from excessive perspiration as needed with commercial electrolyte solutions. *Nursing Process:* Planning *Client Need:* Physiological Integrity

8. *Answer:* 3 (Objective: 8) *Rationale:* Avoid using veins that are in areas of flexion (e.g., the antecubital fossa); highly visible, because they tend to roll away from the needle; damaged by previous use, phlebitis, infiltration, or sclerosis; continually distended with blood, or knotted or tortuous; or in a surgically compromised or injured extremity (e.g., following a mastectomy), because of possible impaired circulation and discomfort for the client. *Nursing Process:* Assessment *Client Need:* Physiological Integrity

9. *Answer:* 4 (Objective: 8) *Rationale:* A blood transfusion is the introduction of whole blood or blood components into the venous circulation. To avoid transfusing incompatible red blood cells, both blood donor and recipient are typed and their blood is crossmatched. Stop the transfusion immediately if signs of a reaction develop. Human blood is commonly classified into four main groups (A, B, AB, and O). *Nursing Process:* Assessment *Client Need:* Physiological Integrity

10. *Answer:* 4 (Objective: 8) *Rationale:* Special precautions are necessary when administering blood. When a transfusion is ordered, obtain the blood from the blood bank just before starting the transfusion. Do not store the blood in the refrigerator on the nursing unit; lack of temperature control may damage the blood. Once blood or a blood product is removed from the refrigerator, there is a limited amount of time to administer it (e.g., packed RBCs should not hang for more than 4 hours after being removed from the refrigerator). Follow agency policies for verifying that the unit is correct for the client. The Food and Drug Administration (FDA) requires blood products to have bar codes to allow for scanning and machine-readable information on blood and blood component container labels to help reduce medication errors. Blood is usually administered through a #18- to #20-gauge intravenous needle or catheter; using a smaller needle may slow the infusion and damage blood cells

(although a smaller-gauge needle may be necessary for small children or clients with small, fragile veins). A Y-type blood transfusion set with an in-line or add-on filter is used when administering blood. One arm of the administration set connects to the blood; normal saline (0.9% NaCl) is attached to the other arm of the Y-type set. Saline is used to prime the set and flush the needle before administering blood. It also provides a means to keep the vein open should a transfusion reaction occur. No other IV solutions should be administered with blood; they may cause the blood cells to clump or cause clotting. A transfusion should be completed within 4 hours of initiation. The risk of sepsis increases if blood hangs for a longer period. Blood tubing is changed after every 4 to 6 units per agency policy; new intravenous tubing is used following a transfusion. *Nursing Process:* Implementation *Client Need:* Physiological Integrity